HANDBOOK
OF
ESSENTIAL
PSYCHOPHARMACOLOGY

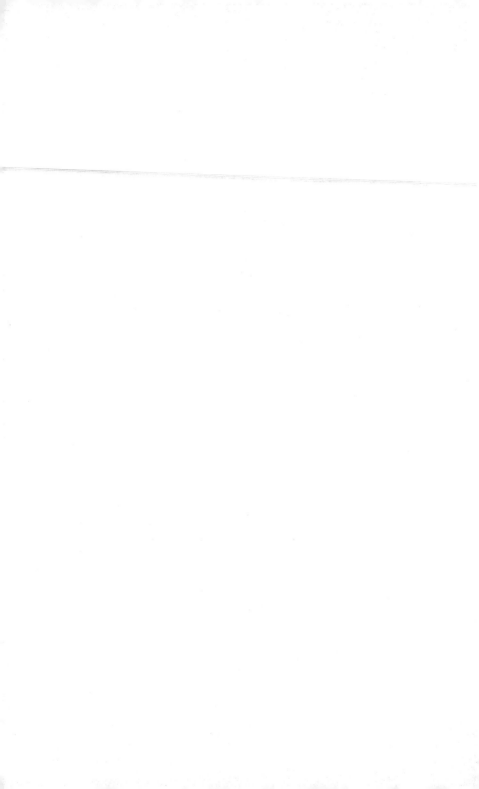

HANDBOOK
OF
ESSENTIAL
PSYCHOPHARMACOLOGY

Ronald W. Pies, M.D.

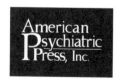

American Psychiatric Press, Inc.

Washington, DC
London, England

Copyright © 1998 American Psychiatric Press, Inc.
ALL RIGHTS RESERVED
Manufactured in the United States of America on acid-free paper
First Edition
01   00   99   98   4   3   2   1

American Psychiatric Press, Inc.
1400 K Street, N.W., Washington, DC   20005
www.appi.org

Library of Congress Cataloging-in-Publication Data
Pies, Ronald W., 1952–
    Handbook of essential psychopharmacology / Ronald W. Pies.
— 1st ed.
      p.   cm.
    Companion v. to : Clinical manual of psychiatric diagnosis and treatment. c1994.
    Includes bibliographical references and index.
    ISBN 0-88048-765-8 (alk. paper)
    1. Psychopharmacology—Handbooks, manuals, etc.   I. Pies, Ronald W., 1952–   Clinical manual of psychiatric diagnosis and treatment.   II. Title.
    [DNLM: 1. Psychotropic Drugs—pharmacology—handbooks.
2. Psychotropic Drugs—pharmacology—examination questions.   QV 39
P624h 1998]
RM315.P495   1998
615′.78—dc21
DNLM/DLC
for Library of Congress   97-24581
                                         CIP

British Library Cataloguing in Publication Data
A CIP record is available from the British Library.

CONTENTS

INTRODUCTION

The mercurial nature of psychopharmacology—a result of our ever-expanding knowledge—creates a daily struggle for those of us who practice and teach it. To cite but one example, information about the cytochrome enzymes, and their complex roles in drug metabolism, seems to multiply almost weekly. This increased information is due not only to the plethora of published research studies, but also to the hundreds of case reports that pour into journals and drug company data bases nearly every day. How can the busy clinician possibly keep up with all this, not to mention the many theoretical papers on drug mechanisms of action, pharmacokinetics, and efficacy studies?

In part, this handbook is an attempt to address these questions. My goal is to provide the busy, practicing psychiatrist with a readily accessible and *interactive* source of up-to-date knowledge. To achieve this goal, I have included dozens of tables summarizing important topics in psychopharmacology, which can be consulted quickly and efficiently "in a pinch." But good teaching requires an active and engaged pupil; it is not enough to bombard one's audience with reams of data. For this reason, I have used a question-and-answer format as one of the pillars of this book. My hope is not only to present the clinician with questions he or she may well be entertaining, but also to *involve* the reader in a give-and-take exercise. In my experience, nothing activates the limbic system of a physician so much as the pointed *clinical question*. Carrying this conviction to its logical conclusion, I have included a number of "clinical puzzles" at the end of each chapter, by which time the reader will have assimilated enough knowledge (one hopes) to attempt to answer these brainteasers. This feature also may aid those preparing for the psychiatry board examination. (In this regard, I see this handbook as a "companion" to my earlier book, *Clinical Manual of Psychiatric Diagnosis and Treatment: A Biopsychosocial Approach* [1994].)

Another feature of this handbook is the introductory overview of each of the four major drug classes. I have always found, in my own learning, that a synopsis of the topic at hand—a sort of "micropedia"—helps build the confidence and motivation required for more detailed study. The overview is also meant to "signal forward" (i.e., to provide the reader with some terse signposts that, in subsequent sections, will lead to longer roads of inquiry). Although some material is deliberately repeated from one section to another, the format and degree of detail are varied in a way that I believe is conducive to learning.

The four chapters of the book cover the antidepressants, antipsychotics, anxiolytics and sedative-hypnotics, and mood stabilizers. I have focused on these groups of psychotropics in order to realize the goal of covering "essential" aspects of psychopharmacology; however, some coverage is given to anticholinergic agents, β-blockers, calcium channel blockers, clonidine, and various adjunctive agents within the relevant chapters. The book as a whole has both a vertical and a horizontal structure. A reader who wanted to learn as much as possible about antidepressants—their indications, mechanisms of action, side effects, and so on—would read "vertically" through the chapter's overview, tables, questions, and vignettes. A reader who wanted to delve generally into pharmacokinetics would best be served by moving "horizontally" across the "Pharmacokinetics" sections of each chapter. That horizontal "cut" may be repeated at the level of the chapters' "Overview," "Tables," and "Questions and Answers" sections. Each chapter concludes with a series of "Vignettes and Puzzlers" designed to challenge the reader and consolidate his or her understanding. As this handbook is adapted for use in the electronic media, such vertical and horizontal browsing should become even easier. I recommend beginning by reading the "Overview" section of a given chapter, browsing the "Tables" and "Questions and Answers" sections, and then using the "Vignettes and Puzzlers" section as a self-test.

I am indebted to many individuals who have contributed to the development of this handbook. Dr. Carol Nadelson prompted the initial project—an outgrowth, as I recall, of her own attempts to find a good, concise source of detailed psychopharmacological information. Dr. David Harnett kindly read over the chapter on antidepressants, and Dr. David Osser provided helpful comments for the chapter on antipsychotics. I also wish to thank Dr. Sara Bolton, who—as a resident rotating through the Solomon Mental Health Center Emergency Service—found time to provide me with a list of questions and problems with which a senior resident might be grappling. I am also greatly indebted to the manuscript reviewers at American Psychiatric Press, Inc., who put in so much time and effort on the first draft. I'd also like to thank Pamela Harley for her editing assistance. Of course, the author alone bears responsibility for the final content of the book. Finally, I want to thank my wife, Nancy Butters, L.I.C.S.W., for her suggestions, technical support, and encouragement as I made my way through the thickets of psychopharmacology.

The first edition of any textbook is, in a sense, an open invitation. I welcome constructive criticism, suggestions, and clinical vignettes from interested readers, in hopes that the next edition will be an improvement upon its predecessor.

Reference

Pies RW: Clinical Manual of Psychiatric Diagnosis and Treatment: A Biopsychosocial Approach. Washington, DC, American Psychiatric Press, 1994

CHAPTER 1

Antidepressants

Overview

■ Drug Class

The class of agents termed "antidepressants" is a very hetero-geneous group. The terminology applied to these agents can be quite confusing, since there is no universally acceptable term for the diverse agents that are *not* monoamine oxidase inhibitors (MAOIs). The term *heterocyclic* is widely used to describe all non-MAOIs, including the tricyclics and many newly introduced agents that have fewer or more than three "rings" (Ayd 1995). Actually, in most cases, it is the nature of the compound's "side chains"—not its cyclical struc-ture—that strongly influences its biochemical function (Pot-ter et al. 1995). We often speak of the "SSRIs" (selective serotonin reuptake inhibitors) as a homogeneous group, even though these agents differ in both structure and phar-macodynamic effect. The recent addition of atypical agents, such as mirtazapine, makes classification even more compli-cated. Although it makes sense to describe antidepressants in terms of their neurotransmitter effects, even this classifica-tion will probably prove superficial as we learn more about the effects of antidepressants on neuronal receptors, second-ary messenger systems, and gene products.

■ Indications

Antidepressants (ADs), including tricyclics, "heterocyclics," and MAOIs, are used in a wide variety of psychiatric disorders besides depression. However, their main indication is in the treatment of major depression and severe dysthymic disorder. Some (essentially serotonergic) ADs are also used in the treatment of obsessive-compulsive disorder (OCD), panic disorder (PD), and posttraumatic stress disorder (PTSD). Both tricyclics and, to some degree, serotonin reuptake inhibitors have been found useful in certain chronic pain disorders. Occasionally, some ADs are used in treating schizoaffective disorder, somatoform disorders, some personality disorders, eating disorders, generalized anxiety disorder, chronic insomnia, and benzodiazepine withdrawal states. Agitated or depressed patients with dementia may also benefit from certain ADs.

▊ Mechanisms of Action

The precise mechanism underlying AD efficacy is not known. The old notion that ADs simply replenish one or more neurotransmitters is inadequate; most likely, ADs optimize the concentrations of several neurotransmitters—particularly serotonin (5-HT) and norepinephrine (NE)—and restore optimal pre- and postsynaptic receptor sensitivity. Some animal data suggest that depression may involve a state of supersensitive catecholamine receptors, secondary to decreased NE availability. ADs may work, in part, by down-regulating (reducing the number of) β-adrenergic receptors. Increased 5-HT_2 binding sites have been found in the platelets and some brain regions of depressed/suicidal patients. Downregulation of 5-HT_2 receptors seems to be a common mechanism in many ADs, but because electroconvulsive therapy (ECT) *increases* the density of 5-HT_2 receptors and is an extremely effective AD, it seems unlikely that 5-HT_2 downregulation is causally related to AD effectiveness. ADs also may work, in part, by normalizing pathological neuroendocrine functions in depressed patients (e.g., hypercortisolemia due to excessive corticotropin-releasing hormone) or by resetting aberrant circadian rhythms (e.g., decreased REM latency in many patients with major depression). Although all of these theories have stimulated useful research, *none* have been consistently verifiable in animal or human models. Furthermore, all of the receptor changes previously mentioned actually may be neuronal *adaptations* to the acute and subacute effects of ADs. The "real" mechanism of AD action probably involves changes below the level of the receptor, in which various secondary messengers ultimately lead to the production of new gene products.

∎ Pharmacokinetics

ADs in general are absorbed from the small bowel, enter the portal blood, pass through the liver where they undergo significant first-pass "extraction" and metabolism, and then enter the systemic circulation. ADs tend to be highly protein-bound and are highly lipophilic. Tricyclic antidepressants (TCAs) generally have elimination half-lives ($t\frac{1}{2}$s) of 16–70 hours, but $t\frac{1}{2}$ may be longer for protriptyline (Vivactil) and for any AD used in elderly patients. Most of the selective serotonin reuptake inhibitors (SSRIs) have $t\frac{1}{2}$s in the range of 12–24 hours, with the exception of the much longer acting fluoxetine.

ADs—like nearly all psychotropics—undergo extensive metabolism in the family of enzymes known as the cytochrome P450 (CYP) system. So-called *xenobiotic* CYP enzymes metabolize "foreign" biological substances, such as drugs and toxins, and are located in the endoplasmic reticulum of brain, liver, and bowel cells. (*Steroidogenic* CYP enzymes, located in the mitochondria of cells, are responsible mainly for the synthesis of steroids.) CYP enzymes in the liver and bowel wall carry out primarily *oxidative metabolism,* a process affecting many psychotropic agents, including ADs. Many ADs are metabolized in the cytochrome P450 2D6 (CYP2D6) system, and about 8% of Caucasians show genetically based reduction of activity in CYP2D6. Many psychotropic and "general medical" drugs also use the CYP2D6 system, and interactions with ADs are common (see the following discussion on "Drug-Drug Interactions"). Tertiary TCAs, and perhaps some metabolites of SSRIs, appear to utilize another cytochrome enzyme system known as 3A4. Tertiary TCAs (e.g., amitriptyline, imipramine) are demethylated to related secondary amines (nortriptyline, desipramine), and the parent-to-metabolite ratio varies widely from patient to patient. SSRIs also use CYP2D6 and may increase plasma levels of other compounds using this pathway.

Several studies suggest that therapeutic response to some TCAs may be related to plasma levels, and "therapeutic windows" (optimal dosage/plasma level ranges) have been postulated for several TCAs; the window for nortriptyline (approximately 60–150 ng/mL) is widely accepted. Plasma TCA levels also may be correlated with toxicity. Plasma levels seem to be far less useful with the SSRIs and other non-TCAs.

▌ Main Side Effects

Side effects of TCAs are of three main types, which overlap on a neurochemical level: 1) cardiac/autonomic, 2) anticholinergic, and 3) neurobehavioral. Cardiac/autonomic effects include orthostatic hypotension and dizziness; less commonly, hypertension, tachycardia, and prolonged intracardiac conduction manifest as prolonged Q-T intervals and sometimes "heart block." Anticholinergic side effects include dry mouth, urinary retention, blurry vision, constipation, confusion/memory impairment, and tachycardia. Neurobehavioral side effects include exacerbation of psychosis or mania, memory impairment (especially with highly anticholinergic agents), psychomotor stimulation (especially with desipramine and protriptyline), myoclonic twitches (including nocturnal myoclonus), tremors, and, rarely, extrapyramidal symptoms (amoxapine may cause extrapyramidal symptoms, and even neuroleptic malignant syndrome in rare cases, because of its dopamine-blocking metabolite). The effects of TCAs on seizure threshold are inconsistent, although high-dose clomipramine (and perhaps other tricyclics) appears to increase the risk of seizures through undetermined mechanisms (Edwards et al. 1986; Peck et al. 1983). Other side effects seen with TCAs (and other ADs) include significant sedation (especially with tertiary amines), weight gain, hepatic dysfunction, and sexual dysfunction (anorgasmia, impaired ejaculation). The SSRIs (fluoxetine, sertraline, paroxetine, fluvoxamine) are less likely to cause anticholinergic and cardiac/autonomic side effects than are the TCAs but are associated with frequent gastrointestinal (GI) side effects (nausea, diarrhea), headache, sexual dysfunction, insomnia, psychomotor agitation, and extrapyramidal reactions. Newer agents such as nefazodone and venlafaxine have side effect profiles that resemble the SSRIs but with some TCA-like effects as well (see Table 1–11).

▌ Drug-Drug Interactions

As noted, most ADs have the potential for interacting with a wide variety of hepatically metabolized drugs, as well as with each other. Both pharmacokinetic and pharmacodynamic interactions may occur. TCAs, heterocyclic ADs, and "atypical" ADs such as trazodone may interact with, for example, antihypertensive agents, anticonvulsants, various steroid hormones, antiarrhythmic agents, and sympathomimetic amines. Fluoxetine and paroxetine can significantly affect the metabolism of other non-SSRI ADs, leading to markedly elevated levels of some TCAs. SSRIs also may affect metabolism of some antipsychotic agents, barbiturates, triazolo-type benzodiazepines, and anticonvulsants. Pharmacodynamic interactions may occur between SSRIs and various psychotropics (antipsychotics, buspirone, and lithium). A serious toxic syndrome (termed the *serotonin syndrome*) may result from the

combination of an SSRI and an MAOI. MAOIs also may interact adversely with TCAs, antihypertensive agents, opioids,
and sympathomimetic amines. The new serotonin antago-
nist/reuptake inhibitor (SARI) nefazodone can inhibit the cytochrome 3A4 system and thus can reduce metabolism of
triazolobenzodiazepines, terfenadine, cisapride, and many
other substrates of this enzyme.

■ Potentiating Maneuvers

Many so-called treatment-resistant depressed patients actually have received inadequate doses of ADs, achieved insufficient plasma levels, or been on the agent for too little time.
Others have comorbid diagnoses (such as borderline personality disorder [BPD] or a psychotic disorder) that diminish response to standard ADs. Numerous strategies may be used to
augment the effects of ADs. The addition of lithium to a TCA
or an SSRI may convert some nonresponders to responders.
Thyroid hormone or psychostimulants such as methylphenidate also may potentiate TCAs and SSRIs. The combination of
a TCA (such as nortriptyline) with an SSRI (such as sertraline)
also may benefit some patients with refractory depression.
MAOIs may be combined with TCAs (not with SSRIs) in selected cases, if the procedure is done carefully (e.g., by beginning the two agents simultaneously, using very low doses of
the MAOI, and avoiding imipramine or clomipramine).
When depression is accompanied by psychosis, the addition
of an antipsychotic agent is usually necessary; AD treatment
alone may lead to incomplete response or even worsening of
the patient's condition.

■ Use in Special Populations

The elderly require special precautions when TCAs or a
long-acting SSRI such as fluoxetine is used. The elderly are
especially sensitive to the anticholinergic and cardiovascular
side effects of the tertiary TCAs and must be monitored care-

fully for postural hypotension, cardiac conduction abnormalities, and cognitive side effects. Elderly patients with ventricular arrhythmias and/or ischemic heart disease *may not* be good candidates for TCAs (Glassman et al. 1993). Elderly patients with dementia may be severely affected by the anticholinergic effects of TCAs. In general, the *non-TCAs*, including bupropion, nefazodone, sertraline, paroxetine, and venlafaxine, are the ADs of choice in the elderly. Fluoxetine also may be useful if dosage and drug-drug interactions are monitored carefully; however, fluoxetine-related weight loss and syndrome of inappropriate secretion of antidiuretic hormone (SIADH) have been reported in the elderly. (SIADH also has been seen with sertraline [Goldstein et al. 1996] and may occur with other SSRIs.) There are few well-designed, controlled studies of AD use in very young populations, in which placebo responsiveness may be high. Several reports of apparent "sudden death" linked to desipramine use in children necessitate caution in prescribing TCAs in children. The ADs as a group seem relatively safe in pregnancy, with little firm evidence of teratogenesis; nevertheless, it is preferable to avoid AD use during the first trimester, unless the risks to mother and fetus are clearly outweighed by the benefits. A recent study of fluoxetine in pregnancy suggests that it has very low teratogenicity but is correlated with a slight increase in miscarriage rate (possibly associated with depression itself).

Tables

▌ Drug Class

Table 1–1. Maintenance dosage and tablet sizes for non–monoamine oxidase inhibitor antidepressants

Antidepressant	Tablet/ capsule sizes	Usual daily adult dose[a]
Amitriptyline (Elavil, Endep)	10, 25, 50, 75, 100, 150 mg	75–250 mg
Amoxapine (Asendin)	25, 50, 100, 150 mg	200–300 mg
Bupropion (Wellbutrin)	75, 100 mg	150–350 mg
Citalopram (not yet available in U.S.)	20, 40 mg	20–40 mg
Clomipramine (Anafranil)	25, 50, 75 mg	50–200 mg
Desipramine (Norpramin, Pertofrane)	10, 25, 50, 75, 100, 150 mg	75–250 mg
Doxepin (Adapin, Sinequan)	10, 25, 50, 75, 100 mg[b]	75–250 mg[c]
Fluoxetine (Prozac)	10, 20 mg[d]	10–60 mg
Fluvoxamine (Luvox)	50, 100 mg	50–250 mg
Imipramine hydrochloride (Janimine, Tofranil)	10, 25, 50 mg	75–250 mg
Maprotiline (Ludiomil)	25, 50, 75 mg	50–200 mg
Mirtazapine (Remeron)	15, 30 mg	15–45 mg
Nefazodone (Serzone)	100, 150, 200, 250 mg	200–500 mg
Nortriptyline (Aventyl, Pamelor)	10, 25, 50, 75 mg	50–100 mg
Paroxetine (Paxil)	10, 20, 30, 40 mg	10–40 mg

(continued)

Table 1–1. Maintenance dosage and tablet size for non–monoamine oxidase inhibitor antidepressants *(continued)*

Antidepressant	Tablet/ capsule sizes	Usual daily adult dose[a]
Protriptyline (Vivactil)	5, 10 mg	20–45 mg
Sertraline (Zoloft)	50, 100 mg	50–200 mg
Trazodone (Desyrel)	50, 100, 150, 300 mg	50–400 mg[e]
Trimipramine (Surmontil)	25, 50, 100 mg	75–250 mg
Venlafaxine (Effexor)	25, 37.5, 50, 75, 100 mg	75–300 mg

[a]This range reflects the somewhat lower maintenance dosages often used in elderly or medically ill patients. In these populations, however, initial dosing is generally lower than the first number in the ranges. For example, in an elderly patient, one might begin nefazodone at 25–50 mg/day and reach a maintenance dose of 200 mg/day only after several weeks. With TCAs, plasma levels are important in determining the adequacy of dosage, with some elderly patients reaching therapeutic levels at lower daily doses than would younger patients. Upper limits of the therapeutic range may exceed those shown here.
[b]Also available as oral concentrate (10 mg doxepin/mL).
[c]Although most references give similar daily dosage ranges for doxepin and other commonly used tricyclics, Janicak et al. (1993) note that "it is possible that doxepin is less potent than imipramine, and slightly higher doses may be necessary to achieve optimal benefit" (p. 228).
[d]Also available as liquid oral solution (20 mg fluoxetine/5 mL).
[e]Trazodone is probably used most often today as an aid to sleep in patients taking more stimulating antidepressants (e.g., fluoxetine). Its antidepressant properties may not be fully realized until the dosage exceeds 300 mg/day, a dose that causes a prohibitive degree of sedation for many patients.

Table 1–2.   Monoamine oxidase inhibitors: tablet sizes and dosage

Agent	Tablet sizes	Usual daily adult dose[a]
L-Deprenyl (selegiline [Eldepryl])	5 mg	10 mg[c]
Isocarboxazid (Marplan)[b]	10 mg	20–50 mg
Moclobemide (Manerix)[d]	100, 150 mg	150–500 mg
Phenelzine (Nardil)	15 mg	30–75 mg
Tranylcypromine (Parnate)	10 mg	20–40 mg

[a]Ranges reflect the lower dosages often used in elderly or medically ill patients. Uppermost ranges may exceed those shown here.
[b]No longer commercially available in the United States.
[c]L-Deprenyl loses its monoamine oxidase-B selectivity at doses above 10 mg/day but is more effective at higher doses.
[d]Available in Canada but not in the United States.
Source.   Data from Pies and Shader 1994.

Table 1–3. Relative monthly costs of selected antidepressants (low to midtherapeutic dose range)

Agent/daily dose[a]	Approximate monthly cost[b]
Fluoxetine 20 mg/day	$69
Nefazodone 300 mg/day[c]	$58
Nortriptyline 75 mg/day	$31
Paroxetine 30 mg/day	$74
Sertraline 100 mg/day	$69
Venlafaxine 125 mg/day	$82

[a]The dosages used are those that, in my clinical experience, are in the low-moderate end of the therapeutic range for the majority of patients. (See letters by Gammon [1996] and Nemeroff [1996] for discussion of controversy regarding usually effective daily dose of sertraline.)

[b]Based on data from a randomly chosen pharmacy in Boston, Massachusetts, March 1996. Costs are based on use of the capsule/tablet combinations that result in lowest possible cost as per pharmacist's calculation (e.g., combining a 25-mg tablet with a 100-mg tablet of venlafaxine). Costs of agents may vary considerably because of special arrangements between, for example, pharmaceutical companies and health maintenance organizations, hospital pharmacies, and others.

[c]Many patients will require doses between 300 and 500 mg/day for optimal response.

Indications

Table 1–4. Off-label indications for antidepressants

Drug or drug class	Indication	Comments/supporting data
SSRIs	OCD	All SSRIs probably useful in OCD; fluoxetine, paroxetine, fluvoxamine now FDA-labeled for OCD
	PD	Preliminary studies show fluoxetine, paroxetine, fluvoxamine, probably other SSRIs useful; must begin with small doses and increase very gradually to avoid overstimulation (paroxetine labeling indications now include PD)
	PTSD	Preliminary evidence shows fluoxetine useful in PTSD; sertraline useful in comorbid PTSD and major depression
	Generalized anxiety disorder	SSRIs not adequately studied but may be helpful
	Social phobia	Preliminary data suggest SSRIs of benefit
	Chronic pain syndromes	Modest documentation for fluoxetine's efficacy in migraine headache pain; diabetic neuropathy and other chronic pain states may respond to SSRIs (some patients develop headache as side effect of SSRIs)
	Personality disorders	Several small studies suggest efficacy for fluoxetine in BPD (e.g., reduced impulsivity or aggression)

(continued)

Table 1–4. Off-label indications for antidepressants *(continued)*

Drug or drug class	Indication	Comments/supporting data
SSRIs *(continued)*	Eating disorders	Fluoxetine (approximately 60 mg/day) helps with short-term management of binge eating, purging in bulimia nervosa; two uncontrolled studies showed some efficacy of fluoxetine in anorexia nervosa
	Somatoform disorders	SSRIs (fluoxetine, fluvoxamine) may be useful in body dysmorphic disorder but are questionable in hypochondriasis; efficacy may be related to degree of depressive and/or obsessive symptomatology
	Insomnia	SSRIs unreliable for initial insomnia (many patients feel overstimulated at bedtime); fluoxetine can lead to disrupted sleep architecture; when insomnia part of major depression, SSRIs helpful at least in first few months
	Aggressive syndromes	Fluoxetine and sertraline useful in patients whose aggression is associated with brain lesions
	Dementia-related syndromes	SSRIs useful in chronically agitated, aggressive dementia patients
TCAs	OCD	Clomipramine superior to nonserotonergic TCAs in meta-analysis of 10 studies; clomipramine is only TCA FDA-labeled for OCD; nortriptyline, desipramine much less effective in OCD; full response may take more than 6 weeks

(continued)

Table 1–4.   Off-label indications for antidepressants
(continued)

Drug or drug class	Indication	Comments/supporting data
TCAs *(continued)*	PD	In seven studies, TCAs superior to placebo (72% versus 51%, respectively); imipramine most widely studied TCA but efficacy reported with desipramine, nortriptyline, amitriptyline, doxepin
	PTSD	Open studies of TCAs have shown some benefits for PTSD; two double-blind controlled trials (using amitriptyline, desipramine) did not show substantial benefit on core features of PTSD
	Generalized anxiety disorder	Relatively low doses of imipramine may be useful for anticipatory anxiety, but effects may not be evident for more than 1 month
	Social phobia	No systematic data available for TCAs
	Chronic neuropathic pain syndromes	Amitriptyline, desipramine, doxepin, imipramine, nortriptyline all reported useful, particularly in diabetic or other peripheral neuropathy
	Personality disorders	Generally poor response in BPD, plus high potential for lethal overdose
	Eating disorders	Imipramine and desipramine appear effective in short term for bulimia nervosa, in reducing binge eating/purging; long-term use carries risk of weight gain

(continued)

Table 1–4.   Off-label indications for antidepressants
(continued)

Drug or drug class	Indication	Comments/supporting data
TCAs *(continued)*	Somatoform disorders (including DSM-III-R somatoform pain disorder/ DSM-IV pain disorder)	Desipramine may be treatment of choice for chronic pain associated with dysthymia; no specific pharmacological treatment of somatization disorder unless patient has concomitant depression (no convincing data on use of TCAs); avoid tertiary TCAs in hypochondriasis (poor tolerance of anticholinergic side effects)
	Insomnia	Low doses of doxepin or amitriptyline (e.g., 25–50 mg of either) may be useful in chronic insomnia (use cautiously in elderly because of central anticholinergic side effects)
	Aggressive syndromes	Some reports show amitriptyline useful in head-injured or encephalopathic patients; patients with BPD may worsen with amitriptyline
	Dementia-related syndromes	Imipramine, other tricyclics may be effective in depressed Alzheimer's patients; anticholinergic side effects may worsen cognitive symptoms

Note. SSRIs = selective serotonin reuptake inhibitors; OCD = obsessive-compulsive disorder; FDA = Food and Drug Administration; PD = panic disorder; PTSD = posttraumatic stress disorder; BPD = borderline personality disorder; TCAs = tricyclic antidepressants.

Sources. Agras 1995; American Psychiatric Association 1987, 1994; Ayd 1995; Blumer 1987; Janicak et al. 1993; Kline et al. 1993; Phillips 1991; Potter et al. 1995; Shader 1994; Silver 1995; Taylor 1995; Tollefson 1995; Trestman et al. 1995; Yudofsky et al. 1995; Zajecka 1995.

▌ Mechanisms of Action

Table 1–5. Neurotransmitter effects of antidepressants

Agent	Serotonin	Norepinephrine	Dopamine
Amitriptyline	++	+	0
Bupropion	0	+	+[a]
Desipramine	+	+++	+/–
Fluoxetine	+++	0	+/–[b]
Nefazodone	++[c]	+/–	0
Nortriptyline	+	++	0
Sertraline	+++	0	+/–[b]
Venlafaxine	+++	++	+[a]

Note. Values are approximations, derived from in vivo, in vitro, and clinical studies. +++ = marked effects; ++ = moderate effects; + = modest effects; +/– = mimimal effects; 0 = virtually no effects.
[a]Dopaminergic effects probably significant only at higher doses.
[b]SSRIs have variable effects on dopamine, perhaps decreasing dopamine in some brain regions. However, sertraline has substantial dopamine reuptake inhibition compared with the other SSRIs, and this may have implications for its apparently beneficial effects on cognitive function in some patients.
[c]Nefazodone antagonizes the 5-HT$_2$ receptor but shows modest blockade of 5-HT reuptake.
Sources. Ereshefsky et al. 1996; Schatzberg and Cole 1991; Sherman 1996.

Table 1–6. Effects of receptor antagonism or reuptake blockade

Receptor or reuptake blockade	Possible clinical implications
Blockade of NE reuptake at synapse	Antidepressant effect (venlafaxine), tremors, jitteriness, tachycardia, sweating
Blockade of 5-HT reuptake at synapse	Antidepressant effect (SSRIs), GI side effects, sexual dysfunction, decreased appetite, variable effects on anxiety
Blockade of dopamine reuptake at synapse	Psychomotor activation, antiparkinsonian effect; possible worsening of psychosis; sexual arousal, activation of "reward" pathways
Antagonism of 5-HT$_2$ receptors	?Probable antidepressant effect (nefazodone); ?antipsychotic effect (risperidone, clozapine); ?counteract sexual dysfunction, anxiety, insomnia
Antagonism of histaminic (H$_1$) receptors	Sedation, weight gain, potentiation of CNS depressants
Antagonism of muscarinic (cholinergic) receptors	Dry mouth, blurry vision, constipation, urinary retention, tachycardia, cognitive impairment
Antagonism of α_1-adrenergic receptors	Postural hypotension, dizziness, reflex tachycardia, impaired ejaculation, priapism (trazodone)

(continued)

Table 1–6.   Effects of receptor antagonism or reuptake blockade *(continued)*

Receptor or reuptake blockade	Possible clinical implications
Antagonism of α_2-adrenergic (presynaptic) receptors	Antagonism of autoreceptors (which normally mediate negative feedback of NE on presynaptic neuron) leads to increased NE release from presynaptic neuron (yohimbine)

Note.   NE = norepinephrine; 5-HT = serotonin; SSRIs = selective serotonin reuptake inhibitors; GI = gastrointestinal; ? = possible/hypothesized; CNS = central nervous system.
Sources.   Preskorn 1994; Richelson 1994; Segraves 1989.

Table 1–7. Effects of serotonin receptor stimulation

Receptor stimulated	Postulated effect/side effect
5-HT$_{1A}$	Anxiolytic, antidepressant action (buspirone)
5-HT$_2$	Anxiety, insomnia, sexual dysfunction (SSRI side effects)
5-HT$_3$ (receptors in brain stem and gut)	Nausea, GI problems (mechanism of ondansetron in counteracting SSRI-induced nausea involves 5-HT$_3$ antagonism)

Note. SSRI = selective serotonin reuptake inhibitor; GI = gastrointestinal.
Source. Stahl 1997a, 1997b.

▌ Pharmacokinetics

Table 1–8. Pharmacokinetics of selected antidepressants

Drug	$t_{1/2}$ of parent cpd/main active metabolites	Main route of elimination/ CYP metabolism	Degree of inhibition by parent cpd/ metabolite on CYP3A4	Degree of inhibition by parent cpd/ metabolite on CYP2D6	Degree of inhibition by parent cpd/ metabolite on CYP1A2
Bupropion (Wellbutrin)	8–24 hours	?3A4, 2B	?	?	?
Hydroxybupropion (one of three active metabolites)	At least one metabolite has $t_{1/2}$ of 24 hours	?2D6	?	?	?
Fluoxetine (Prozac)	24–72 hours	2D6 NonL	+	+++	+
Norfluoxetine[a]	7–15 days	2D6	++ to +++	+++	+
Fluvoxamine (Luvox)	15 hours	?	++	+	+++
Imipramine (Tofranil)	11–24 hours	2D6 (hydroxylation); 1A2, 3A4 (demethylation)	—	+	—
Desmethylimipramine[a] (Norpramin)	12–24 hours	2D6 (hydroxylation)	—	+	—

	$t_{1/2}$				
Mirtazapine (Remeron)	20–40 hours	1A2, 3A4, 2C9, 2D6	?	?	?
Nefazodone (Serzone)	3 hours	3A4 NonL	+++	+	—
OH-Nefazodone/Triazoledione[b]	3 hours/18–33 hours	?	?	?	?
Nortriptyline (Pamelor)	18–44 hours	2D6 (hydroxylation)	—	+	—
Paroxetine (Paxil)	20 hours	2D6 NonL	+	+++	+
Sertraline (Zoloft)	25 hours	3A4	++	+	+
Desmethylsertraline	80 hours	?	++	+	+
Venlafaxine (Effexor)	5 hours	2D6	+/–	+	+/–
O-Desmethyl-venlafaxine	11 hours	3A4	?	?	?

Note. $t_{1/2}$ = half-life; cpd = compound; CYP = cytochrome P450; — = none or none reported; ? = insufficient data; +/– = minimal degree; + = modest degree; ++ = significant degree; +++ = substantial degree; NonL = nonlinear pharmacokinetics (implies that dosage increase may lead to higher-than-expected increase in plasma levels and/or clinical effect, particularly in higher dose ranges).

[a] A metabolite of imipramine also marketed as antidepressant, desipramine.

[b] The compound m-CPP (*m*-chlorophenylpiperazine), which is a significant metabolite of nefazodone. m-CPP may be anxiogenic in some patients.

Sources. Data from Ciraulo et al. 1995b; DeVane 1995; Drug Facts and Comparisons 1996; Gelenberg 1995; Goff and Baldessarini 1995; Golden et al. 1995; Ketter et al. 1995; Nemeroff et al. 1995–1996; Pollock et al. 1996; Preskorn 1996; Tollefson 1995.

Table 1–9.   Effect of selective serotonin reuptake inhibitors on cytochrome P450 2C family

SSRI	Inhibition of CYP2C9/10	Inhibition of CYP2C19
Fluoxetine	?	Moderate
Fluvoxamine	?	Substantial
Paroxetine	NCS	?
Sertraline	NCS	NCS
Clinical implications	CYP2C9/10 metabolizes phenytoin, the active S-enantiomer of warfarin (Coumadin), and tolbutamide. Fluvoxamine can cause buildup of warfarin via indirect effect on CYP2C9/10.[a] Other three SSRIs do not have significant effect on warfarin plasma levels.	CYP2C19 metabolizes clomipramine, imipramine, barbiturates, propranolol, and diazepam (along with CYP3A4). Fluoxetine can produce 50% increase in diazepam levels; fluvoxamine can produce ± 300% increase in diazepam levels.

Note.   SSRI = selective serotonin reuptake inhibitor; CYP = cytochrome P450; NCS = not clinically significant; ? = contradictory data.
[a]Via inhibition of CYP1A2, which metabolizes the R-enantiomer of warfarin; this in turn inhibits the CYP2C9/10 system (Preskorn 1996).
Source.   Data from Preskorn 1996.

Table 1–10. Putative optimal plasma levels for tricyclic
antidepressants

Agent	Optimal plasma level
Amitriptyline (parent compound)	?80–150 ng/mL
Desipramine (as single agent)	> 125 ng/mL or 110–160 ng/mL (unclear whether relationship is linear or curvilinear)
Imipramine (including metabolite, desipramine)	> 225 ng/mL (linear relationship in adults)
Nortriptyline	50–160 ng/mL

Note.   ? = conflicting results regarding linear, curvilinear, or no relationship to efficacy.
Sources.   Data from Arana and Hyman 1991; Janicak et al. 1993.

▌Main Side Effects

Table 1–11.   Side effect profiles of commonly used antidepressants

Drug	Anti-cholinergic (blurry vision, dry mouth, constipation)	Sedation/drowsiness	Insomnia/agitation	Orthostatic hypotension	Cardiac arrhythmia	Gastro-intestinal distress/diarrhea	Weight gain
Amitriptyline (Elavil)	4	4	½	4	3	½	4
Bupropion (Wellbutrin)	0	½	2	0	½	1	0
Desipramine (Norpramin)	1	1	1	2	3	½	1
Doxepin (Sinequan)	3	4	½	3	2	½	3
Fluoxetine (Prozac)	0	½	2	0	½	3	0[a]
Imipramine (Tofranil)	3	3	1	4	3	1	3

Nefazodone (Serzone)	½	½	0	2	½	2	½
Nortriptyline (Pamelor)	1	2	½	1	2	½	2
Paroxetine (Paxil)	½	½	1	0	½	3	0[a]
Sertraline (Zoloft)	0	½	1	0	½	3	0[a]
Venlafaxine (Effexor)	½	½	2	0	½	3	0

Note. All values are rough guidelines and may vary according to dose, duration of treatment, and age of patient. 4 = high; 3 = moderately high; 2 = significant; 1 = modest; ½ = minimal; 0 = virtually none.

[a]Despite published data showing little or no weight gain with the SSRIs, clinical experience has shown that some patients, often after an initial period of weight loss, may gain substantial weight with fluoxetine, paroxetine, and perhaps other SSRIs (see Gelenberg 1997).

Sources. Data from Depression Guideline Panel 1993; Preskorn 1995; and my clinical experience.

Table 1–12. Side effects: tricyclics versus nontricyclics (% of patients reporting, placebo adjusted)

	Imipramine[a]	Bupropion	Fluoxetine	Nefazodone	Paroxetine	Sertraline	Venlafaxine
Cardiac/autonomic							
Dizziness	17.5	6.8	4	23	7.8	5	12
Palpitations	2[b]	4.7	-0.1	—	1.5	1.9	2
Sweating	15	7.7	4.6	—	8.8	5.5	9
Gastrointestinal/sexual							
Dry mouth	50	9.2	3.5	12	6	7	11
Constipation	26.5	8.7	1.2	6	5.2	2.1	8
Nausea	3.5	4	11	11	16.4	14.3	26
Diarrhea	1[b]	-1.8	5.3	1	4	8.4	1
Sexual dysfunction[c]	15[b]	1	15	8	15	15	10
Neurobehavioral							
Drowsiness	25.5	0.3	5.9	11	14.3	7.5	14
Insomnia	8[b]	5.3	6.7	2	7.1	7.6	8
Nervousness	20[b]	13.9	10.3	—	4.9	4.4	12

Headache	2[b]	3.5	4.8	3	0.3	1.3	1
Global average	**16.8[b]**	**5.4**	**6**	**6.4**	**7.6**	**6.6**	**9.5**

Note. — = drug effect was equal to or less than placebo effect.
[a]For imipramine, numbers represent average of imipramine-placebo difference based on two studies (see Branconnier et al. 1983; Dunbar et al. 1991).
[b]Numbers based on my clinical experience and Branconnier et al. 1983; Dunbar et al. 1991.
[c]Reports of sexual dysfunction vary with the type and number of questions asked; these figures may well represent underestimates of the actual prevalence.
Source. Preskorn 1995.

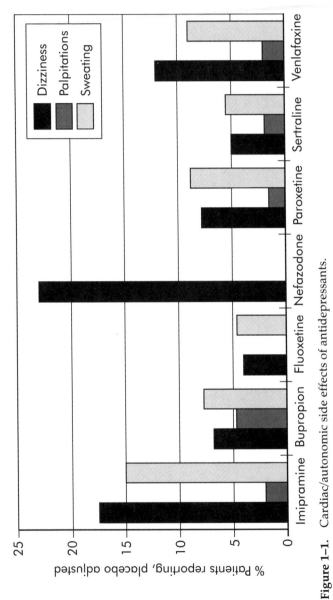

Figure 1–1.   Cardiac/autonomic side effects of antidepressants.
Source.   Data from Preskorn 1995.

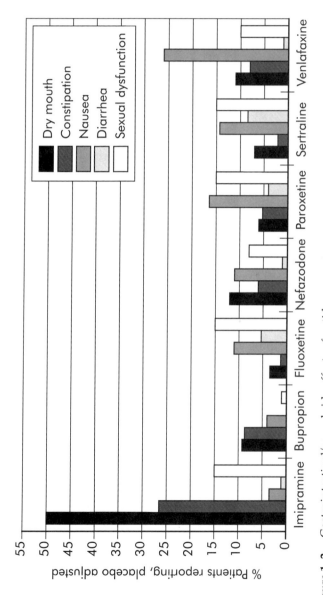

Figure 1–2. Gastrointestinal/sexual side effects of antidepressants.
Source. Data from Preskorn 1995.

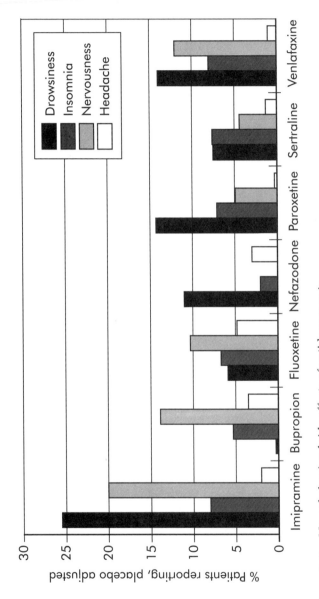

Figure 1–3. Neurobehavioral side effects of antidepressants.
Source. Data from Preskorn 1995.

Table 1–13. Some comparative side effects of selective serotonin reuptake inhibitors (% patients reporting, placebo adjusted)

Side effect	Fluoxetine	Sertraline	Paroxetine	Fluvoxamine
Headache	4.8	1.3	0.3	2
Nervousness	10.3	4.4	4.9	7
Insomnia	6.7	7.6[a]	7.1	11
Drowsiness	5.9	7.5	14.3	14
Fatigue	5.6	2.5	10.3	8[a]
Diarrhea	5.3	8.4	4.0	4
Nausea	11.0	14.3	16.4	26
Constipation	1.2	2.1	5.2	2
Dry mouth	3.5	7.0	6.0	4

[a]Asthenia.
Source. Data from Preskorn 1995; Physicians' Desk Reference 1996.

Table 1–14.   Basic management of antidepressant side effects

Type of side effect	Management strategies
Anticholinergic	Reduce dose
	Wait for tolerance
	Sugar-free candies, "artificial saliva," fluoride lozenges for dry mouth
	Increase fluid, fiber, bulk-forming agents for constipation
	Bethanechol 10–50 mg tid to qid
	Pilocarpine solution for dry mouth, blurry vision
Cardiovascular	
Orthostatic hypotension from TCAs	Switch to less hypotensive agent
	Warn and instruct patients (e.g., rising slowly) regarding orthostasis
	Ample fluid intake, support stockings, abdominal binder for orthostasis
	Supplemental sodium chloride (1–3 g/day), small doses of caffeine for orthostatic hypotension; fludrocortisone (0.1–0.3 mg/day) in refractory cases
Sinus tachycardia, conduction delays, arrhythmias with TCAs	Dosage reduction, splitting dose, "watchful waiting" may help with tachycardia; pretreatment and follow-up ECG now standard of care for all patients taking TCAs[a]; presence of new conduction delay (e.g., second-degree heart block) usually contraindicates continued use of agent

(continued)

Table 1–14. Basic management of antidepressant side effects *(continued)*

Type of side effect	Management strategies
Cardiovascular *(continued)*	
Hypertension with venlafaxine	Monitor blood pressure; adjust venlafaxine dosage
Hypotension with MAOIs	Monitor blood pressure periodically (hypotension can occur after several weeks of MAOI treatment); strategies similar to those for TCAs
Hypertensive crisis with MAOIs	Avoid tyramine and other pressor substances on written list of foods/medications given to patient
	Some clinicians have advised carrying *nifedipine* 10-mg tablet for use in case of known tyramine reaction; if used, the pill should be *crushed and swallowed,* not used sublingually (the drop in blood pressure with sublingual nifedipine may be unpredictable or delayed). However, recent studies have cast doubt on the safety of either sublingual or oral nifedipine for hypertensive emergencies (E. Grossman et al. 1996). Thus, it is probably best for the patient to go to the emergency room after presumed tyramine reaction; IV phentolamine (Regitine) may be used in emergency room.

(continued)

Table 1–14.   Basic management of antidepressant side effects *(continued)*

Type of side effect	Management strategies
Excessive sedation	
Daytime somnolence, psychomotor slowing	"Start low, go slow" with dose
	Wait to see whether tolerance develops
	Consider change to less sedating agent
	Bedtime dosing
	Add small amount of caffeine, psychostimulant,[b] or bupropion
Insomnia	Rule out hypomania/mania, mixed states, worsening of underlying mood or anxiety disorder, akathisia, nocturnal myoclonus
	Wait for tolerance
	Administer all medication in morning
	Add trazodone (25–300 mg qhs) if insomnia due to SSRI
	Add benzodiazepine (especially for nocturnal myoclonus) or zolpidem (5–10 mg qhs)
	Add small dose of sedating TCA (amitriptyline, clomipramine) if insomnia due to SSRI
	If insomnia associated with fluoxetine, consider change to nefazodone

(continued)

Table 1–14. Basic management of antidepressant side effects *(continued)*

Type of side effect	Management strategies
Agitation/ "jitteriness"	Rule out worsening of depression, anxiety, akathisia, hypomania/mania, or mixed states
	Start low, go slow (especially with SSRIs, venlafaxine, bupropion)
	Wait for tolerance to develop
	Reduce dose
	Switch to less activating agent (e.g., nefazodone)
	Add benzodiazepine
	Add β-blocker (e.g., propranolol 10–20 mg bid) if no medical contraindication

Note. TCAs = tricyclic antidepressants; ECG = electrocardiogram; MAOIs = monoamine oxidase inhibitors; IV = intravenous; SSRI = selective serotonin reuptake inhibitor.
[a]Although many clinicians and textbooks continue to advocate baseline ECGs only for patients older than age 40 years or for those with known cardiac conditions, the evolving standard of care seems to point toward baseline (and perhaps follow-up) ECGs for *all* patients taking TCAs. As Stoudemire et al. (1995) note, "A prolonged Q-T interval presents a relative contraindication to [TCA] treatment because of the hazard of malignant ventricular arrhythmias . . . prolonged Q-T intervals may . . . occur on a congenital basis and present problems in using TCAs. Such patients may not be symptomatic and may only be detected on a routine ECG" (p. 784).
[b]Caution: theoretical risk of hypertension with concomitant MAOI.
Sources. McElroy 1995; Pies and Shader 1994.

▌ Drug-Drug Interactions

Table 1–15. Drug-drug interactions with tricyclic antidepressants

Drug added to TCA	Interaction
Anticholinergic agents	Urinary retention, dry mouth
Cimetidine, neuroleptics, SSRIs, oral contraceptives, isoniazid, acetaminophen, chloramphenicol, verapamil, quinidine, epinephrine, disulfiram, methylphenidate, methadone	Increased TCA blood levels, potential toxicity
Concomitant sympathomimetic use	Hypertension
Coumarin anticoagulants	Prolonged bleeding
L-Dopa	Increased agitation; decreased plasma level of antidepressants
Guanethidine, clonidine	Reduced antihypertensive effect
MAOIs	CNS toxicity, hyper-pyrexia, serotonin syndrome (greatest risk is with MAOI plus *clomipramine, imipramine,* and perhaps *desipramine*) (see also Table 1–17)
Phenytoin, barbiturates, carbamazepine, phenylbutazone, rifampin, doxycycline	Decreased level/effect of antidepressants

(continued)

Table 1–15. Drug-drug interactions with tricyclic antidepressants *(continued)*

Drug added to TCA	Interaction
Quinidine, procainamide	Prolonged cardiac conduction
Sedatives, tranquilizers (including benzodiazepines)	CNS depression

Note. TCA = tricyclic antidepressant; SSRIs = selective serotonin reuptake inhibitors; MAOIs = monoamine oxidase inhibitors; CNS = central nervous system.

Sources. Ciraulo et al. 1995a; Krishnan et al. 1996; Pies and Weinberg 1990.

Table 1–15a. Some drugs used in general medicine that may interact with antidepressants via cytochrome systems as substrates or inhibitors

CYP1A2	CYP2C9/10	CYP2C19	CYP2D6	CYP3A3/4
Acetaminophen	Cimetidine	Hexobarbital	Alprenolol	Acetaminophen
Caffeine	Diclofenac	Mephenytoin	Bufuralol	Amiodarone
Cimetidine[a]	Ibuprofen	Omeprazole	Cimetidine	Astemizole
Phenacetin	Naproxen	Propranolol	Codeine	Cimetidine
Propranolol	Phenytoin		Dextromethorphan	Cisapride
Tacrine	Tolbutamide		Encainide	Cortisol (and other steroids)
Theophylline	S-Warfarin		Flecainide	Cyclosporine
R-Warfarin			Metoprolol	Diltiazem
			Propafenone	Erythromycin
			Propranolol	Ethinyl estradiol
			Timolol	Felodipine
				Lidocaine
				Nifedipine

			Propafenone
			Quinidine
			Terfenadine
			Verapamil

Note. CYP = cytochrome P450. The cytochrome systems have not been determined for many agents used in general medicine, and some (e.g., digoxin) do not show extensive hepatic metabolism. Cytochrome systems shown are those that mediate metabolism of the drugs listed beneath them. Note that a given drug may be metabolized via more than one CYP system. Potential interactions with antidepressants are not quantitatively indicated. *This table should not be construed as an exhaustive list.*

[a]Some agents, such as cimetidine, may act as inhibitors across virtually the entire spectrum of cytochrome systems but have not been characterized with respect to their *own* hepatic metabolism.

Sources. Ciraulo et al. 1995a; Ereshefsky 1996; Ereshefsky et al. 1996; Preskorn 1996.

Table 1–16. Drug-drug interactions with monoamine oxidase inhibitors

Drug added to MAOI	Interaction
Atropine compounds	Increased anticholinergic effects
L-Dopa	Hypertension when used with nonselective or MAO-A inhibitor; appears to be safe with selective MAO-B inhibitor selegiline at 10 mg/day
Fenfluramine	Confusional state (?hyperserotonergic effect)
Guanethidine, reserpine, clonidine	Reversal of antihypertensive effect; reserpine + MAOI may lead to hypomania
Insulin	Dangerous hypoglycemia
Meperidine, fentanyl	Toxic brain syndrome/serotonin syndrome, autonomic nervous system collapse, death; codeine safer but not risk free
Methadone	Minimal interaction but needs careful monitoring
Methyldopa	CNS excitation, hypertension
Morphine	Hypotension
Other antihypertensive agents	Hypotension
Other MAOIs, sympathomimetic agents (including ephedrine, phenylephrine, phenylpropanolamine, dopamine, amphetamines), and tyramine	Hypertensive crisis when used concomitantly
Phentermine	Hypertensive reaction

(continued)

Table 1–16. Drug-drug interactions with monoamine oxidase inhibitors *(continued)*

Drug added to MAOI	Interaction
Succinylcholine +phenelzine	Phenelzine may reduce cholinesterase levels, leading to increased levels of succinylcholine and prolonged apnea during ECT; tranylcypromine does not seem to have this effect
Sumatriptan	Increased sumatriptan effects
Thiazide diuretic	Increased risk of hypotension
Tricyclics (especially imipramine, clomipramine), SSRIs, buspirone, other serotonergic agents, dextromethorphan	Hyperserotonergic syndrome, severe confusional states, coma possible

Note. ? = hypothesized; MAOI = monoamine oxidase inhibitor; MAO-A = monoamine oxidase-A; MAO-B = monoamine oxidase-B; CNS = central nervous system; ECT = electroconvulsive therapy; SSRIs = selective serotonin reuptake inhibitors.
Sources. Ayd 1995; Creelman and Ciraulo 1995; Krishnan et al. 1996; Pies and Weinberg 1990.

Table 1–17. Food restrictions for patients taking conventional monoamine oxidase inhibitors

Type of food	Should avoid entirely	Probably safe in moderation
Cheese, dairy products	All matured or aged cheese; casseroles made with these cheeses (all cheeses except those in "probably safe" column)	Fresh cottage cheese, cream cheese, ricotta cheese, processed cheese slices; all fresh milk products, including sour cream, yogurt, ice cream, if stored properly
Meat, fish, poultry	Aged/cured meats (e.g., fermented/dry sausage, pepperoni, salami, mortadella, summer sausage); improperly stored meat, fish, poultry, pickled herring	All fresh/properly refrigerated packaged or processed meat, fish, poultry
Fruits, vegetables	Fava[a] or broad bean pods, overripe figs, banana peel	All fruits and vegetables (except those in "should avoid" column); banana pulp
Alcoholic beverages	All tap beers, red wine[a]	No more than one (1-ounce) glass of vodka or gin per day; no more than one (4-ounce) glass of white wine per day; no more than one bottle or can of beer per day, including nonalcoholic type
Miscellaneous	Marmite concentrated yeast extract, sauerkraut, soy sauce, other soybean condiments	Brewer's yeast, breads, soy milk

[a]Some disagreement in published literature. Patients are generally best advised to err on the side of caution, because identical foods vary widely in tyramine content from region to region.
Sources. Gardner et al. 1996; Shader 1994.

Table 1–18. The serotonin syndrome: differential diagnosis

Core symptoms	5-HT syndrome	Neuroleptic malignant syndrome	Malignant hyperthermia	Lethal (pernicious) catatonia	Central anticholinergic syndrome
	Variable temperature elevations (37.4°C–42.5°C)[a]	Hyperthermia	Hyperthermia (core temperature >41°C)	Hyperthermia	Hyperthermia
	Mental status changes	Severe muscle rigidity (usually "lead pipe")	Muscle rigidity	Muscle rigidity	Decreased sweating[a]
	Hypomania[a]	Diaphoresis	Ischemia	Diaphoresis	Hot, dry skin[a]
	Restlessness	Delirium	Hot skin	Delirium	Dilated, sluggish pupils[a]
	Myoclonus	Muteness	Mottled cyanosis[a]	Extreme hyperactivity[a] (often early in syndrome) or stupor	Tachycardia

(continued)

Table 1–18. The serotonin syndrome: differential diagnosis (*continued*)

	5-HT syndrome	Neuroleptic malignant syndrome	Malignant hyperthermia	Lethal (pernicious) catatonia	Central anticholinergic syndrome
Core symptoms (*continued*)	Hyperreflexia	Incontinence	Hypotension[a]	Psychotic prodrome[a]	Constipation [a]
	Diaphoresis	Rhabdomyolysis	Rhabdomyolysis	Mutism[a]	Urinary retention [a]
	Shivering/teeth chattering[a]	Autonomic instability (fluctuating blood pressure, pallor/flushing)[a]		Posturing[a]	Confusion
	Tremor	Tremulousness		Stupor alternating with excitement[a]	Impaired memory
	Diarrhea	Tachycardia		Hypertension	Delirium

	Incoordination	Tachypnea		Tremulousness	Hallucinations
		EPS Most common temporal sequence[a]: mental status change, rigidity, autonomic dysfunction, hyperthermia			
Laboratory findings	No specific findings	Elevated CPK[a], WBC, LFTs, myoglobinuria	Disseminated intravascular coagulation[a]; respiratory/ metabolic acidosis[a]; hyperkalemia[a]; hyper-magnesemia[a]	No specific findings	No specific findings

(continued)

Table 1–18. The serotonin syndrome: differential diagnosis *(continued)*

	5-HT syndrome	Neuroleptic malignant syndrome	Malignant hyperthermia	Lethal (pernicious) catatonia	Central anticholinergic syndrome
Causes/mechanisms	Activation of 5-HT$_{1A}$ receptors in brain stem, spinal cord; enhancement of overall 5-HT neurotransmission; most commonly due to interaction between MAOI and serotonergic agent (L-tryptophan, SSRI), but may occur with any 5-HT drug	Presumed: blockade of dopaminergic pathways in basal ganglia and hypothalamus; also may result from sudden withdrawal of dopamine agonist ?Lithium may precipitate ?Low serum iron	Inherited disorder; triggering anesthetic (halothane, methoxyflurane) causes calcium release from sarcoplasmic reticulum, leading to activation of myosin ATPase, heat production	Manic and depressed mood states; schizophrenia (also secondary to infection and metabolic, other medical disorders)	Blockade of central and peripheral muscarinic receptors (e.g., due to tricyclic phenothiazine)

Management	Discontinue suspected agent; supportive measures (cooling blanket for hyperthermia); propranolol, methysergide, cyproheptadine may help	Supportive measures (cooling); stop neuroleptic; no clear treatment of choice but dopamine agonists (bromocriptine 5 mg tid), dantrolene, ECT may help	Dantrolene sodium 1 mg/kg via rapid IV infusion; 100% oxygen; sodium bicarbonate; external cooling	Some recommend ECT as therapy of choice (within first 5 days); lorazepam 1–2 mg po or IM up to qid also useful; neuroleptics generally best withheld	Remove offending agent; physostigmine usually not indicated (?unless cardiac arrhythmia present)

Note. ? = data incomplete/hypothesized; 5-HT = serotonin; EPS = extrapyramidal symptoms; CPK = creatine phosphokinase; WBC = white blood cell count; LFTs = liver function tests; MAOI = monoamine oxidase inhibitor; SSRI = selective serotonin reuptake inhibitor; ATPase = adenosinetriphosphatase; ECT = electroconvulsive therapy; IV = intravenous; IM = intramuscular.
[a]Features that help differentiate syndromes. Some authors believe that neuroleptic malignant syndrome and lethal catatonia are closely related syndromes.
Sources. Ayd 1995; Castillo et al. 1989; Fink 1996; Fink et al. 1993; Jenkins and Hansen 1995; Pearlman 1986; Petersdorf 1991; Sternbach 1991; Theoharides et al. 1995; Velamoor et al. 1995.

Table 1–19.   Serotonin syndrome

Symptom	% of patients reporting symptoms (n = 38)
Confusion	42
Hypomania	21
Restlessness	45
Myoclonus	34
Hyperreflexia	29
Diaphoresis	26
Shivering	26
Tremor	26
Diarrhea	16
Incoordination	13

Source.   Data derived from Sternbach 1991.

▌ Potentiating Maneuvers

Table 1–20. Agents used to potentiate/augment antidepressants

Agent	Rationale/comments
Antipsychotic	Almost always necessary in treatment of psychotic depression; also may raise plasma levels of concomitant antidepressant
Buspirone	In high doses (> 50 mg/day), buspirone has antidepressant properties; may be useful as augmenting agent for ongoing tricyclic or SSRI (buspirone, a partial 5-HT agonist, in some cases undermines effects of SSRIs)
Dopaminergic agonists (e.g., pergolide)	Augmenting dopaminergic function may be necessary in some patients with atypical depression or in those taking SSRIs (which may reduce dopamine in some brain regions)
Estrogen	Data are not yet convincing, but estrogen may augment central noradrenergic and/or serotonergic activity; could be used in refractory cases after other augmenters have failed
Lithium	Probably enhances serotonergic function; lithium augmentation is sustained and may reduce relapse rate; response to lithium augmentation may be within first week but usually takes longer
Psychostimulant (e.g., methyl-phenidate)	May enhance dopaminergic function, reduce drowsiness, counteract sexual side effects of SSRIs

(continued)

Table 1–20.   Agents used to potentiate/augment
                antidepressants *(continued)*

Agent	Rationale/comments
Thyroid hormone (usually T_3)	Some depressed patients have subclinical hypothyroidism (e.g., normal T_3, T_4, slightly elevated TSH); even euthyroid patients, however, may benefit; T_3 may be better than T_4 for unipolar depression; T_4 may be better as mood stabilizer in rapid-cycling bipolar disorder; usual dose of T_3 is 15–50 μg/day

Note.   SSRI = selective serotonin reuptake inhibitor; 5-HT = serotonin;
TSH = thyroid-stimulating hormone.
Source.   Data derived from Charney et al. 1995.

Table 1–21. Psychostimulants: main features

Agent	$t\frac{1}{2}$	Peak of clinical effect/ termination of effect	Usual daily dose	Special formulations/ issues	Mechanism of action
Dextro- amphetamine (Dexedrine), methamphet- amine (Desoxyn)	4–7 hours	1–2 hours/ 5 hours	*Children/ adolescents:* 0.3–1.25 mg/kg/day (±5–40 mg/day); dosage usually bid or tid	Dexedrine Spansules may or may not provide 6- to 8-hour effect; Desoxyn Grad- umets do have 8- to 10-hour effect but are expensive	Increases norepi- nephrine and dopamine in cleft; releases dopamine from newly synthe- sized pools and increases dopamine diffusion from vesi- cles to cytoplasm; in high doses may have MAOI action
			Adults: 0.4 mg/kg/day (±20–45 mg/day); dosage usually bid or tid		

(continued)

Table 1–21.   Psychostimulants: main features *(continued)*

Agent	T½	Peak of clinical effect/ termination of effect	Usual daily dose	Special formulations/ issues	Mechanism of action
Methyl-phenidate (Ritalin)	2–3 hours	1–2 hours/ 4 hours (adults with ADHD report shorter duration)	*Children/adolescents:* 0.6–1.7 mg/kg/day (±10–60 mg/day); dosage q 3–5 hours *Adults:* 1.0 mg/kg/day (40–90 mg/day); dosage q 2–3 hours	Ritalin-SR 20 mg; not clear whether effect lasts 8 hours; danger if chewed	?Release of dopamine stored in vesicles

| Pemoline (Cylert) | 7–8 hours (children); 11–13 hours (adults) | Peak levels occur several hours after dosing, and cognitive effects may begin within hours; however, in some children, may take 3–4 weeks for full response | Children/adolescents: 2 mg/kg/day (±56.25–75 mg/day); dosage qd or bid

Adults: 1–1.5 mg/kg/day (±56.25–125 mg/day); usually in one dose but some patients need bid | May cause liver dysfunction; also requires normal renal function | May release stored catecholamines and block reuptake; has few sympathomimetic effects |

Note.   Dosages and dosing schedules have been derived from the literature on treatment of attention-deficit/hyperactivity disorder and are not necessarily applicable when psychostimulants are used as adjuncts in mood disorders. In general, dosages for adjunctive treatment of depression tend to be about 50% of those used in attention-deficit/hyperactivity disorder.

$t\frac{1}{2}$ = half-life; MAOI = monoamine oxidase inhibitor; ADHD = attention-deficit/hyperactivity disorder; ? = presumptive.

Sources.   Data from Bender 1996a; DuPaul and Barkley 1990; Fawcett and Busch 1995; Janicak et al. 1993; Wender 1996; Wender and Shader 1994.

▐ Use in Special Populations

Table 1–22. Selection of nontricyclic antidepressant for patients with special needs or comorbid conditions

Comorbidity	Preferred agents	Rationale
"Atypical" features (hyper-somnia, hyper-phagia)	Bupropion, fluoxetine, venlafaxine	Bupropion, fluoxetine may be more "alerting"; fluoxetine, other SSRIs may decrease carbohydrate craving; venlafaxine is generally less sedating than other agents, does not appear to promote weight gain
Cardiac disease	SSRIs, bupropion, nefazodone, venlafaxine	Do not prolong cardiac conduction; rarely associated with arrhythmias (*Note:* Nefazodone can lead to hypotension, whereas venlafaxine can increase blood pressure. Thus, monitor vital signs, and use caution when prescribing these agents.)
Obesity	Bupropion, fluoxetine (?other SSRIs)	Decrease carbohydrate craving (*Note:* Fluoxetine may cause unwanted weight loss in the elderly.)
Diabetes mellitus	Bupropion, venlafaxine, SSRIs	Little effect on blood glucose level (bupropion, venlafaxine) or have hypoglycemic effect (SSRIs)
ADHD	Bupropion, venlafaxine	Some data suggest efficacy in ADHD

Nicotine dependence	Bupropion	May help with smoking cessation (marketed as Zyban[a])
Bulimia	Fluoxetine	Best-studied SSRI for this condition
Severe insomnia	Nefazodone	Relatively sedating given at bedtime; no adverse effects on normal sleep architecture
Parkinson's disease	Tricyclics; ?SSRIs; ?bupropion	Anticholinergic effects of TCAs may be helpful; SSRIs may be well tolerated but in a few patients may decrease dopamine and worsen EPS; in theory, bupropion's dopaminergic effects may be useful, but data are mixed
Seizure disorder	Desipramine, SSRIs, MAOIs	These agents lower seizure threshold less than others; avoid bupropion, maprotiline, clomipramine (relatively high incidence of seizures at doses > 250 mg/day)
Peptic ulcer disease	Tricyclics (e.g., doxepin)	Blockade of histaminic (H_2) receptor reduces gastric acid
Sexual dysfunction	Bupropion	Very rarely associated with sexual dysfunction and may improve it in patients taking SSRIs; avoid SSRIs if possible

(continued)

Table 1–22. Selection of nontricyclic antidepressant for patients with special needs or comorbid conditions *(continued)*

Comorbidity	Preferred agents	Rationale
Angle-closure glaucoma	SSRIs, bupropion, nefazodone	Lack of anticholinergic effects; avoid tricyclics
Anxiety disorder	SSRIs, nefazodone	SSRIs useful for PD, OCD, ?generalized anxiety; preliminary data suggest nefazodone may be helpful for panic attacks

Note. ? = possibly effective for/data equivocal; SSRIs = selective serotonin reuptake inhibitors; ADHD = attention-deficit/hyperactivity disorder; TCAs = tricyclic antidepressants; EPS = extrapyramidal symptoms; MAOIs = monoamine oxidase inhibitors; PD = panic disorder; OCD = obsessive-compulsive disorder.
[a]Comes in 150-mg sustained-release tablets, taken as 150 mg bid.
Sources.   Apter and Kushner 1996; Charney et al. 1995; Cole et al. 1996; Cummings 1992; Cutler and Post 1982; Glassman et al. 1993; Goodnick et al. 1995.

Questions and Answers

■ Drug Class

Q. Are any of the ADs formulated for intramuscular (IM) or intravenous (IV) use? Is there any experience with the latter for treatment of depression or other conditions?

A. IM preparations are available for amitriptyline, imipramine, and doxepin. There is also a long-acting form of injectable imipramine (imipramine pamoate). These IM formulations may sometimes be useful in medically ill patients (see the discussion on "Use in Special Populations" that follows). Clomipramine is available in IV form, and in Europe it has been used to treat both OCD and major depression. At least for OCD, the data suggest that IV clomipramine may reduce symptoms more quickly than oral clomipramine and (surprisingly) is better tolerated (Koran et al. 1997).

■ Indications

Q. What factors are used in choosing a particular AD for a given patient?

A. Because all ADs are roughly equal in efficacy, the choice of agent depends on the patient's personal, medical, and symptomatic profile. *Past response* to a particular agent is an important concern (e.g., if a patient has demonstrated an excellent response to agent A in the past, that is a compelling reason to use agent A for the index episode). To some degree, the *response of a family member* may be useful (e.g., if a first-degree relative has responded well to agent A, it may be a good choice for the patient, all other factors being equal). The patient's *age* and *associated medical conditions* are critical factors in choosing an AD. Thus, the elderly are usually not good candidates for highly sedating, anticholinergic agents, such as tertiary tricyclics. The presence of a *cardiac conduction abnormality, urinary retention,* or *narrow-angle glaucoma* also would be a relative contraindication for using a TCA. A patient's known or presumed *suicide risk* is an important factor because the TCAs are much more toxic in overdose than most newer agents, such as the SSRIs. Among the TCAs, desipramine appears to have higher toxicity in overdose. The *phenomenology of the patient's depression*—although *not* relevant to the ultimate benefits of AD treatment—may influence the choice of agent, based on the patient's comfort during the first few weeks of treatment. Thus, a more sedating/anxiolytic agent (such as nefazodone) initially may be preferable to more "activating" agents (such as desipramine or bupropion) for depressed patients with severe insomnia, anxiety, and agitation. (Bupropion seems to have minimal benefits for anxiety.) *Cost* is also an important consideration for many patients. The tablet-for-tablet cost of TCAs is much less than that for newer agents; however, the *cost-effectiveness* of the newer agents may be greater in the long run. This greater cost-effectiveness for newer agents compared with TCAs is due to the greater likelihood of serious adverse reactions requiring urgent care, more frequent plasma level monitoring, and somewhat higher dropout rate for those taking TCAs. Nevertheless, the overall number of patients completing treatment with TCAs versus SSRIs is relatively similar (Nelson 1994), and the choice of agent must remain a highly individualized decision involving all of the previously mentioned factors (Pies 1995).

Q. When does a patient with unipolar major depression need to be maintained indefinitely on an AD?

A. About 75% of individuals who experience a first episode of major depression will go on to have multiple episodes (Greden 1995–1996). The more episodes a patient has, the more one can expect and the closer together these episodes will occur. Episodes also tend to be longer lasting and more severe over the course of the patient's lifetime (Greden 1995–1996; Post 1994). Greden (1995–1996) believes that the best rule of thumb for the clinician is "three strikes and you're on" (i.e., with three or more episodes of major depression, the patient should remain "on" ADs indefinitely). This strategy will reduce the recurrence rate for most patients. In contrast, about 75% of untreated patients with recurrent major depression will relapse within a year off medication. Of course, the decision to maintain a patient on ADs must be based on informed consent in which *all* of the relevant factors (e.g., actual benefits from the medication, medication side effects, degree of incapacity off medication, and so on) are carefully considered.

Q. Is there a first-choice AD in treating BPD?

A. It could be argued that the indications for *any* psychotropic in BPD are questionable, based on the most rigorous recent studies (see Cornelius et al. 1993). Long-term success is apparently quite limited with the use of ADs in BPD patients, although many reports exist suggesting short-term improvement in some symptoms. On the other hand, amitriptyline may actually *worsen* behavioral dyscontrol in some BPD patients. MAOIs may be helpful in some BPD patients fitting Klein's description of "hysteroid dysphoria" (rejection-sensitivity, histrionic when not depressed, frequent abuse of diet pills/stimulants, hypersomnolent/lethargic when depressed) (Liebowitz and Klein 1979); however, the risks associated with misuse of MAOIs are significant, and some BPD patients will "test out" the dangers of tyramine-rich foods and so forth. A number of recent reports suggest that SSRIs may be helpful in some BPD patients. Because many such patients also fit criteria for PTSD, the SSRIs may make sense, given that serotonergic agents seem to ameliorate some symptoms of PTSD.

Q. Can any AD be used for the treatment of OCD?

A. Those ADs that lack serotonergic properties have little effect in the treatment of OCD. Thus, the recommended agents for OCD are clomipramine or one of the SSRIs. A highly noradrenergic TCA such as desipramine is not likely to be effective in OCD, although it may be effective for comorbid major depression (which often accompanies OCD). Bupropion also has not been shown to be effective in OCD (Zajecka 1995). A case report from Zajecka et al. (1990) found that venlafaxine had antiobsessional effects in a patient with coexisting major depression and OCD. A case report from R. Grossman and Hollander (1996) found venlafaxine useful in a man with OCD alone who had been refractory to paroxetine. Rauch et al. (1996) recently reported the successful use of venlafaxine in a small group of OCD patients; however, minor side effects (especially nausea) were common, and a "troublesome" withdrawal syndrome developed in four patients tapered off venlafaxine over a period of 4–14 days. Nefazodone has not been systematically tested in OCD, although a recent case report noted emergence of obsessive symptoms in a depressed patient whose depression had actually responded to nefazodone (Sofuoglu and DeBattista 1996). Remember that dosage and/or time course differ in OCD versus major depression (i.e., higher doses of ADs for longer periods of time may be necessary in OCD [Taylor 1995]).

Q. What about ADs for PD—do they all work equally well?

A. Imipramine and MAOIs such as phenelzine are the old standbys and are the ADs most thoroughly studied for use in PD. Other TCAs such as desipramine, nortriptyline, clomipramine, and amitriptyline have been found effective in a limited number of studies, but there are few comparative data (Taylor 1995). In contrast, bupropion does *not* seem to have antipanic properties (Zajecka 1995). Several recent studies show that SSRIs such as fluoxetine, fluvoxamine, paroxetine, or sertraline are also effective for PD (see Jefferson 1997). Some early anecdotal data suggest that both venlafaxine and nefazodone are effective antipanic agents, and nefazodone seems useful in the reduction of generalized anxiety and agitation when compared with imipramine (Zajecka 1995). AD agents are not effective acutely (e.g., to abort an attack already under way) and may actually worsen both generalized and panic-type anxiety when first administered; therefore, it is best to begin with very small doses (e.g., 2.5 mg/day fluoxetine or 10 mg/day imipramine, with gradual upward titration).

Q. What is the role of ADs in mixed anxiety-depressive (MAD) states?

A. With the exception of bupropion, most of the available ADs have demonstrated some degree of benefit in MAD states, although controlled studies of well-defined MAD patients are lacking (Zajecka 1995). SSRIs, MAOIs, and nefazodone may be especially effective in MAD patients, although large-scale controlled studies are lacking. Some patients with "atypical depression" clearly overlap with MAD patients, but the definition of *atypical* has varied widely in the literature (Pies 1988). Nevertheless, there is a strong clinical impression that MAOIs may be superior to TCAs for patients with atypical depression with prominent anxiety (Zajecka 1995).

Q. Are the MAOIs especially effective in atypical depression?

A. The term *atypical depression* has had many meanings over the years. Ironically, patients with atypical features, variously defined, are quite common in clinical practice (see Pies 1988; Pies and Shader 1994). Although one meaning of atypical depression has indeed included marked anxiety or panic attacks, that is not the sense in which the term is used in DSM-IV (American Psychiatric Association 1994); there, the specifier "with atypical features" applies to patients who show 1) mood reactivity (i.e., mood brightens in response to positive events) and 2) two or more of the following: significant weight gain or hyperphagia, hypersomnia, "leaden paralysis," and a long-standing pattern of interpersonal rejection sensitivity. These criteria were heavily influenced by the research of the Columbia Group (see Quitkin et al. 1988) and differ somewhat from the "anxious, phobic" patients described in some early British studies (e.g., West and Dally 1959). Although some studies have shown MAOIs to be superior to TCAs in anxious-depressive patients, most of the "pro-MAOI" data stem from studies of patients meeting the Columbia criteria for atypical depression and who underwent treatment with either imipramine or the MAOI phenelzine. To quote J. R. T. Davidson (1992), the Columbia criteria may identify "a type of depression which is somewhat unresponsive to imipramine, although the effects of imipramine would still appear to outweigh those of placebo" (p. 347). Some authors have erroneously concluded from these limited data that MAOIs "don't work" for typical depression (e.g., in patients with major depression and melancholic features), although there is little evidence for this view (see Giller et al. 1984). In short, MAOIs appear more effective for some atypically depressed patients, although these patients are not necessarily those with mixed anxiety and depression, and also may be effective in patients who do not meet criteria for atypicality.

Q. Are ADs useful in treating dysthymic disorder?

A. There have been only six controlled studies of "pure" dysthymia in which ADs were used. Overall, both imipramine and the SSRIs were superior to placebo (Harrison and Stewart 1995). In one large, multicenter study ($N = 416$) of early-onset dysthymic disorder, imipramine and sertraline were shown to be similarly effective and both more so than placebo (Kocsis et al. 1994). The sertraline group had a significantly lower discontinuation rate (due to side effects) than did the imipramine group (25% versus 51%, respectively). In an open study of primary dysthymia using a dichotomy developed by Akiskal et al. (1983), Ravindran et al. (1994) found fluoxetine effective in the *subaffective,* but not in the character spectrum, subtype of dysthymia (77% versus 25% response rate, respectively). The subaffective patients are essentially those who have some melancholic features and a family history of mood disorders. The character spectrum patients are those who show significant character pathology, drug/alcohol abuse, and a family history of alcoholism and personality disorder more so than mood disorder. One interpretation of this study is that the more dysthymic patients resemble "classic" major depressive patients, the better their response to an SSRI. Some patients labeled dysthymic also may respond to MAOIs (Harrison and Stewart 1995). The response of dysthymic patients to SSRIs may take as long as 6–16 weeks. This finding was confirmed by a recent German report (Albert and Ebert 1996) on fluvoxamine used in pure dysthymic patients who had not responded to 6 weeks of a TCA followed by 6 weeks of fluvoxamine. The patients were then kept on fluvoxamine for another 10 weeks at the maximum dose (300 mg/day). By week 8 of fluvoxamine treatment, only 11% were responders. But by week 16, 53% of these refractory patients had responded, based on Hamilton Rating Scale (Hamilton 1960) scores. There was no control group, so conclusions are tentative. However, it seems prudent to extend AD trials in refractory dysthymic patients well beyond the usual 6 weeks deemed adequate for major depression.

▌Mechanisms of Action

Q. What is the role of serotonin receptors in the mechanism of ADs?

A. Although the story is incomplete, it seems likely that 5-HT$_1$ and 5-HT$_2$ receptors are involved. Long-term AD treatment may lead to hypersensitivity of postsynaptic 5-HT$_{1A}$ receptors but *hypo*sensitivity of presynaptic 5-HT$_{1A}$ *autoreceptors*. The latter—when stimulated by 5-HT—normally cause decreased production and release of serotonin. Thus, *decreased sensitivity* of these autoreceptors should lead to enhanced 5-HT outflow from the presynaptic neuron. Coupled with increased sensitivity of postsynaptic 5-HT$_{1A}$ receptors, the net effect of chronic AD treatment would be to enhance serotonergic function (Leonard 1996). Although 5-HT$_2$ receptors appear to be involved in both the etiology of depression and AD effects, it is not clear that they are causally involved in the antidepressant action of most ADs. Thus, downregulation of 5-HT$_2$ receptors seems to be a common mechanism of TCAs and SSRIs. But because ECT may *increase* the density of 5-HT$_2$ receptors (in rodent studies) and is an extremely effective AD, it seems unlikely that 5-HT$_2$ downregulation is causally related to AD effectiveness (Leonard 1996).

Q. What about the role of noradrenergic and dopaminergic function in ADs' mechanism of action?

A. In animal studies, chronic AD treatment leads to decreased activity and density of cortical β-adrenoreceptors, increased density of cortical α$_1$-adrenoreceptors, and decreased functional activity of cortical α$_2$-autoreceptors (Leonard 1996). (These autoreceptors normally exert an inhibitory influence on NE outflow.) It is difficult to subsume these changes under a simple increase or decrease model of noradrenergic function; rather, these changes, if applicable in humans, seem to indicate a subtle reconfiguring of noradrenergic function, perhaps favoring a net increase. Chronic AD treatment also leads to decreased functional activity of dopamine autoreceptors in the rat brain cortex, implying a net increase in dopaminergic function (Leonard 1996). This finding would be consistent with the apparent dopaminergic effects of bupropion and venlafaxine, although these effects seem to occur at rather high doses (Golden et al. 1995).

Q. Are there ADs now under development that work via new biochemical mechanisms?

A. Many agents now being tested (e.g., idazoxan, mianserin, and the recently released mirtazapine [Remeron]) act as α_2-adrenoreceptor antagonists. Antagonism of this autoreceptor leads to enhanced noradrenergic outflow from the presynaptic neuron. A number of new agents also combine noradrenergic and serotonergic effects. For example, mirtazapine may indirectly stimulate 5-HT$_{1A}$ receptors via antagonistic effects on inhibitory α_2-*heteroreceptors* located on serotonergic nerve terminals (Leonard 1996). (Heteroreceptors are receptors on one type of neuron [e.g., serotonergic] that receive input from a different type of neuron [e.g., noradrenergic].) By antagonizing such inhibitory heteroreceptors, mirtazapine leads to increased 5-HT output. In essence, mirtazapine's effect of increasing NE leads indirectly to increased 5-HT function. This finding highlights a principle that is becoming increasingly important in neuropharmacology, that is, the interdependence of neurotransmitter systems. It is doubtful, on a neurochemical level, that there are pure effectors of only one neurotransmitter system among the available ADs.

Q. Is there any way to predict which patients will respond to serotonergic versus noradrenergic ADs based on some biochemical test?

A. No. Attempts have been made to relate differential drug response to factors such as urinary 3-methoxy-4-hydroxy-phenylglycol (MHPG; a metabolite of NE), cerebrospinal fluid levels of 5-hydroxyindoleacetic acid (5-HIAA; a serotonin metabolite), or the ratio of serum tryptophan to other amino acids. These attempts have generally foundered, with too much variability in the results to prove clinically useful (Charney et al. 1995). Thus, selection of an AD is based primarily on the factors discussed previously in "Indications."

Q. Are there ways of speeding up the mechanism of action of ADs?

A. This question remains unsettled (Pies 1997). Despite claims of some new ADs, there are few data showing that any such agent has a faster onset of action than standard tricyclics, which usually require 2–4 weeks for therapeutic effects (Leonard 1996). ("Pushing" the dose of venlafaxine to high levels during the first week of treatment may accelerate response in some patients, but the accompanying GI side effects often make this strategy counterproductive in my experience.) Recently, studies have used the β-adrenoreceptor antagonist pindolol to reduce the "lag time" and/or to potentiate the AD effects of various SSRIs (Artigas et al. 1994). Pindolol apparently acts as an antagonist at the 5-HT_{1A} autoreceptor, thereby increasing serotonergic outflow from the presynaptic neuron. Local clinical experience with pindolol has yielded less impressive results, and large-scale, controlled studies will be needed to determine whether pindolol's acceleration effect can be replicated (Leonard 1996). As Chester A. Pearlman, M.D., has observed, "the often rapid improvement of responders to any antidepressant or ECT creates false hopes for [a] generally rapid response" (personal communication, February 1997).

▌ Pharmacokinetics

Q. What happens to AD metabolism in the various age groups?

A. As a broad generalization, neonates have relatively low rates of hepatic metabolism, whereas children have very high rates. Older adolescents and young adults are not far from the neonatal range, and elderly patients may have reduced metabolism for at least some ADs (Nemeroff 1995–1996). However, in the elderly, much depends on the particular agent. Demethylation of tertiary amines is reduced in the elderly (e.g., conversion of amitriptyline to nortriptyline [Dubovsky 1994]), whereas metabolism of desipramine seems minimally affected by age (Dunner 1994; von Moltke et al. 1993). (Decreased renal function, however, may lead to higher levels of desipramine's hydroxylated metabolite.) Nortriptyline metabolism seems largely unaffected by age in elderly patients without concurrent medical illness (Dunner 1994; von Moltke et al. 1993), but again, one would expect its hydroxylated metabolite to increase if renal excretion were reduced. Fluoxetine metabolism does not seem to be markedly affected by aging, although more information is needed regarding norfluoxetine (von Moltke et al. 1993). Paroxetine metabolism, in contrast, *does* seem to be reduced in the elderly, with therapeutic plasma levels achieved at about half the young adult dose (10 mg/day versus 20 mg/day, respectively [Dunner 1994]). Steady-state pharmacokinetics of venlafaxine does not seem to be altered in healthy elderly subjects; however, clearance of desmethylvenlafaxine may be about 15% less in those older than age 60 years, probably because of slightly decreased renal function (G. Magni, cited in "Academic Highlights: Venlafaxine" 1993).

Q. What is known about the metabolic pathways for bupropion metabolism?

A. We are just beginning to understand bupropion's metabolism, based mainly on clinical reports of drug-drug interactions and findings in patients with genetically aberrant cytochrome systems. Thus, high plasma levels of bupropion's *metabolite* (hydroxybupropion) have been found in three patients with genetically low levels of CYP2D6 activity, whereas carbamazepine (but not valproate) appears to decrease bupropion levels (Ketter et al. 1995; Pollock et al. 1996). Taken together, these findings suggest that bupropion itself may be metabolized (in part) via CYP3A4 (which is sensitive to carbamazepine), although its metabolite may be broken down by CYP2D6. The latter finding suggests caution when combining inhibitors of CYP2D6 (e.g., fluoxetine, paroxetine) with bupropion.

Q. Is it necessary to taper off ADs before discontinuing them, and if so, does the $t\frac{1}{2}$ of the agent influence the rate of tapering?

A. As a general rule, it is rarely wise to stop any psychotropic suddenly, except in cases of severe drug toxicity, anaphylactic reaction, or other life-threatening conditions arising from the agent's use. Most ADs may be discontinued over brief periods (3–7 days) without serious withdrawal reactions. However, with highly anticholinergic ADs, especially when used in high doses, rapid discontinuation of the drug can lead to a "cholinergic rebound" syndrome, characterized by hypersalivation, diarrhea, urinary urgency, abdominal cramping, and sweating. Some authorities (e.g., Schatzberg and Cole 1991) advise a tapering schedule no more rapid than 25–50 mg every 2–3 days for TCAs. Should GI symptoms develop during TCA withdrawal, treatment with propantheline bromide (15 mg tid prn) is recommended. (It may be just as useful to restart the TCA at a low dose [e.g., 15–25 mg/day amitriptyline].) In general, sudden discontinuation of any psychotropic with a short $t\frac{1}{2}$ is associated with more rapid, if not more intense, withdrawal symptoms than would be seen with longer-acting agents. Most of the TCAs have similar $t\frac{1}{2}$s, in the range of 24–70 hours. Therefore, likelihood of withdrawal symptoms may depend more on how anticholinergic the TCA is and how high the dose was at the time of discontinuation. With the SSRIs, fluoxetine has a markedly longer $t\frac{1}{2}$ than do the other agents in this class (see Table 1–8); in theory, sudden discontinuation of fluoxetine should not pose a high risk of withdrawal symptoms, and clinical experience generally confirms this. Sertraline has a shorter $t\frac{1}{2}$ than fluoxetine (about 24 hours versus 3–5 days, respectively), but sertraline's metabolite, desmethylsertraline, has modest clinical activity and a $t\frac{1}{2}$ of about 3 days, which may act as a buffer against withdrawal symptoms to some extent. In contrast, rather severe withdrawal reactions have been reported even with relatively gradual discontinuation of paroxetine (Paxil), which has a $t\frac{1}{2}$ of only 24 hours and no active metabolites. Withdrawal from paroxetine may present as a flulike syndrome characterized by nausea, vomiting, fatigue, myalgia, vertigo, headache, and insomnia (Barr et al. 1994). These symptoms have occurred even when paroxetine was tapered over 7–10 days. Venlafaxine-induced withdrawal has been treated with fluoxetine, probably because of the latter's long-lasting serotonergic action (Giakas and Davis 1997).

Q. What are the effects of hepatic and renal disease on the pharmacokinetics of ADs?

A. Hepatic damage leads to reduced first-pass extraction of most psychotropic drugs, with resultant higher plasma levels of the parent compound after oral administration. TCAs such as amitriptyline and imipramine will be less readily demethylated to nortriptyline and desmethylimipramine, respectively, when hepatic damage is significant (e.g., in severe cirrhosis). This may result in more side effects related to the parent compounds, such as sedation or hypotension.

SSRIs undergoing demethylation (e.g., fluoxetine to nor-fluoxetine; sertraline to desmethylsertraline) also will be affected by significant hepatic dysfunction. In cirrhotic patients, the mean $t\frac{1}{2}$ of fluoxetine may increase from 2–3 days to 7.6 days and for norfluoxetine, from 7–9 days to 12 days (Physicians' Desk Reference 1996). The clearance of sertraline also is decreased in cirrhotic patients. Although paroxetine has a short $t\frac{1}{2}$ and no active metabolites, increased plasma levels can occur in patients with severe hepatic impairment (Physicians' Desk Reference 1996). (*Note:* Hepatotoxicity is associated with the MAOIs isocarboxazid [no longer available in the United States] and phenelzine; tranylcypromine is less hepatotoxic.)

With respect to renal impairment, it appears that mild-to-moderate renal disease has little impact on AD pharmacokinetics. However, severe renal impairment may increase plasma levels of virtually all ADs. In particular, *water-soluble metabolites* of ADs (e.g., 11-hydroxynortriptyline, O-desmethyl-venlafaxine) may show reduced excretion in cases of significant renal dysfunction.

Q. How do alterations in plasma-binding proteins alter the clinical effects of ADs?

A. Reduced hepatic production of plasma-binding proteins is often said to produce increased levels of "free drug" and thus more side effects. Although changes in binding proteins can affect the *measurement of total drug* (free plus bound) and the *free fraction* (percent of unbound drug), the *absolute amount* of free drug (free drug concentration) is a function of *drug dosage* and *elimination,* not the amount of binding proteins (see Greenblatt et al. 1982 for a thorough explanation of this much-confused topic). In practice, changes in binding proteins usually affect the *therapeutic* and *toxic* ranges for a given agent, not the patient's real exposure to the unbound drug. (See "Vignettes and Puzzlers" for a clinical example.)

Q. Should ADs be taken with or without food?

A. In general, food is not an important factor in the efficacy of AD therapy. However, sertraline plasma levels may be higher if it is taken with food, whereas nefazodone levels may be decreased (Nemeroff 1995–1996).

Q. When are plasma levels (therapeutic drug monitoring [TDM]) of ADs necessary or useful?

A. For the most part, only nortriptyline has demonstrated a strong relationship between a well-defined plasma level and therapeutic efficacy, although data exist for other TCAs (see Table 1–10). Most of the newer agents—SSRIs, bupropion, nefazodone—have not yet been studied sufficiently to generate such correlations. Nevertheless, obtaining plasma levels (TDM) of ADs can be important in the following circumstances: to assess the patient's compliance, to confirm that the patient is a rapid or slow hepatic metabolizer, to monitor changes in AD levels when other hepatically metabolized agents are coadministered (e.g., an SSRI is added to ongoing TCA therapy), to help confirm the clinical diagnosis of drug toxicity, to document that adequate plasma levels have been attained before terminating a trial, and to justify an unusually low or high AD dosage (Arana and Hyman 1991; Ayd 1995). This last point is relevant when 350 mg/day desipramine, for example, is required to achieve a plasma level of 110 ng/mL, which represents the lower end of the putative therapeutic range.

■ Main Side Effects

Q. What are the relative rates of AD-induced seizures among the various tricyclic and nontricyclic agents?

A. In general, ADs are not highly epileptogenic. In one study in which the mean follow-up period was *28 months*, the overall incidence of seizures during imipramine or amitriptyline therapy was approximately 0.5% in nonepileptic patients; thus, the cumulative *yearly* incidence of seizures during TCA therapy would be estimated at approximately 0.2% (Lowry and Dunner 1980). Some data indicate a seizure rate around 0.45% for imipramine at effective doses (Rosenstein et al. 1993). Predisposing factors for AD-related seizures appear to include history of personal or familial seizure disorder, abnormal pretreatment electroencephalogram (EEG), postnatal brain damage, cerebrovascular disease, head trauma, sedative or alcohol withdrawal, and multiple concomitant medications (Lowry and Dunner 1980; Rosenstein et al. 1993). Seizure risk for most ADs appears to increase with dose and/or blood level (Rosenstein et al. 1993). Among the TCAs, amitriptyline may be more likely to aggravate seizures (Edwards et al. 1986). Although bupropion in high doses (more than 450 mg/day) may have a greater likelihood of inducing seizures than do other ADs, a recent 102-site study of bupropion at doses up to 450 mg/day showed an overall incidence of seizures of 0.36%; this finding was interpreted as comparable to other ADs (Johnston et al. 1991). (Maprotiline [Ludiomil], a rarely used AD, does appear to have a higher risk of inducing seizures than do the TCAs.) The SSRIs appear to have around a 0.2% incidence of seizures (Johnston et al. 1991)—somewhat lower than the incidence for TCAs (Rosenstein et al. 1993). A recent uncontrolled study suggested that fluoxetine actually had *anticonvulsant* effects in a small group of patients with complex partial seizures (Favale et al. 1995). However, these patients were also maintained on their usual anticonvulsants. MAOIs also seem to have a lower risk of inducing seizures than do TCAs (Rosenstein et al. 1993). Although there is less postmarketing information regarding nefazodone and venlafaxine, it appears that both agents have a low rate of associated seizures. During clinical trials with nefazodone, the overall incidence of seizures was only 0.04%; however, patients with a history of seizures had been excluded from these studies (Bristol-Myers-Squibb, data on file with company). In a similar population treated with venlafaxine, premarketing testing showed a seizure rate of 0.26% (8 of 3,082) (D. L. Albano, Wyeth-Ayerst Laboratories, personal communication, February 1996). This finding was comparable to the rate of seizures seen in the placebo group and less than that for comparator drugs, including imipramine, trazodone, clomipramine, fluoxetine, and amitriptyline. It is important to keep in mind that postmarketing reports do not necessarily establish a cause-and-effect relationship between the index drug and the occurrence of a seizure. In summary, all ADs, with the exception of maprotiline (and perhaps high-dose therapy with bupropion), have a relatively low rate of associated seizures. Of available AD agents, nefazodone may prove to have the lowest rate, but more clinical data are needed.

Q. Do SSRIs affect hemostasis?

A. A few case reports have implicated two SSRIs (fluoxetine and paroxetine) in abnormal bleeding (Aranth and Lindberg 1992; Ottervanger et al. 1994), but the frequency of this reaction is unknown. It has been attributed to SSRI-induced depletion of platelet serotonin and may be associated with *normal* values for platelet count, prothrombin time, and partial thromboplastin time (Ottervanger et al. 1994). Hyperserotonemia also can cause dilated capillaries or telangiectasia, possibly leading to ecchymoses without hemostatic defect.

Q. What are the main side effects of mirtazapine (Remeron)?

A. The most common side effects are *somnolence, increased appetite, weight gain,* and *dizziness.* SSRI-like side effects (nausea, insomnia, sexual dysfunction) seem to be minimal (Kehoe and Schorr 1996).

Q. What is the risk of agranulocytosis with mirtazapine (Remeron), and how should it be managed?

A. Preclinical experience with mirtazapine indicated that agranulocytosis occurred in 2 of 2,796 patients, leading the manufacturer to estimate the risk as roughly 1.1 per 1,000. (One of the two patients had a rare autoimmune disease, so it is not clear that this incidence will hold up in clinical studies.) Although the manufacturer advises informing the patient of this risk, no specific guidelines for blood monitoring are given. In its 1996 package insert, Organon does state that "if a patient develops a sore throat, fever, stomatitis or other signs of infection, along with a low white blood cell (WBC) count, treatment with Remeron should be discontinued and the patient . . . closely monitored." In my opinion, mirtazapine must be considered a second-line treatment for depression until more is known about its risk of agranulocytosis. I also would recommend advising patients to report sudden onset of sore throat, fever, stomatitis, or other signs of infection. A baseline complete blood count and at least one follow-up during the first month of treatment would seem a prudent medicolegal strategy, although—if experience with clozapine is any clue—it is by no means clear that this would increase the pickup rate of agranulocytosis.

Q. Can ADs induce mania or "rapid cycling" in bipolar patients? If so, what is the best strategy for dealing with depressed bipolar patients?

A. *Rapid cycling* is defined in DSM-IV as "at least four episodes of a mood disturbance in the previous 12 months that meet criteria for a Major Depressive, Manic, Mixed, or Hypomanic Episode" (p. 391). In DSM-IV, "episodes" are demarcated either by partial or full remission for at least 2 months or by a switch to an episode of the opposite polarity. Persad et al. (1996) have reviewed the pharmacological and nonpharmacological factors involved in rapid cycling bipolar disorder, which occurs in about 17% of all patients suffering from bipolar disorder, usually late in the course of illness. It is not clear whether this pattern reflects the natural evolution of bipolar illness or the unintended consequence of various "cyclogenic" drugs. Citing work by Cutler and Post (1982), Persad et al. (1996) note that rapid cycling was seen in some patients even before the era of pharmacological treatment. Persad et al. (1996) list TCAs, piribedil (a dopamine agonist), MAOIs, conjugated estrogen, amphetamines, and (surprisingly) *lithium* as agents that can induce rapid cycling. It is unclear whether drug-induced rapid cycling is a *dose-related* phenomenon or whether some bipolar patients will cycle rapidly with *any* dose of certain cyclogenic agents. Among nonpharmacological factors in rapid cycling, Persad et al. (1996) cite pregnancy, multiple sclerosis, Graves' disease, right hemisphere stroke, and (again, somewhat surprisingly) *ECT*. They also note the association among hypothyroidism, female gender, and rapid cycling and suggest a possible association between rapid cycling in women and postpartum thyroid dysfunction. Persad et al. (1996) consider the use of ADs in rapid cycling "inadvisable." However, it is hard to demonstrate a causal link between any of the aforementioned drugs/factors and rapid cycling.

In my experience, there is little evidence that lithium alone can induce rapid cycling; however, there are at least two case reports in which manic symptoms followed *addition of lithium to AD treatment* (Delisle 1986; Price et al. 1984). Similarly, the claim that ECT can induce rapid cycling requires strong qualification. Although ECT occasionally may induce hypomania or mania, there is no compelling evidence that it increases manic episode frequency over time, as may tricyclics (Wehr and Goodwin 1987; Zornberg and Pope 1993). There is evidence that *unilateral* ECT may worsen mania in some cases, leading to the recommendation of bilateral ECT for mania (Milstein et al. 1987). However, subsequent research has suggested that the poor response to unilateral ECT in mania may be due to inadequate stimulus intensity (Mukherjee et al. 1994). Srisurapanont et al. (1995) recommend adding an *MAOI* to lithium for anergic bipolar depression unresponsive to lithium alone. They recommend adding either an *SSRI* or *bupropion* to lithium (in preference to a tricyclic) for nonanergic bipolar depression. These recommendations are based on the assumption that MAOIs, bupropion, and SSRIs are somewhat less likely than tricyclics to induce a switch into mania or to promote cycling. A recent retrospective study of treatment-refractory bipolar patients did not find a significant difference between "heterocyclic" ADs (undefined) and MAOIs, in terms of inducing mania or cycle acceleration (Altshuler et al. 1995). However, this study did not sort out rapid-cycling patients from other refractory bipolar patients. Altshuler et al. (1995) found an association between AD-induced *cycle acceleration* and the following factors: AD-induced mania, younger age at first treatment intervention, bipolar II diagnosis, and female gender. The study by Altshuler et al. could not confirm the clinical impression that mood stabilizers (e.g., lithium, valproate) "protect" patients from a drug-induced switch into mania. A recent study by Robinson et al. (1996) reviewed the adverse effects of nefazodone in approximately 3,500 patients, of whom a subset had bipolar depression. For the index period, the rate of manic episodes with nefazodone was 1.6% (2 of 125) versus 5.1% (2 of 39) for tricyclic-treated patients. This finding suggests that like bupropion, nefazodone has a relatively low potential for inducing mania in bipolar patients. The bottom line is avoid ADs in all rapid-cycling patients, if possible, and use them judiciously in any bipolar patient. In my experience, *low-dose bupropion*—sometimes as little as one-fourth of a 75-mg tablet of bupropion per day—may be effective and well tolerated in depressed bipolar patients, in combination with divalproex. It remains to be seen whether this clinical impression is borne out in large-scale, prospective studies.

Q. What are the best strategies for managing anti-depressant-induced sexual dysfunction (AISD)?

A. AISD contributes to both noncompliance with medication and decreased quality of life. AISD may take the form of *decreased libido, erectile dysfunction, delayed orgasm, anorgasmia, impaired or painful ejaculation, penile or clitoral anesthesia,* or *penile or clitoral priapism.* AISD tends to be more common with the tricyclics (particularly clomipramine), the SSRIs, MAOIs, and venlafaxine. Trazodone is disproportionately associated with priapism, although it occurs in only about 1 in 6,000 male patients. Curiously, this often occurs at doses *less* than 150 mg/day and during the first month of treatment (Golden et al. 1995; Thompson et al. 1990). AISD seems to be less common with both bupropion and nefazodone (McElroy 1995). Feiger et al. (1996), using a detailed sexual function questionnaire, found that nefazodone-treated patients had low rates of sexual complaints. AISD may begin early or late in the course of treatment and can be dose related. General management includes careful questioning as to specific sexual problems (which patients may be reluctant to discuss), careful differential diagnosis (e.g., sexual dysfunction may be an integral part of major depression), reducing the dosage, and waiting for tolerance to occur. If the problem persists, switching to bupropion or nefazodone, or adding an agent to enhance sexual function, is an appropriate strategy. Case reports have noted success with the addition (to ongoing antidepressant) of any one of the following: *yohimbine* (5.4–16.2 mg/day), *bupropion* (75–150 mg/day), *trazodone* (50–200 mg/day), *bethanechol* (10–50 mg tid to qid), *cyproheptadine* (4–12 mg qhs), *amantadine* (100–300 mg/day), or *buspirone* (15–60 mg/day), or low doses of dextroamphetamine (McElroy 1995). However, the use of cyproheptadine, a 5-HT antagonist, has sometimes been associated with recurrence of depression or decreased efficacy of concomitant SSRI treatment (Feder 1991b). Anecdotal data also suggest that the herbal extract ginkgo biloba (60–120 mg bid) may be useful in reversing AISD (Goldman 1997).

Q. What is the mechanism for SSRI-induced "apathy," and how is this best managed?

A. It has been observed that after a period of weeks or months, some patients taking SSRIs develop a syndrome of apathy, loss of initiative, lack of emotional responsiveness, or (less commonly) "disinhibition" (Hoehn-Saric et al. 1991). Although this "frontal lobe syndrome" has been reported with fluoxetine and fluvoxamine, it can occur with the other SSRIs, in my experience. In the case reported by Hoehn-Saric et al. (1991), this syndrome was associated with decreased cerebral blood flow in the frontal lobes and neuropsychological changes associated with frontal lobe impairment; clinical manifestations disappeared about a month after discontinuation of fluoxetine. Although the mechanism underlying these frontal lobe symptoms is unclear, it is possible that serotonin's ability to decrease dopaminergic tone in some brain regions (Roth and Meltzer 1995) may be involved. In my experience, the use of the dopaminergic agent methylphenidate (10–20 mg/day) may help restore normal mood and affect in some patients with this syndrome, but controlled studies of this maneuver are lacking.

Q. With respect to TCA toxicity in an overdose, which is more useful: a TCA plasma level or an electrocardiogram (ECG)?

A. Some patients with relatively low plasma TCA levels may still have complete heart block; conversely, some patients with high TCA levels (e.g., greater than 400 ng/mL) show no cardiac arrhythmias. Thus, an ECG is the more relevant and useful test in an overdose situation (Nemeroff 1995–1996), with a QRS duration greater than 0.10 seconds being a particularly useful index of toxicity (Janicak et al. 1993). Nevertheless, tricyclic levels in excess of 1000 ng/mL are associated with increased cardiac and neurological morbidity (Janicak et al. 1993).

▌ Drug-Drug Interactions

Q. What are the most serious drug-drug interactions with TCAs and non-TCAs?

A. The drug-drug combinations that may cause serious or life-threatening interactions include the following: 1) combination of an MAOI and SSRI, which may lead to severe serotonergic syndrome (fever, myoclonus, confusion, coma); 2) combination of an MAOI with meperidine (Demerol), which may lead to fatal hyperthermia and serotonin syndrome (dextromethorphan also may be dangerous in combination with an MAOI); 3) combination of an MAOI and a sympathomimetic, such as amphetamine, which may provoke a hypertensive reaction; and 4) combination of an MAOI with a TCA, which also provokes a serotonergic syndrome (less commonly, a hypertensive reaction). Potentially dangerous reactions also may result from a combination of an SSRI and a TCA, which may lead to markedly increased levels of the TCA, and from a combination of a TCA with a type-1A antiarrhythmic agent such as quinidine, leading to dangerous conduction abnormalities. Despite the risks associated with these various combinations, certain cases of refractory depression may warrant such polypharmacy. Thus, when carefully controlled and monitored, TCAs may be combined with MAOIs and SSRIs with TCAs (see the following discussion on "Potentiating Maneuvers").

Q. What are the risks of combining ADs with antipsychotics and anticonvulsants? Which combinations are safest?

A. Complex interactions often occur when hepatically metabolized psychotropics are combined. This is especially true when two or more agents use the same enzymatic pathway of metabolism (e.g., the CYP2D6 pathway). As a rule, TCAs increase plasma levels of some antipsychotic agents (e.g., imipramine and nortriptyline increase chlorpromazine levels). Fluoxetine impairs haloperidol metabolism and virtually any other psychotropic using the CYP2D6 pathway. Conversely, haloperidol, thiothixene, perphenazine, and chlorpromazine inhibit the metabolism of TCAs (Ciraulo et al. 1995a). When TCAs and phenothiazine-type antipsychotics are given together, higher plasma levels of both types of agent often occur, leading to increased sedation, anticholinergic effects, and perhaps cardiac toxicity because of quinidine-like effects. Anticonvulsants may affect metabolism of both ADs and antipsychotic agents (Ciraulo et al. 1995a). Carbamazepine tends to be an enzymatic inducer, leading to reduced levels of other psychotropics (e.g., haloperidol). Valproate tends to inhibit metabolism of other psychotropics, but the effects are sometimes modest (e.g., valproate raised plasma clozapine levels only about 6% in one study [Centorrino et al. 1994] and actually decreased clozapine levels by 15% in another study [Longo and Salzman 1995]).

Q. What drugs used in general and internal medicine are likely to have pharmacokinetic interactions with ADs?

A. Because many such drugs use the same cytochrome systems as do ADs, there is significant potential for interaction. *Analgesics* such as acetaminophen, ibuprofen, naproxen, and codeine; *anticonvulsants,* such as phenytoin and mephenytoin; *calcium channel blockers; β-blockers; corticosteroids; androgens; estrogens;* and *macrolide antibiotics* all may interact with ADs metabolized via CYP1A2, 2C19, 2C9, 2D6, and 3A3/4. Other agents that may interact with ADs include theophyl-

line, barbiturates, omeprazole, warfarin, quinidine, tamoxifen, and ketoconazole (Ereshefsky 1996; Ereshefsky et
al. 1996). (See Table 1–15a for specific cytochrome systems involved.)

Q. Can the antiobesity agent fenfluramine interact with
ADs?

A. Fenfluramine inhibits reuptake and promotes release of
5-HT and is thus capable of interacting adversely with SSRIs
to produce a serotonin syndrome (Krishnan and Hamilton
1997). (Actually, fenfluramine [Pondimin] is a racemic mix-
ture of the dextro and levo forms of fenfluramine and has
augmenting effects on 5-HT, NE, and dopamine; *dex*fenfluramine [Redux] primarily affects 5-HT.) Moreover, a recent
report suggests that fenfluramine may markedly increase
plasma levels of imipramine (Fogelson 1997) and other TCAs.
Thus, fenfluramine and dexfenfluramine must be used cautiously, if at all, in patients taking ADs. These two agents
were recently removed from the United States market because of their cardiopulmonary side effects.

Q. Can foods or beverages interact pharmacokinetically
with ADs?

A. *Grapefruit juice* appears to be a significant inhibitor of
CYP3A3/4 and may increase plasma levels of clomipramine
and its metabolite, desmethylclomipramine (Oesterheld and
Kallepalli 1997). In principle, other ADs metabolized via this
cytochrome system—as well as triazolam, calcium channel
blockers, and other drugs—could be affected by unusually
high intake of grapefruit juice.

▌ Potentiating Maneuvers

Q. What constitutes an adequate trial duration on an AD?

A. The old notion that we can reach conclusions about an AD's efficacy after 4 weeks is probably wrong, with 5–6 *weeks* being closer to the minimum time needed to know whether a drug will work. Some patients will continue to show improvement on an AD up to 12 weeks after beginning treatment (Gorman 1995). Geriatric patients sometimes require up to 12–16 weeks to show a full response (Wise 1995). In practical terms, however, if a patient shows absolutely *no* improvement after 3–4 weeks—despite *adequate AD plasma levels*—it is my practice to switch to another agent. If the patient has had a *partial* response to the first agent after 3–4 weeks, it may be reasonable simply to wait—on the premise that a full response might be seen with an additional week or two. However, if a patient is in *significant distress,* even after a partial response by week 3, it is my usual practice to try an augmentation strategy at that point.

Q. Are TCAs more effective for severe depression than SSRIs?

A. This issue remains hotly debated. Although there is modest evidence that TCAs may be more effective in severe melancholic depression in the elderly (Roose et al. 1994), the majority of studies have not established any overall superiority of the TCAs when compared with the SSRIs (Nierenberg 1994). In my experience, however, a TCA often will be effective in older patients who have failed trials on more than one SSRI.

Q. In refractory major depression, when is it appropriate to *potentiate* an ongoing AD, as opposed to *switching* to another class of agent?

A. There are no randomized, controlled studies (to date) *directly* comparing these strategies. Thus, most of the advice given on this question is derived from clinical experience and a few studies examining success rates in depressed patients switched from one agent to another ("crossover monotherapy").

Keller (1995) has suggested that crossover monotherapy for treatment-resistant depression (TRD) may have advantages over the use of combination treatments. With crossover monotherapy (e.g., switching a refractory patient from a tricyclic to an SSRI or vice versa), there is reduced risk of drug-drug interactions and (usually) reduced expense, compared with augmentation therapy. Keller (1995) presented preliminary results of two such crossover studies now in progress, involving patients with "double depression" (major depression plus dysthymia, n = 341) and chronic major depression (n = 294). Keller and his colleagues found that of the 198 patients for whom data were available, only about 27% had actually undergone an adequate trial of an AD prior to the study—defined as at least 150 mg/day imipramine or its equivalent for at least 4 consecutive weeks. In phase 1 (lasting 12 weeks), patients were randomly assigned to either sertraline or imipramine in a 2-to-1 ratio. Among those who completed the 12-week acute treatment phase, *responders* to either drug continued on the same drug in double-blind fashion for 16 weeks. *Nonresponders* to either drug were crossed over to the other drug, also in double-blind fashion (phase 2). Results of the first (12-week) phase showed that slightly more than 60% of patients who completed this phase were responders to either treatment—suggesting that even patients with chronic depression are responsive to adequate medication. With respect to phase 2—the crossover from one agent to the other—results indicate that sertraline treatment of imipramine nonresponders is both effective and well tolerated. Similarly, imipramine treatment of sertraline nonresponders also was effective, although less so than sertraline treatment of imipramine nonresponders. In Keller's study (1995), imipramine was not as well tolerated as sertraline. Interestingly, the response to crossover medication was inversely proportional to the initial drug response: in effect, *the worse the response to the first drug, the more likely the response to the second (crossover) medication.* Other SSRIs (fluoxetine, paroxetine) have been investigated (as crossover therapies) in tricyclic TRD. Overall, studies on outpatients yield a response rate of between 30% and 70% to this strategy. Several inpatient studies of fluvoxamine in TCA-refractory patients have yielded less impressive results; however, outpatient studies using fluvoxamine have shown good results. There are fewer studies of crossover from an SSRI to a tricyclic. One such study by Peselow et al. (1989) investigated the use of imipramine in paroxetine nonresponders and found a 73% response rate after 6 weeks of imipramine treatment (see Thase and Rush 1995 for a full discussion of these studies). In summary, rather than using an augmenting agent, it may be worthwhile first to change from one AD class to another in some TRD patients. In my experience, this strategy makes sense primarily in patients who have *poor* or *minimal* response to the first agent.

Q. What about changing from one SSRI to another SSRI in a TRD patient?

A. Four studies (using varying methods) have focused on this question and reached somewhat different conclusions; however, the change from one SSRI to another *does* make sense in many TRD patients, at least up to a point (Gelenberg 1996). Brown and Harrison (1995) found that 72% of fluoxetine-intolerant outpatients ($n = 113$) responded to sertraline and were generally able to tolerate it (only 10% had adverse reactions). Conversely, Apter and Birkett (1995) found that around 63% of outpatients who had failed treatment with sertraline (due to lack of effect or intolerable side effects) responded well to fluoxetine, with only one patient dropping out because of an adverse event. Zarate et al. (1996) came to a less positive conclusion in their retrospective review of 39 inpatients sequentially treated with fluoxetine and sertraline. They found that of 31 inpatients with major depression or bipolar depression treated with sertraline, only 42% were considered responders; of those, only 26% continued to do well at follow-up. Of 21 patients who had discontinued fluoxetine because of side effects, 43% also discontinued sertraline because of side effects. Twelve of 16 (75%) patients who had side effects during sertraline treatment had the *same* side effects as when taking fluoxetine (including allergic-type reactions). Zarate et al. (1996) concluded that if a patient has not done well on fluoxetine, there is only a modest benefit in changing to sertraline. Looking at the Zarate et al. (1996) data from a different perspective, we can say that at least one in four fluoxetine nonresponders may do quite well on sertraline. Finally, in an open study of 55 patients with major depression who had failed on one of the SSRIs, Joffe et al. (1996b) found that 28 of the 55 had a marked or complete AD response to a second SSRI. In toto, the available data support the utility of switching from one SSRI to another, even though some patients will have similar side effects with each agent. However, in my experience, a patient who has had absolutely no response to two full SSRI trials rarely responds to a third SSRI. At that point, trying an agent with different chemical properties (e.g., bupropion, venlafaxine) may make more sense.

Q. Can SSRIs be combined with bupropion in refractory depression?

A. Large-scale, controlled studies of this combination are not available, but a few case reports suggest that this combination may be safe and effective. In one such case, a depressed woman who had previously been refractory to both paroxetine alone (with intolerable sedation at 50 mg/day) and bupropion alone (with significant agitation at 300 mg/day) responded well to a combination of paroxetine 30 mg/day plus bupropion 225 mg/day, with reduction in the aforementioned side effects (Marshall and Liebowitz 1996). (*Note:* Her concomitant obsessive-compulsive symptoms also improved along with the depression.)

A second case series reported the efficacy of sertraline combined with bupropion in refractory depression (Marshall et al. 1995). Keep in mind that because the metabolic pathway of bupropion is not well defined (see "Pharmacokinetics"), it is possible that some SSRIs may increase plasma levels of bupropion (and its metabolite, hydroxybupropion); in theory, this could increase seizure risk at higher bupropion doses. Indeed, there are now several case reports of anxiety and neurotoxicity (e.g., myoclonus, delirium) following use of combined *fluoxetine* and bupropion (Hopkins 1996). The pharmacodynamic mechanism of bupropion's efficacy is not known, although noradrenergic effects have been implicated.

Q. Can psychostimulants be used to potentiate the effects of SSRIs ?

A. Stoll et al. (1996) recently presented five cases of major depression in which open trials of methylphenidate (10–40 mg/day) were used to augment fluoxetine or paroxetine. Self-reported symptom reduction occurred rapidly in all cases, with few adverse effects. The authors discuss the possibility that methylphenidate and other psychostimulants reverse the dopamine-depleting effect of the SSRIs. Metz and Shader (1991) also have reported that the combination of fluoxetine and pemoline was effective in several cases of refractory major depression.

Q. Can MAOIs be potentiated with either TCAs or stimulants, such as methylphenidate? What about MAOIs plus lithium in refractory depression?

A. The combination of an MAOI and a TCA is somewhat controversial, primarily because of the paucity of controlled outcome studies and the theoretical risk of the serotonin syndrome (Pies and Shader 1994). In general, this combination should be used only after other potentiation strategies and/or ECT have failed; nevertheless, when carried out properly, an MAOI/TCA combination may be safe and effective for appropriately selected patients (Ayd 1995). Among this group are highly refractory patients with anxious, phobic, and somatized (atypical) depressions who have *not* had a history of hypomania, mania, or psychosis (Ayd 1995). Some data implicate *imipramine, clomipramine,* and perhaps *desipramine* as the most likely TCAs to interact adversely with an MAOI, so these agents should be avoided (Ciraulo et al. 1995a). The best approach to MAOI/TCA cotherapy is to begin both agents simultaneously, using small doses of each, or to add a small amount of the MAOI (e.g., 5 mg/day tranylcypromine) to ongoing TCA treatment (Pies and Shader 1994). TCAs should *never* be added to an ongoing MAOI regimen (Ciraulo et al. 1995a). Despite theoretical concerns about hypertensive reactions, MAOIs have been successfully combined with pemoline (Fawcett et al. 1991) in TRD. Methylphenidate also may be combined with an MAOI, although some patients may experience orthostatic hypotension, restlessness, or hypomania (Ayd 1995; Feighner et al. 1985). MAOIs may be combined with lithium in refractory depressed patients. In general, this combination seems to be well tolerated, although some patients may become tremulous or hypomanic. There have been two case reports of dyskinetic movements associated with this combination (Ayd 1995).

Q. Is there a role for the herbal remedy St.-John's-wort in the treatment of depression?

A. There is growing evidence—mainly from the German literature—that St.-John's-wort (*Hypericum perforatum*) is well tolerated and more effective than placebo in mild-to-moderate, nonpsychotic depression (Bender 1996b). Gastrointestinal irritation, allergic reactions, and fatigue are the most common side effects, but each occurs in fewer than 1% of cases. Rarely, cardiac arrhythmias have been reported (J. M. Ellison, M.D., personal communication, September 1997). St. John's-wort is usually taken in tablet form as 300 mg tid, though a tea may also be prepared from the raw herb. The effects of St.-John's-wort in bipolar and psychotic depression are not known, nor are its potential interactions with standard antidepressants. Until more controlled studies are available using standardized preparations of this herb, St.-John's-wort must be considered "investigational" in nature; however, it seems to be relatively benign for most patients and may be of some benefit to those who cannot tolerate conventional treatments.

Q. What is the role of benzodiazepines in the adjunctive treatment of depression?

A. Although benzodiazepines are sometimes used during the initiation of AD therapy—particularly for agitated or insomniac depressed patients whose primary AD is a more "stimulating" type—benzodiazepines have a rather limited role in the long-term treatment of depression. Indeed, benzodiazepines may sometimes exacerbate depression, although this effect does not appear to be common (Smith and Salzman 1991). Summing up the available data, Joffe et al. (1996a) conclude as follows: "benzodiazepines decrease nonspecific symptoms of depression such as insomnia, agitation, and anxiety, but do not have specific or intrinsic antidepressant effects and do not have an enduring therapeutic benefit" (p. 29). (See also Chapter 3 [Table 3–7] for more information on alprazolam as an AD.)

▌ Use in Special Populations

Q. What are the special needs of depressed patients with cancer and other medical illnesses?

A. Major depression may be seen in approximately 5%–15% of cancer patients—higher than the prevalence in the general population (6%) but probably no higher than seen in comparably ill medical patients with other diagnoses (Derogatis et al. 1983; Pies 1996). Depressive symptoms vary along a continuum of severity in cancer patients, ranging from no depression at all in more than 40% of cancer patients to mild, moderate, or severe symptoms in the remainder (Derogatis et al. 1983; Massie and Holland 1990).

Massie and Holland (1990) suggest that the following features should prompt consideration of a psychiatric consultation: *depressive symptoms that last longer than a week, worsening course of depressive symptoms, and depressive symptoms that interfere with the patient's ability to function or to cooperate with treatment.* The *tertiary TCAs* (e.g., amitriptyline, doxepin) or *trazodone* may be especially useful for depressed cancer patients with significant agitation and insomnia. Less sedating *secondary amine tricyclics* (e.g., desipramine, nortriptyline) may be more useful in lethargic patients or those at risk for anticholinergic side effects. There is no convincing evidence, however, that one type of AD is more effective than another in the long-term treatment of cancer patients. Newer, nontricyclic agents—particularly the *SSRIs*—may be of use in depressed cancer patients with significant orthostatic hypotension or cardiac conduction abnormalities, but the side effect profile of the SSRIs is not always suitable for cancer patients. ADs may be used as analgesic adjuncts in cancer-related pain and appear to be effective for pain relief even in the absence of clinical depression. Cancer patients, like most elderly patients, generally require lower total therapeutic dosages of TCAs (about 50–100 mg/day), perhaps as a consequence of altered drug metabolism and absorption (Massie and Holland 1990). (However, *plasma levels* of the tricyclics may still need to be within the usual therapeutic range for the treatment of major depression.) The principal side effects of the TCAs—particularly the tertiary amines—include *anticholinergic, orthostatic, sedative,* and *cardiovascular effects.* Anticholinergic effects (dry mouth, constipation, urinary retention, gastric reflux, blurry vision) are especially to be avoided in cancer patients with xerostomia or stomatitis and in those recovering from GI or genitourinary surgery (Harnett 1994; Massie and Holland 1990). (*Central* anticholinergic side effects include confusion and memory impairment and also should be avoided in patients already prone to neurotoxic drug effects.) Cancer patients (and other medically ill patients) with volume depletion and hypotension are not good candidates for trazodone or tertiary amine tricyclics; nortriptyline, however, in doses of 50–75 mg/day, may be relatively free of hypotensive effects. Because of their quinidine-like properties, all TCAs can cause cardiac conduction abnormalities and generally are contraindicated in patients with preexisting cardiac arrhythmias. The SSRIs have far fewer anticholinergic, hypotensive, sedating, and cardiovascular side effects than the tertiary amine TCAs and are far less toxic in overdose situations; however, they can provoke anorexia, nausea, diarrhea, weight loss, tremor, extrapyramidal effects, and hyponatremia in some patients (Harnett 1994; Massie and Holland 1990). There also have been some case reports of sinus node slowing with fluoxetine (Ellison et al. 1990; Feder 1991a), and this slowing might be particularly likely when SSRIs are used together with β-blockers. Despite these potential drawbacks, fluoxetine and other SSRIs have been used successfully in cancer patients, usually by beginning with a low dose and increasing it slowly. 5-HT$_3$ receptor antagonists, such as ondansetron, may ameliorate SSRI-related nausea (Harnett 1994). Bupropion—a nontricyclic, non-SSRI—also may be safe in this population but is relatively contraindicated in patients with a history of seizures. Data on use of newer ADs (nefazodone, fluvoxamine, venlafaxine) in cancer patients are still incomplete.

Q. What about depressed patients with cancer and other diseases who cannot tolerate oral ADs?

A. Many medically ill patients become too weak to swallow even liquid medications; others cannot take medications orally because of stomatitis or oral, pharyngeal, or esophageal surgery (Massie and Holland 1990). In such cases, the use of IM preparations or rectal suppositories may be considered. Amitriptyline, imipramine, and doxepin can be given IM, and the successful use of rectal doxepin and carbamazepine in patients with cancer has been reported (Massie and Lesko 1989; Storey and Trumble 1992). The rectal administration of amitriptyline (50 mg in cocoa butter twice daily) resulted in clinical improvement in one severely depressed cancer patient (Adams 1982). Doxepin capsules (25 mg) with no suppository base also have been used in a small number of patients, with apparent clinical benefit (Storey and Trumble 1992). Measurements of these drugs in the serum suggest that they are well absorbed per rectum.

Q. Are the psychostimulants useful in depressed cancer patients and other depressed, medically ill populations?

A. The *psychostimulants* (methylphenidate, pemoline, and dextroamphetamine) also may be useful in depressed cancer patients, promoting a sense of well-being, decreased fatigue, and improved appetite (when used in low doses) in cancer patients (Massie and Holland 1990). These agents have a rapid onset of AD action and are not abused in the medically ill population; however, tolerance may sometimes develop. The psychostimulants, like the ADs, also potentiate the pain-relieving effects of narcotic analgesics and help counteract their sedating effects. Some clinicians regard the psychostimulants as first-line treatments of depression in the medical setting because of their rapid therapeutic effect and low frequency of adverse reactions.

Q. What drug-drug interactions have importance in medically ill patients taking ADs?

A. Because most medically ill patients will be taking several nonpsychotropic medications, the issue of drug-drug interactions often becomes critical (Ciraulo et al. 1995a, 1995b; Gelenberg 1995). Keep in mind that the SSRIs are strong inhibitors of the CYP system, which is responsible for the metabolism of numerous "nonpsychiatric" drugs and medications. The CYP2D6 system—which is strongly inhibited by *paroxetine* and *fluoxetine*—metabolizes many antiarrhythmics (encainide, propafenone), β-blockers, opiates, and terfenadine. CYP3A4—which is strongly inhibited by *fluvoxamine, nefazodone,* and, to a lesser degree, *sertraline*—metabolizes lidocaine, quinidine, carbamazepine, calcium channel blockers, erythromycin, steroids, cisapride, and the nonsedating antihistamines astemizole and terfenadine (*Note:* The latter is also metabolized by CYP2D6).

To cite one example of a potentially dangerous interaction, coadministration of the new AD *nefazodone* with the drugs *terfenadine* or *astemizole* could provoke dangerous cardiac arrhythmias (Gelenberg 1995). The clinician is well advised to assume a drug-drug interaction, until proven otherwise, when combining psychotropics with any medications metabolized by the liver (see Table 1–15a).

Q. What are the risks of AD use during pregnancy and the postpartum period? What special concerns arise when dosing ADs in the pregnant patient?

A. With respect to ADs, most data come from studies of tricyclics and fluoxetine (Prozac); there is only a modicum of information about newer agents such as sertraline (Zoloft), paroxetine (Paxil), venlafaxine (Effexor), and nefazodone (Serzone) (Altshuler et al. 1996; Pies 1994; Stowe and Nemeroff 1995). The tricyclics (e.g., desipramine [Norpramin], imipramine [Tofranil], nortriptyline [Pamelor]) appear to have little potential for teratogenicity. Similarly, a study by Pastuszak et al. (1993) found no evidence of teratogenicity in 128 women taking fluoxetine during the first trimester, compared with matched control subjects. Although there was a trend toward higher *miscarriage* rates in the fluoxetine group compared with control subjects taking known nonteratogens, the risk was small (relative risk, 1.9) and comparable to that of tricyclics. (Interestingly, depression itself also may raise the risk of miscarriage.) A recent study by Chambers et al. (1996) found no significant differences between fluoxetine-treated pregnant women and control subjects in number of spontaneous pregnancy losses or major structural anomalies; however, the incidence of three or more minor anomalies was significantly higher in the fluoxetine cohort, and women who took fluoxetine during the third trimester were at increased risk for perinatal complications. The study by Chambers et al. (1996) has been criticized on a variety of methodological grounds, including its failure to control for coexisting diseases (Nulman et al. 1997). Nulman et al. (1997) found that in utero exposure to either tricyclics or fluoxetine does *not* affect global IQ, language development, or behavioral development in preschool children. The more anticholinergic tricyclics (e.g., amitriptyline, doxepin) can occasionally induce fetal tachyarrhythmias, urinary retention, or intestinal obstruction. Clomipramine (Anafranil)—a tricyclic used mainly in the treatment of OCD—also has substantial anticholinergic effects and would be expected to produce similar effects in the neonate. With respect to dosing, Wisner et al. (1993) found that the doses of TCAs required to achieve remission actually increased during the second half of pregnancy, reaching 1.6 times the mean dose required when the patients were not pregnant. This increase was attributed, in part, to enhanced hepatic metabolism of ADs during pregnancy and to increased volume of distribution. Neonatal irritability, tachypnea, tremor, and hypotonia may result from either tricyclic toxicity or withdrawal. It is therefore prudent to monitor maternal blood levels of tricyclics throughout pregnancy and gradually to reduce the dosage during the week before delivery. A recent comprehensive review by Altshuler et al. (1996) concludes that "use of psychotropic medications during pregnancy is appropriate in many clinical situations and should include thoughtful weighing of risk of prenatal exposure versus risk of relapse following drug discontinuation" (p. 592). Finally, the clinician should keep in mind that ECT appears to be a safe and effective alternative for the pregnant patient with severe depression.

Q. Is there an AD of first choice during pregnancy?

A. There are probably insufficient data from well-designed studies to allow such a determination. Miller (1994) concludes that the *tricyclics* of choice during pregnancy are desipramine and nortriptyline because of the comparative wealth of data about them, the ability to monitor serum levels, and a favorable side effect profile. Among newer agents, fluoxetine (Prozac) may be a reasonable choice for the pregnant patient with major depression in light of the data from Pastuszak et al. (1993) and Nulman et al. (1997) and notwithstanding the data from Chambers et al. (1996).

Q. How safe is breast-feeding while taking an AD?

A. Little is known about the excretion of ADs into breast milk or the effects of this on the nursing infant. Some studies indicate that several ADs or their metabolites can accumulate in breast milk, possibly peaking at about 4–6 hours after an oral dose. It is not clear to what extent ADs accumulate in the blood of the nursing infant or whether significant adverse effects result from such accumulation; nevertheless, some clinicians believe that breast-feeding is best avoided when the mother is taking ADs postpartum. A recent report by Spigset et al. (1996), however, found no adverse effects in an infant whose mother was breast-feeding while taking paroxetine. This report notes that accumulation of paroxetine in breast milk may be lower than that seen with fluoxetine or fluvoxamine. Finally, the psychological importance of breast-feeding to the mother also must be weighed in the decision.

Vignettes and Puzzlers

Q. An elderly depressed patient is taking 75 mg/day nortriptyline, with a plasma level of 120 ng/mL (therapeutic, 50–150 ng/mL). Her hepatic and renal functions are normal. Her primary physician notes her presenting symptoms as a 1-week history of fever, dysuria, and malaise. Urine culture at that time reveals evidence of infection, but blood urea nitrogen (BUN), creatinine, and liver functions are at baseline. She shows no evidence of postural hypotension, tachycardia, new-onset anticholinergic side effects, or confusion. An ECG shows no evidence of conduction abnormality. A nortriptyline level at that time comes back at 170 ng/mL. Does the patient have a "toxic" nortriptyline level, and should her dose be reduced?

A. This apparent elevation of nortriptyline level most likely reflects elevation of *total* serum nortriptyline levels (free plus protein-bound) and not increased or toxic levels of the free drug. Many psychotropic medications are bound to α_1-acid glycoprotein, termed an acute phase reactant, because levels may increase in response to myocardial infarction, shock, severe burns, or *infectious processes* (Friedman and Greenblatt 1986). This increase in α_1-acid glycoprotein causes increased binding of some basic (nonacidic) drugs, *without* increased clinical or toxic effects. Therefore, the clinician's therapeutic range for a given drug may shift such that—in the present case—a plasma level of 170 ng/mL is likely well within the therapeutic range for nortriptyline (Friedman and Greenblatt 1986). It is possible, but quite expensive, to order levels of only the free drug. In the present case, no adjustment of the patient's nortriptyline dose is necessary, particularly because there is no clinical evidence of tricyclic toxicity.

Q. A 40-year-old woman with bipolar II disorder had been taking fluoxetine 10 mg/day during her depressed phase. When she became hypomanic, she began taking carbamazepine (800 mg/day) and achieved a plasma level of 5 μg/mL after 1 week. After 9 days, she developed a rash on her legs, sore throat, general malaise, conjunctivitis, and a temperature of 103°F. Intraoral ruptured bullae and "target" lesions of the skin were observed on the patient's hands and feet. What is the most likely diagnosis?

A. Stevens-Johnson syndrome, a potentially lethal form of erythema multiforme, is probably a hypersensitivity reaction due to various drugs, including barbiturates, meprobamate, *fluoxetine,* and—as in this case—*carbamazepine.* About 24 cases have been reported with carbamazepine, making this quite a rare side effect (Pagliaro and Pagliaro 1993) but one with severe consequences.

Q. A 67-year-old woman with major depression was begun on nortriptyline 25 mg hs, with subsequent increases to 50 mg hs. Her plasma level was 74 ng/mL. After about 2 weeks, the patient complained of severe eye and face pain, nausea, vomiting, loss of visual acuity, and "colored halos" in her visual field. What is the most likely diagnosis?

A. This case strongly suggests *narrow-angle glaucoma* precipitated by the anticholinergic effects of nortriptyline. The most common adult form of glaucoma—chronic, open-angle type—is not usually worsened by anticholinergic agents. Narrow-angle or angle-closure glaucoma may be worsened by psychotropics with anticholinergic properties, leading to blockage of aqueous humor flow and an acute rise in intraocular pressure. Thus, a careful medical and ophthalmological history is necessary prior to prescribing a TCA or similar agents (Gelenberg 1994).

Q. An elderly patient with recurrent depression had responded only to nortriptyline. This drug worked well at 75 mg/day hs, but the patient noted "a funny feeling in my chest" when the total dose was given at bedtime. ECGs done in the morning showed second-degree atrioventricular block. The patient was converted to a 25 mg bid and 25 mg hs schedule. Both the chest discomfort and the ECG abnormalities disappeared. What is the pharmacokinetic explanation?

A. Whereas the average steady-state plasma drug level does not change whether the total dose is given once a day or in divided doses, the "height" of Cmax (peak plasma drug concentration after a dose) does increase when a drug is given in a single large dose. This increase may be associated with greater direct quinidine-like effects of nortriptyline on cardiac nerve fibers and thus greater conduction delay and arrhythmias (see Preskorn 1993).

Q. A 64-year-old woman with severe major depression began taking venlafaxine at 75 mg po bid. The patient also was taking cimetidine (Tagamet) 200 mg bid for peptic ulcer and quinidine sulfate 200 mg tid for occasional premature ventricular contractions. Because of ongoing psychotic symptoms, haloperidol 1 mg po bid was added 5 days after beginning the venlafaxine. Four days later, the patient complained of severe nausea, somnolence, and dizziness. What is the likely cause?

A. Venlafaxine is metabolized by the CYP2D6 system. All of the other medications noted (quinidine, haloperidol, and cimetidine) inhibit CYP2D6 and probably raised plasma venlafaxine levels into a toxic range for this patient—nausea being a clue. (*Note:* Quinidine is itself *metabolized* via CYP3A4 but is an inhibitor of CYP2D6.)

Q. A bipolar patient maintained on carbamazepine 200 mg tid with a plasma level of 7.0 µg/mL is admitted to the hospital with severe depression. He begins taking nefazodone 100 mg bid, increased to 150 mg bid. Four days later, the patient is ataxic, with slurred speech and nystagmus. A carbamazepine level comes back at 12 µg/mL, which is within the putative therapeutic range (5–12 µg/mL). What is a likely explanation for the patient's clinical picture?

A. Nefazodone is an inhibitor of CYP3A4, which is the pathway involved in metabolism of carbamazepine. The 10,11-epoxide of carbamazepine can cause neurotoxicity even when the parent compound is within the therapeutic range. Most likely, this epoxide metabolite has increased to toxic levels in this case.

Q. A 73-year-old woman with major depression had a partial response to nefazodone, 250 mg/day, and was tolerating it without significant side effects. Because the effective dosage range is usually between 300 and 600 mg/day, the patient's psychiatrist increased the nefazodone (over a period of 5 days) to 400 mg/day. Two days after the final dosage adjustment, the patient complained of somnolence, nausea, dizziness, and confusion. What is the explanation?

A. Nefazodone exhibits nonlinear pharmacokinetics at steady state (i.e., an increase in dose results in a greater-than-proportional increase in plasma levels). Thus, mean peak plasma levels following daily doses of 100, 200, and 400 mg are 270, 730, and 2,050 ng/mL, respectively (DeVane 1995). In this case, the patient probably experienced a marked increase in plasma levels, leading to side effects, despite the dosage being well within the usual therapeutic range; her advanced age may well have been a factor (De-Vane 1995).

Q. A 23-year-old man with major depression began taking sertraline 50 mg bid. He responded well to this dosage and experienced no significant side effects. One month later, during hay fever season, the patient complained of "itchy, watery eyes" and sneezing. He was placed on astemizole (Hismanal), a nonsedating antihistamine, 10 mg/day. Four days later, the patient complained of muscle twitches, shivering, diarrhea, and confusion. He was disoriented to day and date and had difficulty with short-term memory. What is the likely syndrome, and what is the etiology?

A. This patient probably has serotonin syndrome (see Table 1–18) due to elevated levels of sertraline. Sertraline is metabolized via CYP3A4, as is astemizole. However, astemizole is also an *inhibitor* of CYP3A4 (Gelenberg 1995) and may lead to significantly elevated levels of sertraline, resulting in the patient's complaints.

Q. A 45-year-old man with major depression, panic attacks, and asthma begins taking fluvoxamine 50 mg qd, which is increased over the next 5 days to 100 mg bid. He is also taking 200 mg bid theophylline (Theo-Dur) and 1 mg tid alprazolam. Five days after beginning the fluvoxamine, the patient is tachycardic and anxious yet also *drowsy with mildly slurred speech*. What explains this?

A. Fluvoxamine is an inhibitor of CYP1A2, which metabolizes theophylline. Fluvoxamine also inhibits CYP3A4, which metabolizes the triazolobenzodiazepines (including alprazolam). Most likely, this patient developed toxic levels of both theophylline (leading to tachycardia and anxiety) *and* alprazolam (leading to drowsiness and slurred speech).

References

Academic highlights: venlafaxine: a new dimension in antidepressant pharmacotherapy. J Clin Psychiatry 54:119–126, 1993

Adams F: Amitriptyline suppositories (letter). N Engl J Med 306:996, 1982

Agras WS: Treatment of eating disorders, in The American Psychiatric Press Textbook of Psychopharmacology. Edited by Schatzberg AF, Nemeroff CB. Washington, DC, American Psychiatric Press, 1995, pp 725–734

Akiskal HS: Dysthymic disorder: psychopathology of proposed chronic depressive subtypes. Am J Psychiatry 140:11–20, 1983

Albert R, Ebert D: Full efficacy of SSRI treatment in refractory dysthymia is achieved only after 16 weeks (letter). J Clin Psychiatry 57:176, 1996

Altshuler LL, Post RM, Leverich GS, et al: Antidepressant-induced mania and cycle acceleration: a controversy revisited. Am J Psychiatry 152:1130–1138, 1995

Altshuler LL, Cohen L, Szuba MP, et al: Pharmacologic management of psychiatric illness during pregnancy: dilemmas and guidelines. Am J Psychiatry 153:592–606, 1996

American Psychiatric Association: Diagnostic and Statistical Manual of Mental Disorders, 3rd Edition, Revised. Washington, DC, American Psychiatric Association, 1987

American Psychiatric Association: Diagnostic and Statistical Manual of Mental Disorders, 4th Edition. Washington, DC, American Psychiatric Association, 1994

Apter JT, Birkett M: Fluoxetine treatment in depressed patients who failed treatment with sertraline. Presentation at the 34th annual meeting of the American College of Neuropsychopharmacology, San Juan, Puerto Rico, December 1995

Apter JT, Kushner SF: A guide to selection of antidepressants. Primary Psychiatry 3:14–16, 1996

Arana GW, Hyman SE: Handbook of Psychiatric Drug Therapy, 2nd Edition. Boston, Little, Brown, 1991

Aranth J, Lindberg C: Bleeding, a side effect of fluoxetine (letter). Am J Psychiatry 149:412, 1992

Artigas F, Perez V, Alvarez E: Pindolol induces a rapid improvement of depressed patients treated with serotonin reuptake inhibitors. Arch Gen Psychiatry 51:248–251, 1994

Ayd FJ: Lexicon of Psychiatry, Neurology, and the Neurosciences. Baltimore, MD, Williams & Wilkins, 1995

Barr LC, Goodman WK, Price LH: Physical symptoms associated with paroxetine discontinuation (letter). Am J Psychiatry 151:289, 1994

Bender KJ: Maintaining psychostimulant ADHD mainstay beyond childhood. Psychiatric Times, February 1996a (suppl)

Bender KJ: St-John's-wort evaluated as herbal antidepressant. Psychiatric Times 13:58, 1996b

Blumer D: The Dysthymic Pain Disorder: Chronic Pain as Masked Depression. Biomedical Information Corporation, 1987

Branconnier RJ, Cole JO, Ghazvinian S: Clinical pharmacology of bupropion and imipramine in elderly depressives. J Clin Psychiatry 44:130–133, 1983

Brown WA, Harrison W: Are patients who are intolerant to one serotonin selective reuptake inhibitor intolerant to another? J Clin Psychiatry 56:30–34, 1995

Castillo E, Rubin RT, Holsboer-Trachsler E: Clinical differentiation between lethal catatonia and neuroleptic malignant syndrome. Am J Psychiatry 146:324–328, 1989

Centorrino F, Baldessarini RJ, Kando J, et al: Serum concentrations of clozapine and its major metabolites: effects of cotreatment with fluoxetine or valproate. Am J Psychiatry 151:123–125, 1994

Chambers CD, Johnson KA, Dick LM, et al: Birth outcomes in pregnant women taking fluoxetine. N Engl J Med 335:1010–1015, 1996

Charney DS, Miller HL, Licinio J, et al: Treatment of depression, in The American Psychiatric Press Textbook of Psychopharmacology. Edited by Schatzberg AF, Nemeroff CB. Washington, DC, American Psychiatric Press, 1995, pp 575–601

Ciraulo DA, Creelman WL, Shader RI, et al: Antidepressants, in Drug Interactions in Psychiatry, 2nd Edition. Edited by Ciraulo DA, Shader RI, Greenblatt DJ, et al. Baltimore, MD, Williams & Wilkins, 1995a, pp 29–63

Ciraulo DA, Shader RI, Greenblatt DJ: SSRI drug-drug interactions, in Drug Interactions in Psychiatry, 2nd Edition. Edited by Ciraulo DA, Shader RI, Greenblatt DJ, et al. Baltimore, MD, Williams & Wilkins, 1995b, pp 64–89

Cole SA, Woodard JL, Juncos JL, et al: Depression and disability in Parkinson's disease. J Neuropsychiatry Clin Neurosci 8:20–25, 1996

Cornelius JR, Soloff PH, Perel JM, et al: Continuation pharmacotherapy of borderline personality disorder with haloperidol and phenelzine. Am J Psychiatry 150:1843–1848, 1993

Creelman W, Ciraulo DA: Monoamine oxidase inhibitors, in Drug Interactions in Psychiatry, 2nd Edition. Edited by Ciraulo DA, Shader RI, Greenblatt DJ, et al. Baltimore, MD, Williams & Wilkins, 1995, pp 90–128

Cummings JL: Depression and Parkinson's disease: a review. Am J Psychiatry 149:443–454, 1992

Cutler NR, Post RM: Life course of illness in untreated manic-depressive patients. Compr Psychiatry 23:101–114, 1982

Davidson JRT: Monoamine oxidase inhibitors, in Handbook of Affective Disorders, 2nd Edition. Edited by Paykel ES. New York, Guilford, 1992, pp 345–358

Delisle JD: Rapid switch in a bipolar patient during lithium-tricyclic therapy. Am J Psychiatry 143:1326–1327, 1986

Depression Guideline Panel: Depression in Primary Care, Vol 2: Treatment of Major Depression (Clinical Practice Guideline) (DHHS Publ No 93-0551). Rockville, MD, Agency for Health Care Policy and Research, U.S. Department of Health and Human Services, 1993

Derogatis LR, Morrow GR, Fetting J, et al: The prevalence of psychiatric disorders among cancer patients. JAMA 249:751–757, 1983

DeVane CL: Nefazodone—pharmacology and efficacy of a new antidepressant agent: formulary considerations. Pharmacy and Therapeutics, June 1995, pp 363–374

Drug Facts and Comparisons. St. Louis, MO, Facts and Comparisons, 1995

Dubovsky SL: Geriatric neuropsychopharmacology, in The American Psychiatric Press Textbook of Geriatric Neuropsychiatry. Edited by Coffey CE, Cummings JL. Washington, DC, American Psychiatric Press, 1994, pp 596–631

Dunbar GC, Cohn JB, Feighner JP, et al: A comparison of paroxetine, imipramine and placebo in depressed outpatients. Br J Psychiatry 159:394–398, 1991

Dunner DL: Treating depression in the elderly. J Clin Psychiatry 55 (suppl):48–58, 1994

DuPaul GJ, Barkley RA: Medication therapy, in Attention Deficit Hyperactivity Disorder. Edited by Barkley RA. New York, Guilford, 1990, pp 573–612

Edwards JG, Long SK, Sedgwick EM, et al: Antidepressants and convulsive seizures: clinical, electroencephalographic, and pharmacologic aspects. Clin Neuropharmacol 9:329–360, 1986

Ellison JM, Milofsky JE, Ely E: Fluoxetine-induced bradycardia and syncope in two patients. J Clin Psychiatry 51:385–386, 1990

Ereshefsky L: Drug interactions of antidepressants. Psychiatric Annals 26:342–350, 1996

Ereshefsky L, Overman GP, Karp JK: Current psychotropic dosing and monitoring guidelines. Primary Psychiatry 3:21–45, 1996

Favale E, Rubino V, Mainardi P, et al: Anticonvulsant effect of fluoxetine in humans. Neurology 45:1926–1927, 1995

Fawcett J, Busch KA: Stimulants in psychiatry, in The American Psychiatric Press Textbook of Psychopharmacology. Edited by Schatzberg AF, Nemeroff CB. Washington, DC, American Psychiatric Press, 1995, pp 417–435

Fawcett J, Kravitz HM, Zajecka JM, et al: CNS stimulant potentiation of monoamine oxidase inhibitors in treatment-refractory depression. J Clin Psychopharmacol 11:127–132, 1991

Feder R: Bradycardia and syncope induced by fluoxetine (letter). J Clin Psychiatry 52:139, 1991a

Feder R: Reversal of antidepressant activity of fluoxetine by cyproheptadine in three patients. J Clin Psychiatry 52:163–164, 1991b

Feiger A, Kiev A, Shrivastava RK: Nefazodone versus sertraline in outpatients with major depression: focus on efficacy, tolerability, and effects on sexual function and satisfaction. J Clin Psychiatry 57 (suppl 2):53–62, 1996

Feighner JP, Herbstein J, Damlouji N: Combined MAOI, TCA, and direct stimulant therapy of treatment resistant depression. J Clin Psychiatry 46:206–209, 1985

Fink M: Response to "Neuroleptic malignant-like syndrome due to cyclobenzaprine?" J Clin Psychopharmacol 16:97–98, 1996

Fink M, Bush G, Francis A: Catatonia: a treatable disorder, occasionally recognized. Directions in Psychiatry 13:1–7, 1993

Fogelson DL: Fenfluramine and the cytochrome P450 system (letter). Am J Psychiatry 154:436–437, 1997

Friedman H, Greenblatt DJ: Rational therapeutic drug monitoring. JAMA 256:2227–2233, 1986

Gammon GD: Incentive bias? (letter) J Clin Psychiatry 57:265, 1996

Gardner DM, Shulman KI, Walker SE: The making of a user friendly MAOI diet. J Clin Psychiatry 57:99–104, 1996

Gelenberg AJ: Angle-closure glaucoma and tricyclic antidepressants. Biological Therapies in Psychiatry Newsletter 17:35–36, 1994

Gelenberg AJ: The P450 family. Biological Therapies in Psychiatry Newsletter 18:29–31, 1995

Gelenberg AJ: Switching SSRIs. Biological Therapies in Psychiatry Newsletter 19:9–10, 1996

Gelenberg AJ: Can an SSRI lower cholesterol? Biological Therapies in Psychiatry Newsletter 20:6, 1997

Giakas WJ, Davis JM: Intractable withdrawal from venlafaxine treated with fluoxetine. Psychiatric Annals 27:85–92, 1997

Giller E, Bialos D, Harkness L, et al: Assessing treatment response to the monoamine oxidase inhibitor isocarboxazid. J Clin Psychiatry 45:44–48, 1984

Glassman AH, Roose SP, Bigger JT: The safety of tricyclic antidepressants in cardiac patients: risk-benefit reconsidered. JAMA 26:2673–2675, 1993

Goff DC, Baldessarini RJ: Antipsychotics, in Drug Interactions in Psychiatry, 2nd Edition. Edited by Ciraulo DA, Shader RI, Greenblatt DJ, et al. Baltimore, MD, Williams & Wilkins, 1995, pp 129–174

Golden RN, Bebchuck JM, Leatherman ME: Trazodone and other antidepressants, in The American Psychiatric Press Textbook of Psychopharmacology. Edited by Schatzberg AF, Nemeroff CB. Washington, DC, American Psychiatric Press, 1995, pp 195–214

Goldman EL: Ginkgo eases drug-induced sex dysfunction. Clinical Psychiatry News, July 1997, p 5

Goldstein L, Barker M, Segall F, et al: Seizure and transient SIADH associated with sertraline (letter). Am J Psychiatry 153:732, 1996

Goodnick PJ, Henry JH, Buki VMV: Treatment of depression in patients with diabetes mellitus. J Clin Psychiatry 56:128–136, 1995

Gorman JM: Special considerations in switching antidepressants. Teleconference (chaired by Keller MB), Providence, RI, August 18, 1995

Greden J: Maintenance antidepressant treatment. Progress Notes, Fall/Winter 1995–1996, pp 28–34

Greenblatt DJ, Sellers EM, Koch-Weser J: Importance of protein binding for the interpretation of serum or plasma drug concentrations. J Clin Pharmacol 22:259–263, 1982

Grossman E, Messerli FH, Grodzicki T, et al: Should a moratorium be placed on sublingual nifedipine capsules given for hypertensive emergencies and pseudoemergencies? JAMA 276: 1328–1331, 1996

Grossman R, Hollander E: Treatment of obsessive-compulsive disorder with venlafaxine (letter). Am J Psychiatry 153:576–577, 1996

Hamilton M: A rating scale for depression. J Neurol Neurosurg Psychiatry 23:56–62, 1960

Harnett DS: Psychopharmacologic treatment of depression in the medical setting. Psychiatric Annals 24:545–551, 1994

Harrison WM, Stewart JW: Pharmacotherapy of dysthymic disorder, in Diagnosis and Treatment of Chronic Depression. Edited by Kocsis JH, Klein DN. New York, Guilford, 1995, pp 124–145

Hoehn-Saric R, Harris GJ, Pearlson GD, et al: A fluoxetine-induced frontal lobe syndrome in an obsessive-compulsive patient. J Clin Psychiatry 52:131–133, 1991

Hopkins HS: Fluoxetine-bupropion interaction. Biological Therapies in Psychiatry Newsletter 19:31–32, 1996

Janicak PG, Davis JM, Preskorn SH, et al: Principles and Practice of Psychopharmacotherapy. Baltimore, MD, Williams & Wilkins, 1993

Jefferson JW: Antidepressants in panic disorder. J Clin Psychiatry 58 (2, suppl):20–24, 1997

Jenkins SC, Hansen MR: A Pocket Reference for Psychiatrists, 2nd Edition. Washington, DC, American Psychiatric Press, 1995

Joffe RT, Levitt AJ, Sokolov STH: Augmentation strategies: focus on anxiolytics. J Clin Psychiatry 57 (suppl 7):25–31, 1996a

Joffe RT, Levitt AJ, Sokolov STH, et al: Response to an open trial of a second SSRI in major depression. J Clin Psychiatry 57:114–115, 1996b

Johnston JA, Lineberry CG, Ascher JA: A 102-center prospective study of seizure in association with bupropion. J Clin Psychiatry 52:450–456, 1991

Kehoe WA, Schorr RB: Focus on mirtazapine. Formulary 31: 455–469, 1996

Keller M: Depression in adults. Data presented at the Eighth Annual U.S. Psychiatric and Mental Health Congress, New York City, November 18, 1995

Ketter TA, Jenkins JB, Schroeder DH, et al: Carbamazepine but not valproate induces bupropion metabolism. J Clin Psychopharmacol 15:327–333, 1995

Kline NA, Dow BM, Brown SA, et al: Sertraline efficacy in depressed combat veterans with post-traumatic stress disorder. Paper presented at the 146th annual meeting of the American Psychiatric Association, San Francisco, CA, May 1993

Kocsis JH, Thase M, Koran L, et al: Pharmacotherapy of pure dysthymia: sertraline vs. imipramine and placebo. Eur Neuropsychopharmacol 4:204–206, 1994

Koran LM, Sallee FR, Pallanti S: Rapid benefit of intravenous pulse loading of clomipramine in obsessive-compulsive disorder. Am J Psychiatry 154:396–401, 1997

Krishnan KRR, Hamilton MA: Obesity. Primary Psychiatry 4:49–53, 1997

Krishnan KRR, Steffens DC, Doraiswamy PM: Psychotropic drug interactions. Primary Psychiatry 3:21–49, 1996

Leonard BE: New approaches to the treatment of depression. J Clin Psychiatry 57 (suppl 4):26–33, 1996

Liebowitz MR, Klein DF: Hysteroid dysphoria. Psychiatr Clin North Am 2:555–575, 1979

Longo LP, Salzman C: Valproic acid effects on serum concentrations of clozapine and norclozapine (letter). Am J Psychiatry 152:650, 1995

Lowry MR, Dunner FJ: Seizures during tricyclic therapy. Am J Psychiatry 137:1461–1462, 1980

Marshall RD, Liebowitz MR: Paroxetine/bupropion combination treatment for refractory depression (letter). J Clin Psychopharmacol 16:80–81, 1996

Marshall RD, Johannet CM, Collins PY, et al: Bupropion and sertraline combination treatment in refractory depression. Journal of Psychopharmacology 9:284–286, 1995

Massie MJ, Holland JC: Depression and the cancer patient. J Clin Psychiatry 51 (suppl 7):12–17, 1990

Massie MJ, Lesko L: Psychopharmacological management, in Handbook of Psychooncology: Psychological Care of the Patient With Cancer. Edited by Holland JC, Rowland JH. New York, Oxford University Press, 1989, pp 470–491

McElroy SL : Clinical management of antidepressant side effects. Paper presented at the Eighth Annual U.S. Psychiatric and Mental Health Congress, New York City, November 18, 1995

Metz A, Shader RI: Combination of fluoxetine with pemoline in the treatment of major depressive disorder. Int Clin Psychopharmacol 6:93–96, 1991

Miller LJ: Psychiatric medication during pregnancy: understanding and minimizing risks. Psychiatric Annals 24:69–75, 1994

Milstein V, Small JG, Klapper MH, et al: Uni- versus bilateral ECT in the treatment of mania. Convuls Ther 3:1–9, 1987

Mukherjee S, Sackheim HA, Schnur DB: Electroconvulsive therapy of acute manic episodes: a review of 50 years' experience. Am J Psychiatry 151:169–176, 1994

Nelson JC: Are the SSRIs really better tolerated than the TCAs for treatment of major depression? Psychiatric Annals 24:628–631, 1994

Nemeroff CB: Drug interactions in perspective. Progress Notes, Fall/Winter 1995–1996, pp 35–37

Nemeroff CB: Dr. Nemeroff replies (letter). J Clin Psychiatry 57:267–268, 1996

Nemeroff CB, Devane CL, Pollack BG: Summary and review of antidepressants and the cytochrome P450 system. Progress Notes, Fall/Winter 1995–1996, pp 38–40

Nierenberg AA: The treatment of severe depression: is there an efficacy gap between SSRI and TCA antidepressant generations? J Clin Psychiatry 55 (suppl A):55–59, 1994

Nulman I, Rovet J, Stewart DE, et al: Neurodevelopment of children exposed in utero to antidepressant drugs. N Engl J Med 336:258–262, 1997

Oesterheld J, Kallepalli BR: Grapefruit juice and clomipramine: shifting metabolic ratios. J Clin Psychopharmacol 17:62–63, 1997

Ottervanger JP, Stricker BHCH, Huls J, et al: Bleeding attributed to the intake of paroxetine (letter). Am J Psychiatry 151:781–782, 1994

Pagliaro LA, Pagliaro AM: Carbamazepine-induced Stevens-Johnson syndrome. Hospital and Community Psychiatry 44:999–1000, 1993

Pastuszak A, Schick-Boschetto B, Zuber C, et al: Pregnancy outcome following first-trimester exposure to fluoxetine (Prozac). JAMA 269:2246–2248, 1993

Pearlman CA: Neuroleptic malignant syndrome: a review of the literature. J Clin Psychopharmacol 6:257–273, 1986

Peck AW, Stern WC, Watkinson C: Incidence of seizures during treatment with tricyclic antidepressant drugs and bupropion. J Clin Psychiatry 44:197–201, 1983

Persad E, Oluboka OJ, Sharma V, et al: The phenomenon of rapid cycling in bipolar mood disorders: a review. Can J Psychiatry 41:23–27, 1996

Peselow ED, Filippi AM, Goodnick P, et al: The short- and long-term efficacy of paroxetine HCl: data from a double-blind cross-over study and from a year-long trial vs. imipramine and placebo. Psychopharmacol Bull 25:272–276, 1989

Petersdorf RG: Hypothermia and hyperthermia, in Harrison's Principles of Internal Medicine, 12th Edition. Edited by Wilson JD, Braunwald E, Isselbacher KJ, et al. New York, McGraw-Hill, 1991, pp 2194–2200

Phillips KA: Body dysmorphic disorder: the distress of imagined ugliness. Am J Psychiatry 148:1138–1149, 1991

Physicians' Desk Reference, 50th Edition. Montvale, NJ, Medical Economics, 1996

Pies R: Atypical depression, in Handbook of Clinical Psychopharmacology, 2nd Edition. Edited by Tupin JP, Shader RI, Harnett DS. Northvale, NJ, Jason Aronson, 1988, pp 329–356

Pies R: Psychotropic medication during pregnancy: what weighs in the balance? Psychiatric Times 11:30–31, 1994

Pies R: One foot on the bandwagon? (editorial) J Clin Psychopharmacol 15:303–305, 1995

Pies R: Psychotropic medications and the oncology patient. Cancer Practice 4:1–3, 1996

Pies R: Time and the art of psychopharmacology. Harvard Review of Psychiatry 5:36–39, 1997

Pies R, Shader RI: Approaches to the treatment of depression, in Manual of Psychiatric Therapeutics, 2nd Edition. Edited by Shader RI. Boston, Little, Brown, 1994, pp 217–246

Pies R, Weinberg AD: Quick Reference Guide to Geriatric Psychopharmacology. Branford, CT, American Medical Publishing, 1990

Pollock BG, Sweet RA, Kirshner M, et al: Bupropion plasma levels and CYP2D6 phenotype. Ther Drug Monit 18:581–585, 1996

Post RM: Mechanisms underlying the evolution of affective disorders: implications for long-term treatment, in Progress in Psychiatry: Severe Depressive Disorders. Edited by Grunhaus L, Greden JF. Washington, DC, American Psychiatric Press, 1994, pp 23–65

Potter WZ, Manji HK, Rudorfer MV: Tricyclics and tetracyclics, in The American Psychiatric Press Textbook of Psychopharmacology. Edited by Schatzberg AF, Nemeroff CB. Washington, DC, American Psychiatric Press, 1995, pp 141–160

Preskorn SH: Pharmacokinetics of psychotropic agents: why and how they are relevant to treatment. J Clin Psychiatry 54 (suppl):3–7, 1993

Preskorn SH: Advances in Antidepressant Therapy: The Pharmacologic Basis. San Antonio, TX, Dannemiller Memorial Educational Foundation, 1994

Preskorn SH: Comparison of the tolerability of bupropion, fluoxetine, imipramine, nefazodone, paroxetine, sertraline, and venlafaxine. J Clin Psychiatry 56 (suppl 6):12–21, 1995

Preskorn SH: Clinical Pharmacology of Selective Serotonin Reuptake Inhibitors. Caddo, OK, Professional Communications, 1996

Price LH, Charney DS, Henniger GR: Manic symptoms following addition of lithium to antidepressant treatment. J Clin Psychopharmacol 4:361–362, 1984

Quitkin FM, Stewart JW, McGrath PJ: Phenelzine versus imipramine in the treatment of probable atypical depression: defining syndrome boundaries of selective MAOI responders. Am J Psychiatry 145:306–311, 1988

Rauch SL, O'Sullivan RL, Jenike MA: Open treatment of obsessive-compulsive disorder with venlafaxine: a series of ten cases. J Clin Psychopharmacol 16:81–83, 1996

Ravindran AV, Bialik RJ, Lapierre YD: Therapeutic efficacy of specific serotonin reuptake inhibitors (SSRIs) in dysthymia. Can J Psychiatry 39:21–26, 1994

Richelson E: Pharmacology of antidepressants: characteristics of the ideal drug. Mayo Clin Proc 69:1069–1081, 1994

Robinson DS, Roberts DL, Smith JM, et al: The safety profile of nefazodone. J Clin Psychiatry 57 (suppl 2):31–38, 1996

Roose SP, Glassman AH, Attia E, et al: Comparative efficacy of selective serotonin reuptake inhibitors and tricyclics in the treatment of melancholia. Am J Psychiatry 151:1735–1739, 1994

Rosenstein DL, Nelson JC, Jacobs SC: Seizures associated with antidepressants: a review. J Clin Psychiatry 54:289–299, 1993

Roth BL, Meltzer HY: The role of serotonin in schizophrenia, in Psychopharmacology: The Fourth Generation of Progress. Edited by Bloom FE, Kupfer DJ. New York, Raven, 1995, pp 1215–1227

Schatzberg AF, Cole JO: Manual of Clinical Psychopharmacology, 2nd Edition. Washington, DC, American Psychiatric Press, 1991, pp 313–318

Segraves RT: Effects of psychotropic drugs on human erection and ejaculation. Arch Gen Psychiatry 46:275–284, 1989

Shader RI: Dissociative, somatoform, and paranoid disorders, in Manual of Psychiatric Therapeutics, 2nd Edition. Edited by Shader RI. Boston, MA, Little, Brown, 1994, pp 15–24

Sherman C: SSRIs benefit cognition in elderly who are depressed. Clinical Psychiatry News 24:19, 1996

Silver JM: Clinical update on the management of agitation in the elderly. Paper presented at the Eighth Annual U.S. Psychiatric and Mental Health Congress, New York City, November 16, 1995

Smith BD, Salzman C: Do benzodiazepines cause depression? Hospital and Community Psychiatry 42:1101–1102, 1991

Sofuoglu M, DeBattista C: Development of obsessive symptoms during nefazodone treatment (letter). Am J Psychiatry 153: 577–578, 1996

Spigset O, Carleborg L, Nordstrom A, et al: Paroxetine level in breast milk (letter). J Clin Psychiatry 57:39, 1996

Srisurapanont M, Yatham LN, Zis AP: Treatment of acute bipolar depression: a review of the literature. Can J Psychiatry 40: 533–544, 1995

Stahl SM: Remeron (mirtazapine): designing specific serotonergic actions. Psychiatric Annals 27:138–139, 1997a

Stahl SM: Serotonin pathways: mediators of SSRI side effects. Psychiatric Annals 27:82–84, 1997b

Sternbach H: The serotonin syndrome. Am J Psychiatry 148: 705–713, 1991

Stoll AL, Pillay SS, Diamond L, et al: Methylphenidate augmentation of serotonin selective reuptake inhibitors: a case series. J Clin Psychiatry 57:72–76, 1996

Storey P, Trumble M: Rectal doxepin and carbamazepine therapy in patients with cancer. N Engl J Med 327:1318–1319, 1992

Stoudemire A, Moran MG, Fogel BS: Psychopharmacology in the medically ill patient, in The American Psychiatric Press Textbook of Psychopharmacology. Edited by Schatzberg AF, Nemeroff CB. Washington, DC, American Psychiatric Press, 1995, pp 783–801

Stowe ZN, Nemeroff CB: Psychopharmacology during pregnancy and lactation, in The American Psychiatric Press Textbook of Psychopharmacology. Edited by Schatzberg AF, Nemeroff CB. Washington, DC, American Psychiatric Press, 1995, pp 823–837

Taylor CB: Treatment of anxiety disorders, in The American Psychiatric Press Textbook of Psychopharmacology. Edited by Schatzberg AF, Nemeroff CB. Washington, DC, American Psychiatric Press, 1995, pp 641–655

Thase ME, Rush AJ: Treatment-resistant depression, in Psychopharmacology: The Fourth Generation of Progress. Edited by Bloom FE, Kupfer DJ. New York, Raven, 1995, pp 1081–1097

Theoharides TC, Harris RS, Weckstein D: Neuroleptic malignant-like syndrome due to cyclobenzaprine? J Clin Psychopharmacol 15:79–81, 1995

Thompson JW Jr, Ware MR, Blashfield RK: Psychotropic medication and priapism: a comprehensive review. J Clin Psychiatry 51:430–433, 1990

Tollefson GD: Selective serotonin reuptake inhibitors, in The American Psychiatric Press Textbook of Psychopharmacology. Edited by Schatzberg AF, Nemeroff CB. Washington, DC, American Psychiatric Press, 1995, pp 161–182

Trestman RL, deVegvar M, Siever LJ: Treatment of personality disorders, in The American Psychiatric Press Textbook of Psychopharmacology. Edited by Schatzberg AF, Nemeroff CB. Washington, DC, American Psychiatric Press, 1995, pp 753–768

Velamoor VR, Swamy GN, Parmar RS, et al: Management of suspected neuroleptic syndrome. Can J Psychiatry 40:545–550, 1995

von Moltke LL, Greenblatt DJ, Shader RI: Clinical pharmacokinetics of antidepressants in the elderly: therapeutic implications. Clin Pharmacokinet 24:141–160, 1993

Wehr TA, Goodwin FK: Can antidepressants cause mania and worsen the course of affective illness? Am J Psychiatry 144:1403–1411, 1987

Wender PH: ADHD in adults. Psychiatric Times 13:41–44, 1996

Wender PH, Shader RI: Diagnosis and treatment of attention deficit disorder in children and adults, in Manual of Psychiatric Therapeutics, 2nd Edition. Edited by Shader RI. Boston, Little, Brown, 1994, pp 167–179

West ED, Dally PJ: Effect of iproniazid in depressive syndromes. BMJ 1:1491–1494, 1959

Wise MG: Special considerations in switching antidepressants. Teleconference (chaired by Keller MB), Providence, RI, August 18, 1995

Wisner KL, Perel JM, Wheeler SB: Tricyclic dose requirements across pregnancy. Am J Psychiatry 150:1541–1542, 1993

Yudofsky SC, Silver JM, Hales RE: Treatment of aggressive disorders, in The American Psychiatric Press Textbook of Psychopharmacology. Edited by Schatzberg AF, Nemeroff CB. Washington, DC, American Psychiatric Press, 1995, pp 735–751

Zajecka JM: Treatment strategies for depression complicated by anxiety disorders. Paper presented at the Eighth Annual U.S. Psychiatric and Mental Health Congress, New York City, November 16, 1995

Zajecka JM, Fawcett J, Guy C: Coexisting major depression and obsessive-compulsive disorder treated with venlafaxine (letter). J Clin Psychopharmacol 10:152–153, 1990

Zarate CA, Kando JC, Tohen M, et al: Does intolerance or lack of response with fluoxetine predict the same will happen with sertraline? J Clin Psychiatry 57:67–71, 1996

Zornberg GL, Pope HG: Treatment of depression in bipolar disorder: new directions for research. J Clin Psychopharmacol 13: 397–408, 1993

CHAPTER 2

Antipsychotics

Overview

■ Drug Class

The designation *antipsychotic* is often used synonymously with *neuroleptic* or *major tranquilizer*. The last term should be avoided because these agents do not merely "tranquilize" but have specific effects on core features of psychosis such as auditory hallucinations. *Neuroleptic* implies something that "seizes the nervous system"—a vestige of the belief that effective antipsychotics (APs) were associated with extrapyramidal side effects. Experience with newer, atypical APs has refuted this view (Janicak et al. 1993). Thus, whereas haloperidol may be termed a neuroleptic, clozapine and olanzapine (and other atypical agents) are properly termed antipsychotics. However, we will apply this term (AP) generically to all agents discussed in this chapter. The specific classes of AP agents include the *phenothiazines* (e.g., chlorpromazine), *thioxanthenes* (e.g., thiothixene), *butyrophenones* (e.g., haloperidol), *dihydroindolones* (e.g., molindone), *dibenzoxazepines* (e.g., loxapine), *diphenylbutylpiperidines* (e.g., pimozide), *dibenzodiazepines* (e.g., clozapine), and *benzisoxazoles* (e.g., risperidone).

▌ Indications

It may seem redundant to say that the main indication for an
AP is *psychosis,* but because APs are often used (and misused)
for other conditions (such as "agitation"), the point bears em-
phasizing. The main psychiatric disorders for which an AP is
indicated are *schizophrenia, schizoaffective disorder, schizophreniform disorder,* and *brief psychotic disorder.* The APs also play a
role in the treatment of various *secondary psychotic states* (e.g.,
secondary to cocaine intoxication, Alzheimer's disease, ac-
quired immunodeficiency syndrome [AIDS] dementia), *bipolar states* (manic or depressed) associated with psychosis, and
major depression with psychotic features (Shader 1994a). This list
is not exhaustive, nor is it necessarily inappropriate to use an
AP in a nonpsychotic individual. Thus, APs are used to treat
the tics of *Tourette's syndrome,* certain severe cases of
obsessive-compulsive disorder (OCD) with comorbid schizotypal personality disorder or tics, and—in low doses—*borderline personality disorder* (BPD). The evidence that APs are
effective in OCD or BPD is modest at best, and the risk of tardive dyskinesia (TD) (see "Main Side Effects") must con-
stantly be borne in mind. The same applies to the use of APs
in violent or aggressive *developmentally disabled individuals,* in
whom inappropriately high doses of APs may exacerbate the
unwanted behaviors. Although APs are intended primarily
for psychotic conditions, these agents may be used in various
acute medical contexts, even when the patient does not
manifest psychotic features in the strict sense. For example,
the early tranquilizing effect of the APs may be useful in
calming the severely agitated, delirious patient in the intensive care unit.

▌ Mechanisms of Action

The precise mechanism by which APs exert their antipsychotic effects is not known; however, nearly all compounds
with significant antipsychotic activity block central dopa-

mine receptors of one kind or another (Janicak et al. 1993). Some research suggests that agents without dopamine blockade that antagonize the serotonin-2 (5-HT$_2$) receptor may have antipsychotic properties, but the data are preliminary. (Even these agents, such as amperozide and ritanserin, may indirectly reduce dopamine in certain brain regions but increase it in others [see Pickar 1994]). Dopamine receptors belong to two main "families": 1) the D$_1$ and D$_5$ type, and 2) the D$_2$, D$_3$, and D$_4$ type. The potency of classical neuroleptics such as haloperidol is correlated with their affinity for the D$_2$ receptor. However, some atypical APs such as clozapine (and apparently olanzapine) show less D$_2$ blockade and more blockade of D$_1$ and D$_4$ receptors (Owens and Risch 1995). Clozapine also seems to act more selectively on mesolimbic dopamine receptors (so-called A10 neurons) than on striatal (A9) dopamine receptors, perhaps accounting for its low rate of extrapyramidal side effects (see "Main Side Effects"). Clozapine and most other atypical or near-atypical agents, such as risperidone, also antagonize the 5-HT$_2$ receptor. A ratio of 5-HT$_2$ to D$_2$ receptor blockade (or binding affinity) greater than 1.1 seems to define the "atypicality" of an AP (Meltzer et al. 1989). Neuroleptics and APs have many effects on neurotransmitters and receptors that may be related to their therapeutic effects, such as their effects on norepinephrine (NE) release. These agents also have anticholinergic, antihistaminic, and antiadrenergic effects that contribute to side effects (see "Main Side Effects").

▌Pharmacokinetics

Like the antidepressants, the APs undergo hepatic metabolism via the cytochrome P450 (CYP) system (DeVane 1994). Most APs appear to be metabolized via the CYP2D6 system (e.g., perphenazine, thioridazine, risperidone), whereas others are at least partially metabolized through CYP1A2 (e.g., clozapine). Probably some, but not all, of these APs are also inhibitors of the CYP2D6 pathway (fluphenazine, haloperidol). Their metabolism via CYP2D6 makes the APs "competitors" with several of the tricyclics and selective serotonin reuptake inhibitors (SSRIs), and these classes of drug may mutually inhibit each other's metabolism (see "Drug-Drug Interactions"). APs undergo extensive "first-pass" hepatic extraction with oral dosing, leading to lower initial plasma levels than with intramuscular (IM) injection. Peak plasma levels after oral dosing are reached in about 2–3 hours; with IM injection, they are reached in about 20–30 minutes. Because the IM route avoids first-pass effects, plasma levels are roughly twice as high (initially) as with oral agents; thus, the usual IM dose of an AP is about one-half that of the oral drug. Most APs have elimination half-lives ($t\frac{1}{2}$s) of 20–24 hours, with longer times in the elderly or those with hepatic dysfunction. Some APs (e.g., chlorpromazine) generate dozens of active metabolites; others, such as haloperidol, generate only two or three. Still, these metabolites may have therapeutic implications, as with the potentially neurotoxic *haloperidol pyridinium* (Tsang et al. 1994). Few laboratories report plasma levels of AP metabolites. Moreover, in general there is no well-established relationship between plasma AP concentration and clinical efficacy, although modest evidence supports a "therapeutic window" (roughly 4–15 ng/mL) for haloperidol. Similarly, response to clozapine seems to be correlated with plasma levels around 400 ng/mL, although higher and lower levels may be effective for any given patient. Plasma AP levels may be useful in detecting noncompliance, or in confirming toxicity, and may be prudent to obtain when the patient is taking multiple psychotropics undergoing hepatic metabolism.

∎ Main Side Effects

APs have a variety of side effects, arising from their actions at many different neuronal receptors. *Extrapyramidal symptoms*

(EPS), including acute dystonic reactions, akathisia, and parkinsonism, are seen more commonly with high-potency agents, such as haloperidol and fluphenazine. Lower-potency agents, such as thioridazine and chlorpromazine, are more likely to cause *anticholinergic, antihistaminic,* and *antiadrenergic side effects.* Blockade of peripheral α_1-adrenergic receptors appears to mediate the *hypotensive effects* of some APs. Blockade of α_2-adrenergic autoreceptors seems to occur with clozapine and perhaps risperidone, giving these agents some noradrenergic effects (blockade of the α_2 autoreceptor would result in increased NE release from the presynaptic neuron). The antihistaminic effect of low-potency APs may mediate their sedating and weight-promoting side effects. Other side effects associated with the APs include *hepatic dysfunction* (probably mostly with aliphatic phenothiazines), *sexual dysfunction* (mainly with low-potency agents), *menstrual irregularities* and/or *gynecomastia* with typical agents (dopamine blockade leads to increased prolactin secretion with all APs except clozapine), *skin rash, photosensitivity reactions, decreased seizure threshold, neuroleptic malignant syndrome (NMS),* and *TD.* The cumulative yearly incidence of TD in patients taking classic neuroleptics is about 4%–5% and is much higher (around 20%) in elderly populations. With clozapine, the incidence of *agranulocytosis* is about 0.9% per year; agranulocytosis usually occurs within the first 5 months of treatment. Low-potency APs also have some quinidine-like properties (shared with tricyclic antidepressants [TCAs]) that may occasionally cause cardiac conduction abnormalities. Management of side effects involves dosage reduction, slow increases in dose (especially in the elderly), change of agent class (e.g., from a low- to a high-potency agent), use of antiparkinsonian agents for EPS, use of bethanechol (Urecholine) for peripheral anticholinergic side effects, and use of support stockings or salt tablets for AP-induced postural hypotension.

▋ Drug-Drug Interactions

APs with anticholinergic side effects (dry mouth, blurry vision, urinary retention, constipation, and confusional states) may be potentiated by *other anticholinergic agents,* such as trihexyphenidyl (Artane) or benztropine (Cogentin), which are used to counteract EPS. (Thus, the combination of a low-potency AP with antiparkinsonian agents is often unnecessary and unwise, particularly in elderly and dementia patients.) APs may lead to increased EPS when used concomitantly with *lithium* or *SSRIs* such as fluoxetine (Prozac)—most likely via pharmacodynamic interactions in the brain. Both the *TCAs* and *SSRIs* may elevate plasma levels of some APs by reducing their hepatic metabolism. *Propranolol* may lead to elevation of plasma phenothiazine levels via a similar mechanism and also increases the risk of hypotension in AP-treated patients. *Valproate* may modestly increase plasma AP levels, but this is of doubtful clinical significance. Conversely, *phenytoin* (Dilantin) and *carbamazepine* (Tegretol) may significantly reduce plasma AP levels. *Antacids,* such as Maalox, may impair absorption of APs from the gastrointestinal (GI) tract.

▋ Potentiating Maneuvers

As many as 25% of all psychotic patients do not respond adequately to their first trial of a conventional AP agent (Cole et al. 1964). After issues of incorrect diagnosis, poor compliance, and inadequate dose/bioavailability (Osser 1989) have been ruled out, a variety of potentiation strategies are possible. Combining a standard AP with a *benzodiazepine,* an *antidepressant,* a *mood stabilizer* (lithium, valproate, carbamazepine), or *propranolol* has occasionally been successful, depending on the target symptoms; however, many clinicians are moving more quickly toward *atypical agents* (risperidone, clozapine, olanzapine) rather than using such "potentiating" strategies. Nevertheless, in some schizoaffective patients, the addition of a mood stabilizer (lithium or valproate) may reduce emotional lability or dysphoric manic symptoms. β-Blockers may reduce aggressive/violent or self-injurious behaviors, and benzodiazepines may sometimes improve "negative" symptoms in schizophrenia (Janicak et al. 1993). Recent work by Hogarty et al. (1995) suggests that in female patients with chronic schizophrenia and anxious-depressive symptoms, the addition of a tricyclic (desipramine) may be beneficial after 3 months of treatment. Hogarty et al. (1995) found that lithium also may be beneficial as an adjunct to APs in chronic schizophrenic patients with "anxious depression."

▌ Use in Special Populations

As with all psychotropics, use of APs in elderly and medically ill patients generally requires dosage reduction and careful monitoring of vital signs and side effects. Elderly patients, in general, should not be treated with the highly anticholinergic APs, such as thioridazine or chlorpromazine. (Anticholinergic side effects can include urinary retention, bowel obstruction, and confusional states.) Such low-potency agents also tend to promote postural hypotension. Clozapine may be effective in both geriatric and medically ill older patients (e.g., Parkinson's patients with psychosis) but produces many side effects; thus, clozapine dosage should begin in the extremely low range (6.25 mg/day), with very gradual increases. Risperidone may be effective in the elderly but must be used in low doses to avoid hypotension, EPS, and drug-drug interactions.

The use of APs in children and adolescents is complicated by resistance to medication and both over- and under-medication (Dulcan et al. 1995). Age, weight, and severity of symptoms do not provide clear guidelines; moreover, although children metabolize APs more rapidly than adults, they also may require lower plasma levels for efficacy (Dulcan et al. 1995). The best advice is to begin with a low dose and to increase it gradually (no more than once or twice a week). On the other hand, older adolescents with schizophrenia may require AP doses comparable to those of adults. It is not yet clear which class of AP is safest and most efficacious in children and adolescents (Gelenberg 1994).

The use of APs in the pregnant patient—as with any medication—should be avoided, if possible. Unfortunately, the dangers from untreated psychosis may require aggressive treatment and often outweigh the rather remote risks of teratogenesis or neonatal toxicity from APs (Stowe and Nemeroff 1995). Ideally, one should defer treatment until after the first trimester, when organ formation is most susceptible to teratogenic effects, but this is often impractical. Electroconvulsive therapy (ECT) is a viable option in the acutely psychotic/manic pregnant patient but, despite its safety in such circumstances, is often restricted by the courts.

Tables

▌Drug Class

Table 2–1. Dosages and therapeutic levels of currently available antipsychotics

Class/subclass, generic name	Brand name	Usually effective daily oral dose[a] (mg/day)	Putative therapeutic plasma level (ng/mL)
Butyrophenones Haloperidol	Haldol	2–40	2–12
Dihydroindolones Molindone	Moban	20–225	—
Dibenzoxazepines Loxapine	Loxitane	30–150	—
Diphenylbutyl-piperidines Pimozide	Orap	2–12	—
Dibenzodiazepines Clozapine	Clozaril	50–900	200–350 ng/ml for most patients
Thienobenzodiazepine Olanzapine	Zyprexa	10–20	—
Benzisoxazole Risperidone	Risperdal	1–10	—
Phenothiazines Aliphatic			
Chlorpromazine	Thorazine	150–1,000	30–100
Triflupromazine	Vesprin	20–150	—
Promazine	Sparine	25–1,000	—

(continued)

Table 2–1.   Dosages and therapeutic levels of currently available antipsychotics *(continued)*

Class/subclass, generic name	Brand name	Usually effective daily oral dose[a] (mg/day)	Putative therapeutic plasma level (ng/mL)
Phenothiazines *(continued)*			
Piperazine			
Fluphenazine	Prolixin, Permitil	2–20	0.2–2
Perphenazine	Trilafon	8–40	0.8–3
Trifluoperazine	Stelazine	5–30	1–2.5
Acetophenazine	Tindal	40–80	—
Piperidine			
Mesoridazine	Serentil	75–300	—
Thioridazine	Mellaril	100–800	—
Thioxanthenes			
Aliphatic			
Chlorprothixene	Taractan	30–600	—
Piperazine			
Thiothixene	Navane	6–50	2–15

Note. — = insufficient data.
[a]Doses are based on my clinical experience and consensus of sources listed. Acute doses are generally higher than maintenance doses for many patients. Dosage recommendations vary considerably based on age of patient, diagnosis, and plasma levels attained. Initial doses of APs that induce hypotension (e.g., mesoridazine, chlorpromazine) may need to be significantly lower than the ultimately effective dose. Other examples include the following: 1) initial and final doses of risperidone may need to be lower in elderly versus younger patients or in those with bipolar disorder (because high risperidone doses may exacerbate manic symptoms); 2) Clozaril dose may be substantially lower in elderly Parkinson's patients with psychosis than in young, healthy patients with schizophrenia; and 3) for a patient who achieves a plasma haloperidol level of only 1 ng/mL at 10 mg/day, a dosage increase may be necessary.
Sources.   P. F. Buckley and Meltzer 1995; Janicak et al. 1993; Jenkins and Hansen 1995; Kaplan et al. 1994; Lindenmayer and Apergi 1996; Physicians' Desk Reference 1996; Shader 1994a; VanderZwaag et al. 1996; Van Putten et al. 1990a, 1990b.

Table 2–2. Commonly prescribed antipsychotic tablet sizes and dosage equivalents of 100 mg chlorpromazine

Antipsychotic	Tablet/capsule sizes (mg)	Approximate mg equivalent to 100 mg chlorpromazine[a]
Clozapine	25, 100	100
Fluphenazine	1, 2.5, 5, 10	2
Haloperidol	0.5, 1, 2, 5, 10, 20	2
Loxapine	5, 10, 25, 50	12
Mesoridazine	10, 25, 50, 100	50
Molindone	5, 10, 25, 50, 100	10
Olanzapine	2.5, 5, 7.5, 10	3.5
Perphenazine	2, 4, 8, 16	10
Risperidone	1, 2, 3, 4	1.5
Thioridazine	10, 15, 25, 50, 100, 150, 200	100
Thiothixene	1, 2, 5, 10, 20	4
Trifluoperazine	1, 2, 5, 10	5

[a]Data on equivalent doses vary considerably, depending on whether in vitro or clinical data are used. Equivalent doses also vary from patient to patient. Doses are based on my clinical experience and consensus of sources listed.

Sources. Jenkins and Hansen 1995; Kaplan et al. 1994.

Table 2–3.   Dosage ranges for selected new atypical antipsychotics

Agent	Dosage range (mg/day)
Olanzapine	7.5–20
Quetiapine	150–800
Sertindole	12–24
Ziprasidone	80–160

Source.   Data from Jibson and Tandon 1996; Keck and McElroy 1997.

▎Indications

Table 2–4. Indications for use of antipsychotics

Indications	Special considerations
Schizophrenia	Large data base; dose generally 300 chlorpromazine equivalents per day; haloperidol doses above 10–15 mg/day usually unnecessary; plasma haloperidol levels between 4 and 16 ng/mL may be optimal; plasma haloperidol levels above 30 ng/mL may be associated with increased toxicity and unclear benefit; plasma levels less certain with other APs; clozapine for refractory schizophrenia, negative symptoms; possible correlation between clozapine levels 250–420 ng/mL and efficacy; risperidone useful for negative symptoms, history of marked EPS on typical agents
Schizophreniform disorder, brief psychotic disorder	Limited data base; patients with first onset of acute or subacute psychosis may respond rapidly to lower doses of APs than may patients with schizophrenia; lithium may be effective in a small percentage of patients; use of AP for 3–6 months with gradual tapering off may suffice in many cases of schizophreniform disorder; ECT may be indicated in cases with marked catatonic or depressive features; benzodiazepines (e.g., lorazepam 2–6 mg/day) may suffice in brief psychotic episodes or "brief reactive psychosis"
Delusional disorder	Limited data base; delusional disorder relatively uncommon (incidence 25 times less than that of schizophrenia); subtypes include erotomanic, grandiose, jealous, persecutory, somatic; large-scale studies of APs lacking in these patients; anecdotal reports indicate that some patients do respond to APs, particularly paranoid psychoses of late life; erotomanic and jealous subtypes may be more resistant to AP treatment

(continued)

Table 2–4. Indications for use of antipsychotics (*continued*)

Indications	Special considerations
Paranoid, schizoid, schizotypal, borderline personality disorders	Data base limited; low-dose AP trial may be helpful in some borderline patients, although long-term studies not encouraging (serotonergic agents may be preferable); even more limited data base for paranoid, schizoid, schizotypal personality disorders, for which low-dose APs reported useful in a few studies; patients with paranoid personality disorder often extremely resistant to medication, experience it as coercive, and benefits not clear
Schizoaffective disorder	Moderate data base but variably defined syndrome; "schizomanic" and "schizodepressed" subgroups are probably different disorders, with latter group being heterogeneous; in schizomanic patients, AP + mood stabilizer often used; clozapine seems promising in manic-excited phase of schizoaffective disorder, less useful in schizodepressive patients; risperidone may be useful in schizodepressive patients (can exacerbate manic symptoms in some schizoaffective patients unless mood stabilizer used concomitantly); ECT may be useful in both types of schizoaffective illness
Psychosis secondary to drug/toxin	Psychiatric emergencies with psychotic symptoms due to delirium, street drug abuse (hallucinogens) usually respond to low-to-moderate doses of haloperidol (1–5 mg/day), sometimes in combination with lorazepam (0.5–1.5 mg po, IM, or IV, q 1–2 hours); avoid low-potency APs with anticholinergic effects if phencyclidine toxicity suspected

Psychosis secondary to dementia

Moderately large data base; in patients who have dementia with psychotic features (hallucinations, paranoia), APs more effective than placebo but probably not as effective as in younger patients with schizophrenia; the closer the disruptive behaviors of dementia patient resemble psychotic features of schizophrenia, the more effective the AP will be; low-potency agents generally avoided because of peripheral and central anticholinergic effects (e.g., increased cognitive dysfunction in Alzheimer's patients), but dementia patients with psychosis and EPS (e.g., from Parkinson's disease) may benefit from small dose of low-potency agent (e.g., 25 mg thioridazine); clozapine also of use in psychotic Parkinson's patients (6.25–50 mg/day may suffice); haloperidol 0.5–1.0 mg/day may be alternative in patients with dementia with psychotic features; buspirone, trazodone, anticonvulsant may be alternative to AP in disruptive, aggressive dementia patient without true psychotic symptoms

Bipolar disorder

Moderate data base; five well-controlled trials comparing lithium to APs in acute manic episode; overall, lithium was superior (89% versus 54% response rate, respectively); APs have faster onset of action than lithium and may be useful as adjuncts to lithium or valproate in initial management of mania; benzodiazepines also useful acutely; ideally, AP is tapered and decreased as mood stabilizer gains control

Major depression with psychotic features

Large data base; combination of AP and AD works better than either AP or AD alone (some delusionally depressed patients may worsen on AD alone); ECT is excellent alternative; amoxapine (which has neuroleptic metabolite) also may be effective; combination of AP and AD may lead to increased plasma levels of either or both agents

(continued)

Table 2–4. Indications for use of antipsychotics *(continued)*

Indications	Special considerations
Obsessive-compulsive disorder	Small data base; AP rarely indicated in obsessive-compulsive disorder, except as augmenting agent (with serotonergic drug) in patients with comorbid tic disorder or schizotypal features; clozapine may exacerbate obsessive symptoms in some patients
Mental retardation with behavioral dyscontrol (no psychotic symptoms)	APs widely used in developmentally disabled, but few data from well-controlled trials; APs may exacerbate agitation, akathisia, and/or self-injury in some patients with mental retardation; D_1 blockers, clozapine may have theoretical advantages in patients with self-injurious behavior; use lowest-feasible dose of AP or consider alternatives (valproate, β-blocker, buspirone, SSRI, lithium)
Tourette's syndrome	Large data base; haloperidol (0.2 mg/kg/day), pimozide are effective; rare cardiac arrhythmias associated with pimozide; clonidine is usual first-line treatment; possible role for atypical neuroleptics (limited data base)

Note. APs = antipsychotics; EPS = extrapyramidal symptoms; ECT = electroconvulsive therapy; IM = intramuscularly; IV = intravenously; AD = antidepressant; SSRI = selective serotonin reuptake inhibitor.
Sources.   Cornelius et al. 1991, 1993; Janicak et al. 1993; Kaplan et al. 1994; Keck et al. 1995; Keith and Schooler 1989; Lindenmayer and Apergi 1996; Peterson 1995; Pies and Popli 1995; Raskind 1995; Roth 1989; Schexnayder et al. 1995; Tueth et al. 1995; Zarate et al. 1995.

▌Mechanisms of Action

Table 2–5. Relative receptor affinities of haloperidol and two atypical antipsychotics

Agent	D_1	D_2	5-HT$_{1A}$	5-HT$_{2A}$	α_1	α_2	H_1	M_1
Clozapine[a]	++	++	+	+++	+++	+++	++++	+++++
Haloperidol	+++	++++	+/–	+	++	+/–	+/–	+/–
Risperidone[b]	++	++++	++	+++++	+++	+++	++	+/–

Note. Data are intended only as comparative and do not reflect quantitative receptor affinities. +++++ = very strong; ++++ = strong; +++ =significant; ++ = modest; + = minimal; +/– = negligible.

[a]Clozapine also has marked D_4 receptor affinity.

[b]The status of risperidone as an "atypical" agent is controversial because 1) there is no universally agreed-on definition of atypical, and 2) risperidone shows dose-related extrapyramidal side effects (usually at doses > 6 mg/day).

Source. Adapted from Pickar 1995. Data not directly comparable to values in Table 2–6.

Table 2–6.   Relative receptor antagonism of available or soon-to-be released atypical agents

Receptor	Risperidone (Risperdal)	Clozapine (Clozaril)	Olanzapine (Zyprexa)	Quetiapine (Seroquel)	Sertindole (SerLect)
D_2	1	+/−	½	+/−	4
5-HT_{2A}	3	2	1	+/−	4
M_1 (muscarinic cholinergic)	+/−	3	4	1	+/−
H_1 (histaminic)	½	4	2	1	+/−
α_1 adrenergic	2	1	½	½	4

Note.   Data are semiquantitative comparisons of in vitro affinities for a given receptor. Values should not be compared "vertically"; for example, a "4" on D_2 antagonism may not be quantitatively equivalent to a "4" on α_1 antagonism in the same column. See Richelson 1996 for actual affinities of drugs for a given receptor. In vitro affinities do not always correspond with clinical effects.
4 = marked; 3 = substantial; 2 = moderate; 1 to ½ = slight; +/− = minimal.
Source.   Data from Richelson 1996.

▊ Pharmacokinetics

Table 2–7.   Cytochrome P450 2D6 and antipsychotic
metabolism/interaction

AP substrates for CYP2D6	Inhibitors of CYP2D6	Possible clinical problem/interaction[a]
Clozapine[b] Haloperidol Perphenazine Risperidone Thioridazine	Fluphenazine Haloperidol Quinidine Fluoxetine Norfluoxetine Paroxetine Sertraline (modest) (tricyclics in high concentrations)	Fluoxetine, paroxetine, sertraline may reduce clearance of AP agents; fluoxetine may increase haloperidol plasma concentrations by 20% (possibly leading to increased AP side effects); fluoxetine may increase clozapine, fluphenazine decanoate levels; fluoxetine-induced EPS may be more likely in context of AP treatment

Note.   AP = antipsychotic; CYP = cytochrome P450; EPS = extrapyramidal symptoms.
[a]Tricyclic antidepressants at high plasma concentrations also may elevate plasma levels of APs. Conversely, haloperidol and phenothiazines may elevate plasma levels of tricyclics, probably via inhibition of CYP2D6.
[b]Fluvoxamine (Luvox) may increase clozapine levels via an inhibitory effect on CYP1A2, suggesting that this is an important additional pathway for clozapine metabolism.
Source.   Data derived in part from Goff and Baldessarini 1995.

Table 2–8. Atypical agents: metabolism and pharmacokinetics

Risperidone	Clozapine	Olanzapine	Sertindole
$t\frac{1}{2}$ = 4 hours parent, 22 hours active metabolite (9-OH-RSP); main elimination route via CYP2D6; renal excretion of 9-OH-RSP; decrease dose in patients with decreased renal function	Mean $t\frac{1}{2}$ = 16 hours desmethylclozapine metabolite; main elimination routes CYP1A2, CYP3A4	Mean $t\frac{1}{2}$ = 30 hours; main elimination routes CYP1A2, CYP2D6 (CYP1A2 > CYP2D6); glucuronidation	Mean $t\frac{1}{2}$ = 70 hours; main elimination routes CYP2D6, CYP3A4

Note. $t\frac{1}{2}$ = half-life; CYP = cytochrome P450.
Source. Data from Ereshefsky 1996.

▌ Main Side Effects

Table 2–9. Comparative side effects among available antipsychotics

Agent	Sedation	Extrapyramidal	Anticholinergic	Orthostasis
Chlorpromazine	+++	+	+++	+++
Clozapine	+++	+/−	++[a]	+++
Fluphenazine	+	+++	+	+
Haloperidol	+	+++	+	+
Loxapine	++	++	+	++
Mesoridazine	+++	+	++	++
Molindone	+	++	+	+
Olanzapine	++	+/−	+	+

(continued)

Table 2–9. Comparative side effects among available antipsychotics (continued)

Agent	Sedation	Extrapyramidal	Anticholinergic	Orthostasis
Perphenazine	+	++	+	++
Pimozide	+	+++	+	+
Risperidone	+	+	+	++
Thioridazine	+++	+	+++	+++
Thiothixene	+	+++	+	+
Trifluoperazine	+	+++	+	+

Note.   Effects may differ in acute versus chronic treatment, in young versus elderly patients, and with dose and route of administration. +++ = substantial; ++ = moderate; + = mild; +/− = minimal.

[a]Clozapine has high in vitro affinity for the muscarinic (M_1) receptor (see Table 2–5) but has variable clinical effects (e.g., some patients may experience hypersalivation and/or enuresis, whereas others may experience dry mouth, urinary retention, and other anticholinergic effects). There is some evidence that supposed hypersalivation from clozapine may actually reflect *impaired swallowing mechanism* rather than cholinergic effect.

Sources.   Data from my clinical experience; Casey 1996; Drug Facts and Comparisons 1995; Shader 1994a.

Table 2–10. Side effects of selected atypical agents

Side effect profile[b]	Risperidone	Clozapine[a]	Olanzapine[a]	Sertindole	Quetiapine
Extrapyramidal symptoms[c]	+	+/–	+/–	+/–	+/–
Tardive dyskinesia	?	+/–	?	?	?
Seizures	+/–	+++	+/–	+/–	+/–
Agranulocytosis	+/–	+++	+/–	+/–	+/–
Drowsiness	+	+++	++	+/–	++
Hypotension	+	++	+	+	+
Dizziness	+	++	+	+	+
Dry mouth	+/–	+	+	+/–	+
Constipation	+	++	+	+/–	+
Weight gain[d]	+	+++	+	+	+

Note. +++ = high incidence; ++ =moderate incidence; + = low incidence; +/– = negligible incidence; ? = data too preliminary.
[a]Values for clozapine and olanzapine not directly comparable with those in other tables because data may be derived from different sources.
[b]Based on various dosages of agents, with *no direct drug-to-drug comparisons available.*
[c]Sum of dystonia, parkinsonism, akathisia.
[d]Reports of weight gain are often underestimated during early experience with atypical antipsychotics; thus, weight gain with olanzapine, for example, may well prove to exceed the 5%–7% rates reported thus far.
Sources. Data from my clinical experience; Casey 1996; Jibson and Tandon 1996; Lily Research Laboratories, Zyprexa monograph, September 24, 1996; Physicians' Desk Reference 1996; Small et al. 1997; van Kammen et al. 1996.

Table 2–11. Motor and mental features of neuroleptic-induced extrapyramidal side effects

Syndrome	Motor symptoms	Mental symptoms	Psychiatric differential diagnosis
Akathisia	Restlessness, pacing, fidgeting, shifting from foot to foot	Jitteriness, anxiety, irritability, anger, difficulty concentrating, suicidality	Psychotic agitation, anxiety disorder, agitated depression, mixed manic state
Dystonia	Muscle contractions, tongue protrusion, torticollis, opisthotonos	Fear, distress, paranoia	Catatonic posturing, seizure, conversion disorder
Tardive dyskinesia	Buccolingual-masticatory movements of irregular (*nonrhythmic*) nature; choreiform or athetoid (writhing) movements of fingers, extremities, trunk; rarely, respiratory dyskinesia; not present during sleep: *tardive dystonia* related to tardive dyskinesia and may coexist with it (late onset of twisting movements of limbs, trunk, neck)	In mild, early cases, patient often not aware and not distressed by tardive dyskinesia; more severe cases, interfering with chewing or causing dysphagia, may be very distressing as may be (rare) respiratory dyskinesia	Other choreiform disorders, such as Huntington's chorea, Sydenham's chorea; diseases/lesions affecting basal ganglia; electrolyte or other metabolic disease must be ruled out

| **Parkinsonism** | Tremor (resting), rigidity, bradykinesia, masklike facies | Bradyphrenia (slowed thinking), mental clouding | Negative symptoms of schizophrenia; depression; neuroleptic malignant syndrome |

Sources. Adapted from Ayd 1995; Casey 1995.

Table 2-12. Selected agents for treatment of extrapyramidal side effects of neuroleptics

Generic name	Trade name	Usual daily dosage for extrapyramidal side effects
Amantadine	Symmetrel	100–200 mg bid
Benztropine	Cogentin	0.5–2 mg bid orally; 1–2 mg IM for acute dystonic reaction
Biperiden	Akineton	2–6 mg tid orally; 2 mg IM
Clonazepam	Klonopin	0.5–1 mg bid
Diphenhydramine	Benadryl	25–50 mg bid orally; 25 mg IM for acute dystonic reaction
Procyclidine	Kemadrin	2.5–5 mg tid
Trihexyphenidyl	Artane, Tremin, others	2–5 mg tid

Note. IM = intramuscularly.
Sources. Data from Kaplan et al. 1994; Stanilla and Simpson 1995.

Table 2–13. Neuroleptic malignant syndrome: differential diagnosis

	5-HT syndrome	Neuroleptic malignant syndrome	Malignant hyperthermia	Lethal (pernicious) catatonia	Central anticholinergic syndrome
Core symptoms	Variable temperature elevations (37.4°C to 42.5°C)[a]	Hyperthermia	Hyperthermia (core temperature >41°C)	Hyperthermia	Hyperthermia
	Mental status changes	Severe muscle rigidity (usually "lead pipe")	Muscle rigidity	Muscle rigidity	Decreased sweating[a]
	Hypomania[a]	Diaphoresis	Ischemia	Diaphoresis	Hot, dry skin[a]
	Restlessness	Delirium	Hot skin	Delirium	Dilated, sluggish pupils[a]
	Myoclonus	Muteness	Mottled cyanosis[a]	Extreme hyperactivity[a] (often early in syndrome) or stupor	Tachycardia
	Hyperreflexia	Incontinence	Hypotension[a]		Constipation[a]
	Diaphoresis	Rhabdomyolysis	Rhabdomyolysis	Psychotic prodrome[a]	Urinary retention[a]
	Shivering/teeth chattering[a]	Mutism[a]	Tremulousness	Posturing[a]	Confusion
	Tremor	Autonomic instability (fluctuating blood pressure, pallor/flushing)[a]	Tachycardia	Stupor alternating with excitement[a]	Impaired memory
	Diarrhea		Tachypnea	Hypertension	Delirium
			EPS		Hallucinations

(continued)

Table 2–13. Neuroleptic malignant syndrome: differential diagnosis (*continued*)

	5-HT syndrome	Neuroleptic malignant syndrome	Malignant hyperthermia	Lethal (pernicious) catatonia	Central anticholinergic syndrome
Core symptoms (*continued*)	Incoordination	Most common temporal sequence[a]: mental status change, rigidity, autonomic dysfunction, hyperthermia[a]		Tremulousness	
Laboratory findings	No specific findings	Elevated CPK,[a] WBC, LFTs, myoglobinuria	Disseminated intravascular coagulation[a]; respiratory/ metabolite acidosis[a]; hyperkalemia[a]; hyper- magnesemia[a]	No specific findings	No specific findings

Causes/mechanisms					
Activation of 5-HT$_{1A}$ receptors in brain stem, spinal cord; enhancement of overall 5-HT neurotransmission; most commonly due to interaction between MAOI and serotonergic agent (L-tryptophan, SSRI) but may occur with any 5-HT drug	Presumed: blockade of dopaminergic pathways in basal ganglia and hypothalamus; also may result from sudden withdrawal of dopamine agonist ?Lithium may precipitate ?Low serum iron	Inherited disorder; triggering anesthetic (halothane, methoxyflurane) causes calcium release from sarcoplasmic reticulum, leading to activation of myosin ATPase, heat production	Manic and depressed mood states; schizophrenia (also secondary to infection and metabolic, other medical disorders)	Blockade of central and peripheral muscarinic receptors (e.g., due to tricyclic phenothiazine)

(continued)

Table 2–13. Neuroleptic malignant syndrome: differential diagnosis *(continued)*

	5-HT syndrome	Neuroleptic malignant syndrome	Malignant hyperthermia	Lethal (pernicious) catatonia	Central anticholinergic syndrome
Management	Discontinue suspected agent; supportive measures (cooling blanket for hyperthermia); propranolol, methysergide, cyproheptadine may help	Supportive measures (cooling); stop neuroleptic; no clear treatment of choice, but dopamine agonists (bromocriptine 5 mg tid), dantrolene, ECT may help	Dantrolene sodium 1 mg/kg via rapid IV infusion; 100% oxygen; sodium bicarbonate; external cooling	Some recommend ECT as therapy of choice (within first 5 days); lorazepam 1–2 mg po or IM up to qid also useful; neuroleptics generally best withheld	Remove offending agent; physostigmine usually not indicated (?unless cardiac arrhythmia present)

Note. ? = data uncertain; 5-HT = serotonin; EPS = extrapyramidal symptoms; CPK = creatine phosphokinase; WBC = white blood cell count; LFTs = liver function tests; MAOI = monoamine oxidase inhibitor; SSRI = selective serotonin reuptake inhibitor; ATPase = adenosine triphosphatase; ECT = electroconvulsive therapy; IV = intravenous; IM = intramuscular.
[a]Features that help differentiate syndromes. Some authors believe that neuroleptic malignant syndrome and lethal catatonia are closely related syndromes.
Sources. Ayd 1995; Castillo et al. 1989; Fink 1996; Fink et al. 1993; Jenkins and Hansen 1995; Pearlman 1986; Petersdorf 1991; Sternbach 1991; Theoharides et al. 1995; Velamoor et al. 1995.

Table 2–14. Management of antipsychotic side effects

Side effect	Strategy
Dry mouth, blurry vision, constipation, other anticholinergic effects	Encourage fluid intake (nonsugar); use of sugarless gum; use of high-fiber diet and/or stool softener for constipation; use of bethanechol for peripheral anticholinergic side effects; switch to more potent agent if other strategies unsuccessful
Extrapyramidal symptoms	Reduce dose of AP if possible; add anticholinergic (benztropine, trihexyphenidyl); for akathisia, add β-blocker (propranolol 10 mg tid or atenolol 50 mg bid); for refractory EPS, amantadine 100 mg bid (but may worsen psychosis in some patients); benzodiazepines sometimes helpful
Dizziness, hypotension	Instruct patient to dangle legs, rise slowly from bed; reduce dose of AP and/or divide into smaller amounts (e.g., 100 mg bid and 200 mg hs thioridazine rather than 400 mg hs); increase salt intake (e.g., salt tablets); use of support stockings; in difficult cases, use of fludrocortisone (Florinef)
Sexual side effects	Reduce dose of AP if possible; switch to more potent agent (avoid aliphatic piperidine phenothiazines); add small amount of cyproheptadine (or ?yohimbine); bethanechol

Note. AP = antipsychotic; EPS =extrapyramidal symptoms; ? = possibly (limited data).

Table 2–15.   Clozapine and white blood cell count: managing abnormalities

White cell count (mm³)	Granulocyte count (mm³)	Management
<3,500, or history of myeloproliferative disorder, or previous clozapine-induced agranulocytosis/granulocytopenia	—	Do not initiate clozapine treatment
After initiation of clozapine from normal WBC baseline, WBC is <3,500, drops by 3,000 or more from baseline, or shows cumulative drop of 3,000 or more over 3 weeks	—	Repeat WBC and differential counts; evaluate patient for signs of infection, fever, sore throat, malaise (if signs and symptoms of infection present, consider holding clozapine)
Subsequent WBC is between 3,000 and 3,500	Granulocytes > 1,500	Maintain clozapine but perform twice-weekly WBC and differential count
	Granulocytes < 1,500	Hold clozapine; get daily WBC and differential count; monitor for infection; do not resume clozapine unless/until granulocyte count returns to >1,500 and patient shows no signs of infection; continue to get twice-weekly WBC and differential count until total WBC > 3,500

WBC < 3,000 or	→ Granulocytes < 1,500	Hold clozapine; get daily WBC and differential count; monitor for infection; do not resume clozapine unless/until granulocyte count returns to >1,500 and patient shows no signs of infection; continue to get twice-weekly WBC and differential count until total WBC >3,500
WBC < 2,000 or	→ Granuloctyes < 1,000	Continue to hold clozapine; consider bone marrow aspiration, protective isolation if granulopoiesis deficient; if infection develops, perform cultures, start antibiotics; get daily WBC and differential count; do not rechallenge with clozapine, because agranulocytosis likely to reappear with shorter latency

Note.   WBC = white blood cell count.
Source.   Adapted from Sandoz Pharmaceuticals Corporation labeling information in Physicians' Desk Reference 1996, p. 2150.

▌ Drug-Drug Interactions

Table 2–16. Antipsychotic drug interactions

Medication/drug combined with AP	Effect/interaction
Antacids	Impaired GI absorption of chlorpromazine, ?haloperidol, other APs
Anticholinergics	Additive anticholinergic effects when given with low-potency APs (e.g., ileus); in theory, may worsen tardive dyskinesia but often do not
Anticonvulsants	Effect depends on agent: carbamazepine may lead to significantly lower plasma levels of haloperidol and other APs; valproate may inhibit metabolism of chlorpromazine and (to a modest degree) clozapine, thus raising levels of AP; valproate has little effect on haloperidol; chlorpromazine (but not haloperidol) may inhibit metabolism of phenytoin; phenytoin may reduce levels of haloperidol, clozapine; APs in general lower seizure threshold and antagonize anticonvulsants (*Note:* Increased risk of bone marrow suppression with clozapine plus carbamazepine)
Antihypertensives	Effect depends on agent: with captopril and perhaps other ACE inhibitors, propranolol, and methyldopa, increased hypotensive effect (with chlorpromazine, haloperidol); coadministration of chlorpromazine and methyldopa sometimes produces hypertension; antihypertensive effect of guanethidine may be reduced by chlorpromazine and similar APs; molindone does not have this effect, and haloperidol, thiothixene have less interference

(continued)

Table 2–16. Antipsychotic drug interactions *(continued)*

Medication/drug combined with AP	Effect/interaction
Benzodiazepines	Clozapine plus BZD may lead to respiratory suppression (probably most common with high-dose BZD); alprazolam may increase serum levels of fluphenazine or haloperidol
β-Blockers (e.g., propranolol)	Increased levels of both AP and β-blocker; ?enhanced AP effect
Cimetidine	May impair metabolism of clozapine and lead to toxicity; may impair absorption of some APs
CNS depressants (e.g., opiates, barbiturates)	Increased sedation, confusion, falls, hypotension; phenobarbital may decrease chlorpromazine levels via induction of hepatic metabolism
L-Dopa	Decreased antiparkinsonian effect of L-dopa due to dopamine receptor blockade by AP (*Note:* L-Dopa not effective for AP-induced EPS)
Lithium	Increased extrapyramidal effects; rarely, cases of encephalopathy (lethargy, fever, confusion); not clear this is more common with any one AP, although haloperidol-lithium combination more frequently reported
Other APs	May mutually inhibit each other's metabolism, thus raising plasma level of one or both (see "Questions and Answers," pp. 184–185)

(continued)

Table 2–16. Antipsychotic drug interactions *(continued)*

Medication/drug combined with AP	Effect/interaction
SSRIs (fluoxetine, paroxetine)	Fluoxetine, paroxetine (strong inhibitors of CYP2D6) may inhibit metabolism of APs, including risperidone, clozapine; worsening of EPS in some cases; pharmacodynamically, some schizophrenic patients taking APs will benefit from addition of SSRI (see "Questions and Answers," pp. 184–185
Tricyclic antidepressants	Increased plasma levels of both AP and AD; increase in anticholinergic effects with TCA and low-potency AP

Note. ? = hypothesized; AP = antipsychotic; GI = gastrointestinal; ACE = angiotensin-converting enzyme; BZD = benzodiazepine; CNS = central nervous system; EPS = extrapyramidal symptoms; SSRIs = selective serotonin reuptake inhibitors; CYP = cytochrome P450; AD = antidepressant; TCA = tricyclic antidepressant.
Source. Data from Ciraulo et al. 1989, 1994; Dubovsky 1994.

Table 2–17. Atypical antipsychotics: potential drug-drug interactions

Risperidone	Clozapine	Olanzapine	Sertindole
?Inhibitors of CYP2D6 could reverse ratio of risperidone to 9-OH-RSP (clinical significance not clear); risperidone itself is not strong inhibitor of CYP in vitro	Inhibitors of CYP3A4 (ketoconazole, erythromycin) can increase clozapine levels; inducers of CYP3A4 (carbamazepine) can decrease clozapine levels; fluvoxamine (inhibitor of CYP1A2) can markedly increase clozapine levels	Inhibitors of CYP1A2, such as fluvoxamine, likely to increase olanzapine levels; CYP1A2 inducers (omeprazole, rifampin) could decrease olanzapine levels; olanzapine not strong inhibitor of CYPs	Ketoconazole and other CYP3A4 inhibitors could cause significant elevation of sertindole; carbamazepine can significantly reduce sertindole levels; quinidine, fluoxetine, paroxetine may elevate sertindole levels (risk of Q-T prolongation with quinidine); sertindole inhibits CYP2D6 and weakly inhibits CYP3A4

Note. ? = hypothesized; CYP = cytochrome P450.
Source. Data from Ereshefsky 1996.

▌Potentiating Maneuvers

Table 2–18. Potentiation of antipsychotics

Agent added to antipsychotic	Potential benefits	Potential risks, side effects
Benzodiazepines	May improve comorbid anxiety; perhaps improve negative features (?alprazolam), some core symptoms of psychosis (reduced auditory hallucinations); lorazepam (also clonazepam, diazepam) transiently improves "functional catatonic" symptoms (may or may not be due to schizophrenia); BZDs may permit use of lower doses of APs in treatment of acute psychosis	BZD-related side effects, such as memory impairment, sedation, risk of dependency; high BZD doses may cause respiratory suppression in patients taking clozapine; some reports of behavioral disinhibition, exacerbation of psychosis, anxiety, depression; several controlled studies found tolerance developed by 4th week of BZD treatment
β-Blockers	May reduce aggression, perhaps self-injurious behavior in some psychotic patients; may reduce some core features of psychosis	May alter hepatic metabolism of APs (?increase plasma levels); side effects of β-blockers include hypotension, bradycardia, worsening of COPD, masking of hypoglycemia in diabetic patients; some patients may become depressed; not all studies show efficacy

Carbamazepine	May improve affective lability, aggression in some schizoaffective patients; mania complicated by psychotic features responds to anticonvulsants	May reduce plasma levels of some APs (e.g., haloperidol); increased risk of neurotoxicity; increased risk of hepatotoxicity when carbamazepine combined with phenothiazines; increased risk of bone marrow suppression with carbamazepine + clozapine; side effects of carbamazepine include sedation, GI upset, ataxia, SIADH
Lithium	May improve mood stability, depressive-anxious features in some chronic schizophrenic patients; may be useful in schizophreniform patients (?especially with family history of mood disorders)	Increased EPS, cerebellar symptoms; increased risk of neurotoxicity; lithium-related side effects (polyuria, loose stools, tremor)
Other antipsychotics	May sometimes augment partial response to clozapine or risperidone	APs may mutually raise each other's blood levels; possibly worsen side effects or increase risk of agranulocytosis
Valproate (divalproex)	May improve mood lability in some schizoaffective patients; antiseizure prophylaxis in some patients taking high-dose clozapine	May alter hepatic metabolism of some APs but probably not strong effect (e.g., 6% increase in clozapine levels); increased tremor; GI upset, sedation; transient alopecia

Note. ? = data uncertain; BZDs = benzodiazepines; APs = antipsychotics; COPD = chronic obstructive pulmonary disease; GI = gastrointestinal; SIADH = syndrome of inappropriate secretion of antidiuretic hormone; EPS = extrapyramidal symptoms.
Sources. Data from Csernansky and Newcomer 1995; Hogarty et al. 1995; Janicak et al. 1993, pp. 148–153.

▌ Use in Special Populations

Table 2–19.   Antipsychotics in special populations

Special population	Concerns/recommendations
Children/ young adolescents	Few controlled studies of APs in prepubertal children; haloperidol and loxapine appear superior to placebo in adolescent schizophrenic patients; children, adolescents seem more refractory than adults; are more likely to develop sedation, perhaps earlier TD; acute dystonias may be more common in younger males; laryngeal dystonias especially dangerous; reduction of dose more effective than anticholinergics for EPS in children; children may develop greater hypotensive effects than adults before becoming clinically symptomatic—monitor blood pressure closely during initial titration; children metabolize APs more rapidly than adults (lower plasma level at same dose) but also require lower plasma levels for efficacy; age, weight, severity of symptoms do not provide clear dosage guidelines; recommended dose for haloperidol in children is 0.5–16 mg/day, but initial dose should be very low, with no more than twice-weekly increments; divided doses useful initially, with eventual conversion to mostly at bedtime; monitor closely for "behavioral toxicity" (apathy, cognitive dulling, sedation); older adolescents may require dosage similar to that for adults

Elderly patients Concomitant medical problems, numerous psychiatric and nonpsychiatric drugs increase risk for adverse reactions, drug-drug interactions; elderly have increased sensitivity to anticholinergic properties of APs, may develop confusion, memory impairment, hallucinations; postural hypotension may be problem with low-potency APs, clozapine; also quinidine-like properties of low-potency agents may exacerbate conduction abnormalities; some older patients may develop higher plasma AP levels than younger patients; low-potency APs generally not as well tolerated overall as higher-potency APs (haloperidol, fluphenazine), but high-potency agents have higher risk of EPS; haloperidol in range of 0.25–1.5 mg qd to qid is usual range for psychosis in elderly, although some will require higher doses (dementia patients with psychosis usually respond at lower doses); TD may develop more rapidly and at lower AP doses than in younger patients; "start low, go slow" with dosage; monitor blood pressure, vital signs closely; watch for signs of confusion, dizziness, fever, rigidity (risk of NMS); attempt non-AP treatment of "agitation," if possible (e.g., trazodone, buspirone); use low initial doses of clozapine, risperidone in elderly, dementia patients (6.25 mg qd clozapine or 0.5 mg qd risperidone initially)

(continued)

Table 2–19.   Antipsychotics in special populations (*continued*)

Special population	Concerns/recommendations
Developmentally disabled (mentally retarded) and autistic patients	Autism differs from MR in showing qualitative developmental deviations, not just delays and decreased IQ; several studies have shown that haloperidol, trifluoperazine, pimozide lead to improved behavior in autistic children (e.g., reduced stereotypy, withdrawal, hyperactivity, without cognitive impairment); haloperidol may improve language acquisition when combined with behavioral interventions; avoid highly sedating APs in this population; reassess periodically to see if AP necessary or if causing TD; for patients with MR and schizophrenia, APs are just as effective as they are among patients without MR; use of APs for self-injurious behavior, stereotypies in populations with MR have not been well validated, although some studies suggest mixed D_1/D_2 antagonists useful (?clozapine); better results may be obtained for self-injurious behavior by using serotonergic agents, especially given risks of akathisia, TD, cognitive impairment with APs

Pregnant patients

Risks of untreated psychosis (e.g., command auditory hallucinations to "stab the baby") must be weighed against the relatively rare teratogenic effects of these medications; several studies have shown no increase in fetal malformations after first-trimester exposure to APs, although some have found increases in nonspecific congenital defects after exposure to phenothiazines; APs also can cause anticholinergic side effects in the fetus (constipation, intestinal obstruction, urinary retention) and may increase the risk of jaundice in premature infants; mild, transient syndrome of neonatal hypertonia, tremor, and poor motor maturity can be seen after neuroleptic use in late pregnancy; little evidence of "behavioral toxicity" or impaired IQ in infants born to mothers taking APs during pregnancy; some data suggest haloperidol or piperazine-type agents less teratogenic than aliphatic phenothiazines; fetal tachyarrhythmias may be more likely with maternal use of low-potency (hence, more anticholinergic) APs; to prevent fetal sedation and muscle spasms/tremor, consider tapering off AP a week or two in advance of expected delivery date; because APs are variably excreted in breast milk, breast-feeding is best avoided if mother remains on an AP

Note.   APs = antipsychotics; TD = tardive dyskinesia; EPS = extrapyramidal symptoms; NMS = neuroleptic malignant syndrome; MR = mental retardation; ? = data preliminary.
Sources.   Data from Dulcan et al. 1995; Janicak et al. 1993; McElhatton 1992; Pies and Popli 1995; Salzman et al. 1995; Stowe and Nemeroff 1995.

Questions and Answers

▌ Drug Class

Q. When is it appropriate to use *intravenous* (IV) APs?

A. IV haloperidol has been used safely and effectively in the management of agitated, delirious patients in critical care settings (Janicak et al. 1993) (e.g., a delirious patient in the coronary care unit, who is tearing out his IV lines, says he is "in the wrong hotel room," and appears to be hallucinating). For many such patients, higher-than-usual doses of IV haloperidol may be necessary, with hourly doses of 10 mg IV necessary in severe cases (Adams 1988). Supplemental use of IV lorazepam (in combination with haloperidol) may be effective and may result in lower doses of haloperidol. A typical regimen might begin with 5 mg haloperidol, followed immediately by 0.5 mg lorazepam. If there is no response to the first injection, an additional 10 mg haloperidol and 4 mg lorazepam may be given every 30–60 minutes, until the patient is adequately sedated. In most cases, less than 100 mg/day haloperidol is required. The related compound, *droperidol,* also has been used in the treatment of agitated, delirious patients but has produced troublesome hypotension in doses of 10- to 20-mg boluses (Adams 1988). Keep in mind that delirium is a medical emergency that requires diagnosis and treatment of the underlying condition.

Q. What are the conversion formulas for switching a patient from oral to depot neuroleptics?

A. There are no foolproof "formulas" for such conversions because the clinical goal is always to use the lowest-effective maintenance dose for the specific patient. This dose may vary with his or her tolerance of the medication, hepatic metabolism, and pharmacodynamic response at the level of the neuron. However, there are some rules of thumb and rough conversion for use of fluphenazine and haloperidol decanoate. For most chronic schizophrenic patients maintained on a daily *oral* dose of fluphenazine 10–15 mg/day, an appropriate dose of the *decanoate* would be about *25 mg every 2–3 weeks* (Kaplan et al. 1994). The custom of biweekly injections is probably unnecessary in many cases, given the long $t^1\!/_2$ of fluphenazine decanoate. Some data suggest that a plasma level of 1.0–2.8 ng/mL is optimal for patients maintained on fluphenazine decanoate (Janicak et al. 1993); however, many commercial laboratories do not use assays with sufficient sensitivity to measure fluphenazine levels less than 2 ng/mL.

For conversion from oral haloperidol to the *monthly* decanoate dose, the general rule is to multiply the daily oral dose by a factor of 10–20 (e.g., a patient receiving 10 mg oral haloperidol daily may require around 150 mg monthly of the decanoate). Elderly patients and *those prone to significant EPS* may do better taking lower doses (Freudenreich and McEvoy 1995), whereas some severely ill patients may require up to 300 mg per month. Although the package insert for haloperidol decanoate cites data showing that 200 mg/month provides the most consistent relapse prevention, the relapse rates for maintenance on 200 mg/month versus 50 or 100 mg/month differ by only 8%–10%. Although this difference is quite important from an epidemiological perspective, it still suggests that the lower dose range for haloperidol decanoate may be more appropriate, at least initially, for some patients (Freudenreich and McEvoy 1995). The rate of EPS actually seems to be less with the decanoate form of haloperidol than with oral dosing (Janicak et al. 1993), although this may reflect use of lower decanoate doses than equivalent oral dose (D. Osser, personal communication, December 1996).

■ Indications

Q. What is the role of APs in the management of acute mania?

A. APs are often used as an adjunct to lithium in the early stages of acute mania, before achieving therapeutic blood levels of lithium. Some clinicians continue the AP, even after lithium has reached therapeutic levels, to reduce psycho-motor agitation and grandiose delusions. Results of five controlled studies comparing lithium to APs in acute mania suggest that lithium is superior (89% versus 54% response, respectively), although other studies do show some benefit for APs (Janicak et al. 1993). APs may be preferable to lithium in *schizoaffective disorder*, given their faster onset and broader spectrum of activity, although this condition is undoubtedly quite heterogeneous. Recently, clozapine has proved effective in managing dysphoric mania (Suppes et al. 1992), although the risk of agranulocytosis must be borne in mind. Conventional APs have a relatively greater risk of inducing TD in patients with affective disorders and should be used with caution for long-term management of bipolar disorders. It appears that *low-to-moderate* doses of APs are sufficient to control patients who have acute mania with psychotic features and that adverse effects may be minimized with this strategy (Janicak et al. 1993).

Q. Are there any significant risks in *maintaining* bipolar patients on AP medications (along with a mood stabilizer) if they have shown psychotic features in previous manic or depressive episodes?

A. Conventional APs have roughly double the risk of inducing TD in patients with affective disorders (versus nonaffective populations) and should be used with caution for long-term management of bipolar disorders. Moreover, some data suggest that although a patient taking an AP along with lithium has a much smaller chance of having a manic episode, there appears to be a much *greater* chance that the patient will become *depressed* (Gelenberg 1995a).

Q. What is the role of lithium in the management of psychosis?

A. The answer may depend on the nature of the psychotic disturbance. Hirschowitz et al. (1980) found that patients with DSM-III (American Psychiatric Association 1980) *schizophreniform disorder* and those with so-called *good prognosis schizophrenia* (essentially, those with significant recovery from previous psychotic episodes) tend to be lithium responsive. These authors hypothesized that such patients may have "lithium-responsive affective disorders masquerading phenomenologically as schizophrenic-like illnesses" (p. 919). Recently, Schexnayder et al. (1995) examined a group of 66 psychotic patients treated with lithium alone. Lithium responders showed *fewer negative symptoms* of schizophrenia (apathy, withdrawal) and *lacked a family history of "schizophrenic spectrum" disorders*—defined as schizophrenia, schizoaffective disorder, schizophreniform disorder, and schizotypal personality disorder. (*Note:* The study by Hirschowitz et al. (1980) focused on schizophreniform disorder but did not include it with these other schizophrenic spectrum disorders.) (The response of psychosis to lithium is discussed more fully in Chapter 4.)

Q. Is it helpful to use APs in the treatment of personality disorders?

A. In general, the pharmacological approach to personality disorders should focus on specific target symptoms and comorbid Axis I disorders (Cowdry 1987; Pies 1994b). Thus, some patients with BPD who show mild thought process disorder or paranoid thinking may benefit from a trial on low-dose AP medication (e.g., 2 mg/day of thiothixene [Navane]). Early work by Soloff et al. (1986) suggested that BPD patients show a "broad spectrum" response to haloperidol (i.e., they had positive effects on anxiety, hostility, depression, and schizotypal symptoms). However, long-term (16-week) placebo-controlled data on BPD suggest little benefit from haloperidol in doses up to 6 mg/day, except on measures of irritability (Cornelius et al. 1993). Preliminary data suggest that clozapine may improve some aspects of function in BPD, based on a study of 15 BPD patients with atypical psychotic symptoms and utilizing the Brief Psychiatric Rating Scale (BPRS; Overall and Gorham 1962) and the Global Assessment Scale (GAS; Spitzer et al. 1973) (Frankenburg and Zanarini 1993). Given the risk of agranulocytosis with clozapine, use of this agent for BPD would clearly require a careful risk-benefit discussion. With respect to other personality disorders, there is modest (and mainly anecdotal) evidence that APs may be helpful in some patients with paranoid and schizotypal personality disorders (Ellison and Adler 1990; Goldberg et al. 1986). Keep in mind that some patients with paranoid personality disorder may become more distressed when they feel they are being "experimented on" with medication.

Q. Is it appropriate to treat dementia with APs, and if so, what is the appropriate agent and dose?

A. In general, APs should be used sparingly and conservatively in patients with dementia, particularly when psychosis per se is not the target symptom. APs may have a modest beneficial effect in reducing agitation (a term in need of differential diagnosis), insomnia, irritability, and hostility in patients with dementia, but consequent confusion and motoric side effects (e.g., akathisia, parkinsonism, high incidence of

TD) frequently outweigh their marginal benefits (Dubovsky 1994). On the other hand, APs *should not be withheld in cases of dementia complicated by secondary hallucinations and delusions* (e.g., in Alzheimer's disease or multi-infarct dementia). High-potency APs, such as haloperidol 0.25–2 mg/day, may be effective in such cases. Highly anticholinergic APs (thioridazine, chlorpromazine) may exacerbate Alzheimer's disease symptoms because this disorder already entails decreased brain acetylcholine. Risperidone is generally safe in older populations but has not been systematically tested in patients with *dementia*. Risperidone may provoke hypotension in the elderly and should be started at lower-than-recommended doses (e.g., 0.5 mg/day, with slow titration up to 2–3 mg/day). Recent uncontrolled data (Jeanblanc and Davis 1995) suggest that risperidone in doses of 1.5–2.5 mg/day can be helpful in aggressive patients with dementia with psychotic features. (I am aware of unpublished, anecdotal data implicating risperidone in several incidents of apparent cardiovascular collapse or severe arrhythmias. In two of the three cases reported, risperidone was used concomitantly with SSRIs that *inhibit metabolism in the CYP2D6 pathway.* These concerns await large-scale, controlled studies for confirmation but should foster the use of low doses and careful monitoring in elderly patients taking risperidone.) Clozapine appears to be generally safe and effective—when used in very low doses—in psychotic Parkinson's disease patients with levodopa-induced hallucinations; doses in the range of 12.5–50 mg hs are often used (Koller and Megaffin 1994). In many cases, agitated, aggressive patients with dementia are better treated with trazodone, an SSRI, a β-blocker, buspirone, or divalproex than with an AP (Dubovsky 1994).

Q. Since clozapine was first marketed, the indications seem to be broadening. In what situations would clozapine be the AP of *first choice?*

A. Physicians' Desk Reference (PDR) 1996 states that Clozaril is indicated "for the management of severely ill schizophrenic patients who fail to respond adequately to standard antipsychotic drug treatment . . . either because of insufficient effectiveness or the inability to achieve an effective dose due to intolerable adverse effects from those drugs" (p. 2252). The product labeling information also states that clozapine should be used "only in patients who have failed to respond adequately to treatment with appropriate *courses* of standard antipsychotic drugs" (p. 2252, italics added), with *courses* generally interpreted to mean "two or more." Although clinicians are *not* prohibited by law from going outside Food and Drug Administration (FDA)-approved labeling information, the clinician who does so assumes a burden of medicolegal justification. Thus, using the PDR criteria, clozapine would *never* be the first AP prescribed for a psychotic patient. However, Green and Schildkraut (1995) have hypothesized, based on indirect data, that initial treatment with clozapine may improve long-term outcome in first-episode schizophrenia, perhaps by averting the tolerance that seems to develop when patients are treated with standard neuroleptics. These authors have hypothesized, for example, that attenuated response to haloperidol is associated with postsynaptic D_2 supersensitivity after chronic blockade of these receptors. Clozapine has a relatively weak blocking action at D_2 receptors and does not seem to lose its efficacy over time. Green and Schildkraut (1995) are now performing a double-blind clinical trial of clozapine in first-episode schizophrenic patients. All this, of course, does not provide immediate justification for using clozapine as a first-line AP, given the risk of agranulocytosis; however, it paves the way for less-restrictive use of clozapine. For example, some clinicians would move quickly to clozapine if a patient has had 1) continued, severe positive or negative symptoms of schizophrenia after adequate trial on even a single standard neuroleptic, 2) *severe* EPS with conventional neuroleptics and/or risperidone (remember, risperidone tends to lose its atypical qualities and provoke some EPS in doses greater than 6 mg/day, which are sometimes necessary to achieve good control of psychosis), or 3) NMS and *must* be maintained on an AP. Thus far, NMS seems to be quite rare with clozapine, although at least four cases have been reported (Janicak et al. 1993). Keep in mind that 10%–15% of clozapine-treated patients may develop transient hyperthermia (rarely above 104°F) without the other features of NMS (Janicak et al. 1993). Finally, although olanzapine is by no means a "substitute" for clozapine, most clinicians would favor a trial of olanzapine before moving to clozapine.

Q. Is clozapine useful in psychotic patients with polydipsia and intermittent hyponatremia?

A. Several studies have found a corrective effect of clozapine on polydipsia and hyponatremia (Lee et al. 1991; Spears et al. 1996). Several possible mechanisms have been suggested, including moderate D_1 receptor blockade, α_1 blockade, or effects on angiotensin II sensitivity (Spears et al. 1996).

Q. What factors allow us to predict a patient's response to clozapine (Clozaril), and how soon after initiating treatment with clozapine can one identify responders or nonresponders?

A. This is a fairly straightforward question with no straightforward answers. Honer et al. (1995) studied 61 consecutively admitted refractory schizophrenic patients treated with clozapine in an open-design study. Overall, 31% of the patients were classified as responders by week 32 of treatment, based on Global Assessment of Functioning (GAF; American Psychiatric Association 1994) and Clinical Global Impression (CGI; Guy 1976) Scale scores. This figure is somewhat less than that seen by some European investigators (interestingly, effective doses of clozapine also seem to be lower in Europe than in the United States). The investigators found "few clinical features which differed between the 19 responders and the 42 nonresponders" (Honer et al. 1995, p. 209). Age, sex, substance abuse history, mean GAF or CGI scores, age at first admission, and subtype of schizophrenia (paranoid, undifferentiated, or disorganized) all *failed* to predict response. The best predictor of response was a *history of relatively good function at some time in the previous year*. Around 77% of patients continued to have a GAF score of 40 or less, indicating "persistent psychosis and/or major impairment in multiple areas of functioning." Given the risk of agranulocytosis, it would be helpful to have a screening tool that would permit us to avoid fruitless and potentially dangerous trials on clozapine medication. Some earlier data have indicated that shorter duration of illness, female gender, and younger age are significant predictors of a more favorable response to clozapine (Meltzer 1995); these factors were not confirmed in the study by Honer et al. (1995). Work by Lieberman et al. (1994) also suggests that good response to clozapine is predicted by 1) presence of EPS during treatment with a classic neuroleptic and 2) a subtype of paranoid schizophrenia. *Clozapine plasma levels* may be (retrospectively) related to response, with levels below 350 ng/mL correlated with a less-robust response. Because plasma levels were not obtained in this study, it is impossible to know whether these would have predicted eventual outcome. *Weight gain* while taking clozapine also may predict good response (Meltzer 1996), although it is also a factor in noncompliance. Whereas some data suggest that 6–12 months are necessary to identify clozapine responders, Honer et al. (1995) found that by 4 months, it was clear which patients were ultimately going to respond to clozapine. Of some theoretical interest is the finding by Meltzer (1996) that increased *prefrontal cortical sulcal widening* is related to *poor* response to clozapine, consistent with other data bearing on neuroleptic response in patients with underlying structural brain abnormalities.

Q. Can risperidone be used in the treatment of psychosis in patients with Parkinson's disease?

A. There are conflicting data on the benefits of risperidone in psychotic patients with Parkinson's disease or Lewy body dementia (Gelenberg 1995b). It appears that doses up to about 1 mg/day may improve psychosis without worsening EPS; doses above 1 mg/day may worsen EPS and necessitate switching to clozapine.

Q. What is the role of APs in the treatment of OCD?

A. The addition of low-dose dopamine receptor antagonists, such as haloperidol or pimozide, has been found useful in up to 65% of SSRI-resistant OCD patients, particularly those with chronic tic disorder or schizotypal features (McDougle et al. 1990). In a recent study, risperidone at a dose of 1 mg/day was added to ongoing fluvoxamine therapy (250–300 mg/day) in three OCD patients who had been refractory to the SSRI after 12 weeks. All three patients showed significant improvement in their OCD symptoms (McDougle et al. 1995). Another study found that the addition of risperidone to ongoing fluoxetine treatment led to improvement in a patient with sexual obsessions (Bourgeois and Klein 1996). There is at least one case showing clozapine was useful in a patient with extremely refractory OCD after failure of SSRIs and capsulotomy (Young et al. 1994). However, other studies have suggested that clozapine (and perhaps risperidone)—possibly via antagonism of the D_2 receptor—may *worsen* obsessive-compulsive symptoms in some psychotic patients (Baker et al. 1992). Moreover, the risk of TD and drug-drug interactions must be borne in mind if classic APs are used in the treatment of OCD.

Q. Are APs effective in the treatment of delusional disorder?

A. Delusional disorder—in which a "nonbizarre" delusion has been present for at least 1 month and is not the product of schizophrenia—has not been systematically studied with respect to AP use. Anecdotal data suggest that APs are useful, although perhaps not as effective as in the treatment of schizophrenia (Shader 1994b). The AP pimozide seems to be especially useful in treating the somatic type of delusional disorder, which has affinities with both body dysmorphic disorder and so-called monosymptomatic hypochondriasis (Phillips 1991; Shader 1994b). Anecdotal reports also suggest that SSRIs may be beneficial in delusional disorder, raising the question of whether some patients with this condition may fall along the obsessive-compulsive spectrum. Low doses of risperidone and clozapine also have been found useful in delusional disorder, but again, this finding is based on anecdotal information (Manschreck 1996).

▌ Mechanisms of Action

Q. What is the expected lag time for onset of therapeutic effect, in light of the mechanism of action of APs?

A. Several studies suggest that APs usually require between 2 and 4 weeks for significant effects on core positive and negative features of schizophrenia; negative symptoms (apathy, withdrawal) may lag behind positive symptoms in response to conventional APs such as fluphenazine (Breier et al. 1987). Earlier attempts at using high-loading doses of APs (e.g., more than 40 mg/day haloperidol or the equivalent) to manage acute exacerbations of schizophrenia—so-called rapid neuroleptization—have failed to show superiority to lower-dose strategies of 10–20 mg/day haloperidol, often in combination with a benzodiazepine (Tueth et al. 1995). It is not clear that such acute AP/benzodiazepine effects are mediated through the same mechanism of action as is long-term amelioration of core psychotic symptoms. Although acute blockade of nigrostriatal D_2 receptors by APs may account for *acute dystonic reactions,* it is not clear that the sedative effect of acutely administered APs represents much more than a non-specific action common to other sedative agents. Presumably, blockade of mesolimbic dopamine receptors is merely the first step in a chain of intracellular events resulting in altered gene expression, such as increased messenger RNA coding for various dopamine receptors (Chin et al. 1995). Such long-term alterations correspond more closely to the time course of APs' clinical efficacy than does acute D_2 receptor blockade per se.

Q. How do the receptor profiles for classic neuroleptics differ from the new, atypical agents, such as clozapine and olanzapine?

A. Because most APs affect numerous receptors (see Tables 2–5 and 2–6), only a general response to this question is possible. Classical neuroleptics (such as haloperidol) seem to exert their AP effects primarily via antagonism of the D_2 receptor. Newer agents, such as clozapine, are more effective in blocking the 5-HT_2 receptor than the D_2 receptor, and this high ratio of 5-HT_2 to D_2 may confer atypical properties on these agents. Thus, atypical agents seem to be more effective for negative symptoms in schizophrenia, produce fewer EPS, raise serum prolactin only minimally, and may be less likely to promote TD (Jibson and Tandon 1996). An agent such as olanzapine may be characterized in terms of its receptor affinities as a D_1, D_2, D_3, D_4, 5-HT_2, 5-HT_3, and 5-HT_6 antagonist—not to mention its antagonism of α_1-adrenergic, muscarinic, and histaminic receptors (Jibson and Tandon 1996). These multiple receptor effects make for complicated pharmacodynamic effects, as well as some side effects (see Tables 2–9 and 2–10). Clozapine's unique pharmacodynamic profile may be closely related to its antagonism of the D_4 receptor (Seeman 1992). Risperidone, sertindole, and ziprasidone are more narrowly "focused," antagonizing mainly 5-HT$_2$ and D$_2$ receptors (Keck and McElroy 1997).

▌Pharmacokinetics

Q. Because many APs have elimination $t\frac{1}{2}$s of 24 hours or so, is *once-daily* oral dosing optimal?

A. In theory, once-daily dosing (e.g., all at bedtime) should provide sustained therapeutic blood levels (e.g., 4–15 ng/mL haloperidol) for most patients once steady state has been reached. It is not clear in the first place, however, that there is a close correlation between AP blood levels *on a given day* and therapeutic central nervous system (CNS) effects. Indeed, it is likely that the pharmacokinetics of APs in the plasma may not accurately reflect their action at brain receptor sites (A. Campbell and Baldessarini 1985), meaning that *transiently* low plasma levels (e.g., over the course of 1–2 days) do not necessarily lead to worsening of psychotic symptoms for the average patient. Thus, it is difficult to rationalize multiple dosing (two or three times daily) of APs on the basis of either pharmacokinetics or pharmacodynamics. However, the *acute side effects* of APs in some patients may be correlated with once-daily dosing and/or transient increases in peak plasma levels. Thus, an elderly patient with a tendency toward postural hypotension might develop dizziness (due to peripheral α blockade) if given 300 mg chlorpromazine *in a single dose,* versus as 100 mg qd and 200 mg hs. (Incidentally, chlorpromazine would *not* be the agent of choice in such a patient.) Alternatively, a young male patient might develop an acute dystonic reaction if, on the first day of treatment, he were given 15 mg haloperidol in a single dose versus 5 mg qd and 10 mg hs (in this case, prophylactic anticholinergic medication, or a less potent agent, would probably be indicated).

These variable effects probably relate to the *higher peak plasma levels* obtained when dosing is less frequent, even though—at steady state—the *average* plasma concentration over a 24-hour period is the same, whether the medication is given once, twice, or three times daily (Friedman and Greenblatt 1986). In short, APs may generally be given once daily, but individual differences in side effects may sometimes favor multiple dosing.

Q. What is the relationship between clozapine dose and effective therapeutic blood levels?

A. There is great variability in the ratio of plasma level to dose of orally administered clozapine; clozapine levels may vary more than 45-fold on the same oral dose (which is probably also true for most of the phenothiazines). Factors underlying such variability may include dosing schedule, timing of blood drawing, and individual differences in absorption and metabolism of clozapine (Lindenmayer and Apergi 1996). The review of clozapine levels by Lindenmayer and Apergi (1996) concluded that, for the vast majority of patients, the target blood level may be around 250 ng/mL; however, nonresponders at that level probably warrant a dosage increase to achieve levels of 420–450 ng/mL. Of course, side effects (including sedation and perhaps electroencephalogram [EEG] slowing) are usually greater at such higher levels (McEvoy et al. 1996). Lindenmayer and Apergi (1996) give 500 mg/day as the estimated optimal mean clozapine dose for most patients, assuming an optimal plasma level between 250 and 420 ng/mL. Similar, although not identical, conclusions were reached by VanderZwaag et al. (1996), who studied 56 schizophrenic inpatients randomly assigned to clozapine at one of three serum level ranges. They found superior efficacy for the 200–300 ng/mL and 350–450 ng/mL ranges over the 50–150 ng/mL range; however, there was no advantage seen for the 350–450 ng/mL range over the

200–300 ng/mL range. They found that an average dose of 373 mg/day was needed to keep a patient in the "middle" range of clozapine levels. During the first 6 weeks of treatment, sleepiness was more common in groups with higher serum levels, and the authors suggest that clozapine levels above 350 ng/mL may bring an unnecessary burden of side effects.

▌ Main Side Effects

Q. Should anticholinergic agents be given prophylactically with APs to prevent extrapyramidal side effects?

A. The answer depends on the type of AP, the characteristics of the patient, the risks of using such anticholinergic agents, and the time course of treatment. In general, the prophylactic use of anticholinergic agents for patients taking *low-potency* APs (thioridazine, chlorpromazine) or *clozapine* is of dubious value. Most such patients will not develop acute extrapyramidal side effects, and the addition of benztropine or similar agents will add to the total "anticholinergic burden" carried by the patient, sometimes leading to severe side effects (e.g., dry mouth, dental caries, blurry vision, constipation/bowel obstruction, and confusional states). These side effects occur especially in elderly patients, who are often given several anticholinergic agents along with a low-potency AP. On the other hand, a young male patient starting to take haloperidol may well benefit from a prophylactic anticholinergic; indeed, an acute dystonic reaction in such a case may lead to refusal of further medication for fear of "being poisoned." (Some clinicians, however, prefer to begin such patients on relatively low doses of haloperidol—about 2–4 mg/day—and monitor closely for the earliest signs of extrapyramidal side effects, often avoiding use of anticholinergic agents. See, for example, Osser and Patterson 1996a.) Although the data from various studies are fraught with methodological difficulties, about 40% (10%–70%) of patients whose anticholinergics are discontinued *will* subsequently exhibit extrapyramidal side effects, suggesting that these agents *do* have prophylactic effects (Janicak et al. 1993). Nevertheless, because most acute dystonias occur within the first few days or weeks of treatment, many patients chronically maintained on APs may be weaned from their anticholinergics after a few months (Janicak et al. 1993). A certain percentage of these patients may redevelop dystonic symptoms; show low-grade but uncomfortable parkinsonian symptoms, such as mild cogwheeling or rigidity; or develop akathisia. These patients should have their anticholinergics resumed or be considered for trial of an atypical or low-potency AP. (Akathisia may best be treated with a β-blocker such as propranolol.) Patients taking risperidone in doses of 4–6 mg/day, and clozapine, generally have low rates of extrapyramidal side effects. *Risk factors* for developing acute extrapyramidal side effects also enter into the issue of maintaining anticholinergic treatment for patients (e.g., male gender, age younger than 35 years, history of previous dystonic reaction [Stanilla and Simpson 1995]).

Q. Do anticholinergic agents interfere with the therapeutic effects of APs?

A. Some studies have found that anticholinergics may reduce plasma AP levels, but others have not confirmed this finding (Leipzig and Mendelowitz 1992). Other data indicate that for some patients anticholinergics may exacerbate some positive symptoms of schizophrenia (e.g., hallucinations) or produce other behavioral toxicity (Janicak et al. 1993). On the other hand, anticholinergic agents have been reported to improve some negative features of schizophrenia. It is often difficult to distinguish such negative or "deficit" symptoms from parkinsonian side effects and/or depression. The best strategy is to *prevent* the occurrence of extrapyramidal side effects and negative features in the first place by using low doses of classic APs whenever feasible or by using APs with atypical properties.

Q. Is akathisia an extrapyramidal side effect in the same sense that acute dystonic reactions and parkinsonian symptoms are considered extrapyramidal side effects? What is the best treatment for akathisia?

A. Akathisia is usually defined as motor restlessness accompanied by an urge to move, not explained solely by anxiety, psychosis, or mood disorder (Ovsiew 1992). Typically, the patient demonstrates a marching-in-place phenomenon or, if seated, shuffles or taps his or her feet. Neuroleptic-induced akathisia—which may occur in about 20% of neuroleptic-treated patients (Shader 1994a)—has been linked with higher levels of anxiety, depression, violence, and suicide in schizophrenic patients (Csernansky and Newcomer 1995). One study found that the presence of akathisia appears to predict poor response to fluphenazine (Levinson et al. 1990). However, another study found no correlation between akathisia and higher levels of psychotic symptoms during acute haloperidol treatment of inpatients with schizophrenia (Van Putten et al. 1990a). It is possible that common central neurotransmitter mechanisms underlie both akathisia and poor treatment response to APs (Levinson et al. 1990).

Marsden and Jenner (1980) have suggested that akathisia may be due to *mesocortical* rather than *nigrostriatal* dopamine receptor blockade (unlike "ordinary" extrapyramidal side effects). Several positron emission tomography studies taken together suggest that akathisia occurs at around 60%–65% of D_2 receptor blockade, antipsychotic action occurs at 65%–75% of D_2 receptor blockade, and *extrapyramidal parkinsonian signs* occur at about 90% of D_2 receptor blockade (Farde et al. 1988; Seeman 1995). These findings would suggest merely a quantitative difference in the pathophysiology of ordinary extrapyramidal side effects (such as tremor) and akathisia. (They also imply that akathisia may appear at lower AP doses than needed to produce classic parkinsonian side effects.) However, the pathophysiology of akathisia is not well understood. The effectiveness of β-blockers in treating this condition (Shader 1994a) suggests that *noradrenergic mechanisms* are involved. However, some studies have *not* shown β-blockers to be superior to anticholinergics (e.g., Sachdev and Loneragan 1993), and the agent of choice for akathisia remains somewhat controversial. If a β-blocker is elected, propranolol 20–80 mg/day may be more effective than less-lipophilic agents such as nadolol, but double-blind studies are lacking. Anticholinergic agents or benzodiazepines (e.g., lorazepam 0.5–2.0 mg/day) may be effective in some patients (Shader 1994a).

Q. What are the common sexual side effects seen with APs, and which agents are most likely to cause these?

A. Drug-induced sexual dysfunction can include decreased libido; impaired erectile capacity; delayed, painful, retrograde, or "anhedonic" ejaculation (without orgasm); partial or complete anorgasmia; priapism (painful, prolonged erection); and various neuroendocrine side effects that affect sexuality indirectly (Segraves 1992). Although these side effects are commonly associated with antidepressant use (see Chapter 1), APs may cause ejaculatory disturbance, erectile dysfunction, and priapism. Thioridazine (Mellaril) is probably the most common offending agent, usually causing impaired/retrograde ejaculation in one-third or more of male patients. Decreased libido also has been reported with thioridazine and fluphenazine. Medications causing α-adrenergic blockade are most often implicated in priapism, which must be considered a *urological emergency;* failure to treat this problem promptly may result in permanent penile damage (Thompson et al. 1990). Among the phenothiazines, chlorpromazine and thioridazine seem to account for most of the reported cases of priapism, whereas haloperidol, molindone, and other high-potency agents (with relatively less α-blockade) are less frequently implicated. Priapism has been reported with both risperidone and clozapine (Emes and Millson 1994). All classic APs—as well as the quasi-atypical agent, risperidone—elevate prolactin levels, which may lead to amenorrhea, galactorrhea, or gynecomastia and impotence in males. Clozapine does not provoke hyperprolactinemia (Meltzer 1995).

Q. What are the most common side effects with clozapine, and how are they best managed? What about clozapine-induced enuresis and hypersalivation?

A. Clozapine, although effective in carefully selected patients, is not a user-friendly medication. It produces a rather high incidence of (usually) manageable side effects, including sedation (40% incidence), hypersalivation (31%), tachycardia (more than 25%), dizziness (20%), constipation (14%), hypotension (9%), and hypertension (9%). Seizures occur in a dose-related fashion with clozapine, with a rate of about 3% at 300 mg/day and 6% at 600 mg/day (Meltzer 1995). Less-common side effects include transient benign temperature elevations, nausea, weight gain, enuresis, and leukocytosis. NMS has been reported but appears to be less common than with conventional neuroleptics. The elderly and those with underlying brain damage may be more sensitive to clozapine and may experience side effects (and perhaps clinical efficacy) at significantly lower doses. Hypersalivation is occasionally responsive to anticholinergic medication, clonidine, or dosage reduction. There is a strong possibility, however, that hypersalivation is actually a result of *clozapine-impaired swallowing* (esophageal dysfunction) rather than true cholinergically mediated hypersalivation; if true, anticholinergic agents would not be expected to help. Dosage reduction and

patient education (e.g., instruction in swallowing) may reduce complaints (McCarthy and Terkelsen 1994; Pearlman
1994). Enuresis may be managed by reducing the dosage, if
possible; by dividing the daily dose and giving the nighttime
dose early in the evening so that maximum sedation is over
before maximum likelihood of enuresis (C. A. Pearlman, personal communication, February 1997); and by using oxybu-
tynin (Ditropan) or nasal vasopressin (F. Frankenburg, M.D.,
personal communication, February 1997).

Q. What is the risk of agranulocytosis with clozapine, and
are there factors that help predict this risk?

A. Clozapine has an associated incidence of agranulocytosis
of approximately 0.65% (Sandoz Pharmaceuticals Corporation, personal communication, December 1995). The incidence reflects the average rates for women (0.9%) and men
(0.4%). However, many sources cite an incidence of 1%–2%
(e.g., P. F. Buckley and Meltzer 1995), probably reflecting
earlier deficiencies in monitoring. Because this risk is greatest during the first 4–5 months, monitoring every 2 weeks is
practiced in some European countries after the first 6 months
of exposure; in the United States, however, the standard of
care requires weekly monitoring. Agranulocytosis may occur
more frequently in older patients, in females, and possibly in
individuals of Eastern European Jewish extraction, but there
are no well-established clinical predictors as to which patients are most likely to develop agranulocytosis (Meltzer
1995). However, a pattern of *steadily decreasing neutrophil
count* may herald agranulocytosis and calls for extra monitoring (Meltzer 1996). A patient who has developed clozapine-
induced agranulocytosis should not be rechallenged with
this agent.

Q. What is the risk of withdrawal syndromes associated
with stopping AP medication?

A. All APs can produce withdrawal symptoms if suddenly or rapidly discontinued (e.g., insomnia, headache, nausea, vomiting, and withdrawal-emergent dyskinesia). Specific symptoms are related to the potency of the agent, its dopaminergic blockade, and its anticholinergic effects (Hegarty 1996). Low-potency APs, such as chlorpromazine, are strongly anticholinergic, and sudden withdrawal of these agents can provoke diarrhea, drooling, and insomnia ("cholinergic rebound"). Recent case reports specifically point to clozapine withdrawal as leading to rapid psychotic decompensations, evolving over a few days. These appear to be much more rapid than syndromes seen after stopping conventional APs, perhaps as a result of the rapid clearance of clozapine from plasma and/or the CNS (Hegarty 1996). Alternatively, decompensation may be due to overactivity of (previously antagonized) limbic D_4 receptors when clozapine is discontinued and replaced by an AP that is less selective for D_4 antagonism (most classic neuroleptics). Serotonergic effects also may be involved in clozapine-related withdrawal. There is a nearly twofold difference in relapse risk between abrupt and gradual withdrawal of AP agents (Viguera et al. 1997).

Q. What is the side effect profile of risperidone in contrast to that of clozapine?

A. Risperidone tends to be better tolerated than clozapine when used at or near the recommended dose of 4–8 mg/day; however, a few anecdotal reports have noted cardiovascular and CNS side effects (such as syncope and excessive sedation), even at recommended therapeutic doses of risperidone. The most common side effects of risperidone include insomnia, anxiety, agitation, sedation, dizziness, rhinitis, hypotension, weight gain, and menstrual disturbance (Borison et al. 1992). Again, elderly and dementia patients may be more sensitive to risperidone-related side effects, and the recommended initial dosage in these groups is approximately 0.5 mg qd to bid (Jeanblanc and Davis 1995). As suggested earlier in this chapter, the incidence of extrapyramidal side effects with risperidone is dose related and begins to approach that of haloperidol at risperidone doses of approximately 16 mg/day; some patients will show extrapyramidal side effects even at doses of 4 mg/day. Unlike clozapine, risperidone does not produce agranulocytosis; it may be more likely than clozapine to produce amenorrhea. Mania or exacerbation of preexisting manic symptoms has been reported with use of risperidone, perhaps especially (although not exclusively) when a mood stabilizer has *not* been prescribed concomitantly (Dwight et al. 1994). Schaffer and Schaffer (1996), in a small sample of bipolar patients, found that doses of risperidone less than 1 mg/day may be helpful as an adjunctive antimanic agent (e.g., in combination with lithium or valproate) but that higher doses were associated with overstimulation or worsening of hypomania/mania.

Q. What are the signs and symptoms of NMS, and how is NMS managed?

A. NMS is probably not a single, homogeneous disease entity; rather, NMS may represent a continuum of dysfunction related to dopamine receptor blockade and other poorly characterized physiological mechanisms. NMS typically is characterized by the development of fever, muscular rigidity, autonomic instability, altered level of consciousness, elevated creatine phosphokinase (CPK), and elevated white blood cell count (WBC), in the absence of another medical explanation (P. F. Buckley and Meltzer 1995). One or more of these features may be absent, however, in the presence of serious NMS-like syndromes. Although some data indicate that mental alterations may be the earliest indicator of NMS (Velamoor et al. 1995), this may be too nonspecific to permit reliable diagnosis (C. A. Pearlman, personal communication,

February 1997). Although typically associated with the use of neuroleptics or other dopamine receptor blockers, NMS may also occur after sudden discontinuation of dopaminergic agents, such as bromocriptine. NMS has now been reported in association with both risperidone (Webster and Wijeratne 1994) and clozapine (Sachdev et al. 1995). Clozapine-induced NMS may be somewhat atypical in that fewer EPS and lower levels of CPK may be seen. Clozapine-induced NMS must be distinguished from benign, transient clozapine-related fever, often seen in the 2nd week of treatment. Whenever NMS is suspected, the putative offending agent should be held until a workup is completed, including ruling out *infection superimposed on drug-induced EPS* as the cause of apparent NMS. Supportive measures designed to reduce hyperthermia and stabilize vital signs are critical and usually require transfer of the patient to a medical unit or intensive care unit. Although the evidence supporting specific therapeutic agents is only modest, some clinicians will use bromocriptine (30 mg/day) or dantrolene (300 mg/day) (P. F. Buckley and Meltzer 1995). Anticholinergic agents may *worsen* hyperthermia (due to impaired sweating), and benzodiazepines produce inconsistent effects (Pearlman 1986). Refractory cases may respond to ECT (Fink 1996).

Q. What are the risks of rechallenging a patient with a neuroleptic after an episode of NMS?

A. About 30% of patients will have a recurrence of NMS after neuroleptic rechallenge. The risk may be reduced by waiting at least 2 weeks post-NMS before the rechallenge and by using a low-potency neuroleptic (e.g., thioridazine) (Rosebush and Stuart 1989). ECT may be a viable alternative to rechallenge.

Q. How cardiotoxic are the APs, and are there differences among the various agents?

A. The APs as a group are not highly cardiotoxic agents, especially in comparison with the TCAs (Gelenberg 1996). In one study, abnormally long corrected QT_c interval was found in 23% of 143 patients treated with APs, versus 2% in unmedicated control subjects. Neuroleptic doses greater than 2,000 mg/day chlorpromazine equivalents were more than four times as likely as lower doses to prolong the QT_c interval (Gelenberg 1996; Warner et al. 1996). Thioridazine's effects on the heart resemble those of the tricyclics, probably due to both anticholinergic- and quinidine-like effects. A recent study of AP overdoses showed that thioridazine is three to five times more likely than other APs to prolong cardiac conduction (N. A. Buckley et al. 1995). Risperidone and the new atypical agent, sertindole, also can prolong cardiac conduction, perhaps secondary to their α_1-adrenergic blocking properties (Jibson and Tandon 1996). It does not appear, however, that these effects are clinically significant. Recently, a case of apparent fatal risperidone overdose has been reported (Springfield and Bodiford 1996). In general, high-potency APs, such as haloperidol and thiothixene, are safer than alternative agents for patients with cardiac illness. Using any APs along with another agent that prolongs cardiac conduction time (e.g., quinidine, TCA) must be monitored carefully.

Q. What are the side effect profiles and probable risks with the newer atypical antipsychotics sertindole, quetiapine, and ziprasidone?

A. Although experience is limited with these agents, all three seem to be relatively safe and well-tolerated agents. Sertindole (SerLect) may be associated with nasal congestion and decreased ejaculatory volume; the latter does not appear to be associated with impotence or retrograde ejaculation. The FDA has been closely scrutinizing the effects of sertindole on cardiac conduction, since it can prolong the QT_c (corrected QT) interval; however, at this time, the effect is believed to be within the parameters of normal QT interval variations (Abbott Pharmaceuticals, personal communication, August 1997). Thus, sertindole may prolong the QT_c by 14 to 21 milliseconds, with normal variation being between 35 and 75 milliseconds. No ventricular tachyarrhythmias have been reported with sertindole thus far, and it is not clear that sertindole is more likely to prolong the QT interval than some other antipsychotics such as risperidone. Nonetheless, it may be prudent to obtain a pretreatment electrocardiogram when using sertindole, in order to detect individuals with congenitally prolonged QT intervals. Quetiapine (Seroquel) can cause drowsiness, headache, and weight gain, and may also slightly decrease thyroid functions (T_3 and T_4) with no increase in thyroid-stimulating hormone. The clinical importance of this last finding is unclear, however. Ziprasidone (a brand name has not yet been released, to my knowledge) can occasionally cause drowsiness and postural hypotension, and may be somewhat more likely to provoke extrapyramidal side effects than either sertindole or quetiapine. An excellent review of these new agents is provided by Keck and McElroy (1997).

▌ Drug-Drug Interactions

Q. Is it safe to combine APs with TCAs and/or SSRI antidepressants?

A. Antipsychotic-antidepressant combinations are often safe and effective for the treatment of psychotic depression and some cases of schizophrenia (see the following discussion on "Potentiating Maneuvers"); however, pharmacokinetic and pharmacodynamic interactions may pose problems for some patients. In general, TCAs and APs tend to compete for metabolism in one or more cytochrome systems and may mutually raise each other's plasma levels, leading to, for example, increased anticholinergic effects (e.g., in the case of combining amitriptyline and thioridazine), hypotensive effects, or EPS. Fluoxetine and paroxetine are powerful inhibitors of the CYP2D6 system and may elevate plasma levels of many AP agents, including clozapine. Clozapine levels also can be elevated substantially by concomitant use of fluvoxamine, probably via the latter's inhibition of CYP1A2 (Hiemke et al. 1994). Antipsychotic-antidepressant combinations may have several pharmacodynamic interactions. (For example, SSRIs may decrease dopaminergic activity in some brain regions, leading to exacerbation of EPS induced by an AP alone. This effect of SSRIs also may be responsible for the "flattening" of affective or hedonic capacity in some patients.) On the other hand, some serotonergic agents may enhance overall function in chronically psychotic patients, possibly by relieving comorbid depressive or obsessive features (see the following discussion on "Potentiating Maneuvers").

Q. Given potential pharmacokinetic interactions between carbamazepine and some APs, what is the best way to manage coprescription of these agents?

A. Carbamazepine may substantially reduce plasma haloperidol levels (and probably those of other APs), presumably via stimulation of hepatic metabolism; however, the clinical outcome of this interaction shows considerable variability (Ciraulo et al. 1989, 1994). In one study (Arana et al. 1986), seven patients who failed to respond to either haloperidol alone or haloperidol plus lithium were treated with haloperidol plus carbamazepine. Before the addition of carbamazepine, haloperidol levels were around 8.3 ng/mL; after addition of carbamazepine, haloperidol levels dropped to around 3.4 ng/mL, with clinical deterioration seen in at least two of the patients. On the other hand, patients with initial haloperidol levels of 12–14 ng/mL might be expected to tolerate a drop to, for example, 7 ng/mL. In any case, raising the haloperidol dose should overcome this pharmacokinetic problem, but plasma levels should be followed closely. (Remember that carbamazepine also induces its *own* metabolism over time, leading to lower carbamazepine levels at a fixed dose.) Pharmacodynamic interactions also may be seen when carbamazepine is combined with neuroleptics (e.g., lethargy and confusion [Ciraulo et al. 1989]).

Q. What concerns should the clinician have in combining risperidone with other psychotropics?

A. Local experience, based on a few anecdotal reports, has raised concerns about the combination of risperidone with SSRIs that inhibit metabolism of risperidone via the CYP2D6 system (e.g., fluoxetine and paroxetine). Although large-scale studies would be needed to validate these concerns, the clinician should consider using lower-than-usual doses of risperidone when CYP2D6 inhibitors are coprescribed.

▋ Potentiating Maneuvers

Q. Can psychotic patients with obsessive-compulsive features be treated with adjunctive medication?

A. Obsessive-compulsive symptoms may be seen in as many as 25% of schizophrenic patients, who may respond to adjunctive clomipramine (Berman et al. 1995). It appears that doses of clomipramine up to 250 mg/day may be combined safely with *high-potency* neuroleptics (e.g., haloperidol, fluphenazine), without exacerbation of psychotic symptoms and with improvement in obsessive-compulsive symptoms. (Combining this agent with low-potency neuroleptics increases the risk of hypotension and anticholinergic effects.) However, citing evidence that clomipramine may exacerbate psychotic symptoms in some patients, Berman et al. (1995) advised caution in using this strategy in acutely decompensated or manic psychotic patients. Another antiobsessional agent, fluoxetine, has been shown to improve global function in some chronic schizophrenic patients (Goldmann and Janecek 1990).

Q. What is the role of psychotherapy as a potentiating strategy in the treatment of schizophrenia? Does the evidence suggest an additive effect when psychotherapy is combined with medication?

A. A recent review by Csernansky and Newcomer (1995) notes that "there have been relatively few studies where the interaction of psychosocial treatments and drug treatments has been specifically studied [in schizophrenia]" (p. 1273). Nevertheless, McGlashan (1986) has noted, "the individual clinician remains central to any treatment effort [of the schizophrenic patient], if only to coordinate other treatment modalities and provide ongoing evaluation" (p. 108). The fostering of trust and a sense of safety in the patient is, in my experience, critical in the successful pharmacological treatment of patients with schizophrenia and other psychotic disorders. With respect to additive effects, Harnett (1988), after reviewing the available data, cites several studies suggesting that AP medication may act synergistically with psychosocial therapies. Thus, Falloon et al. (1985) demonstrated that for schizophrenic patients on optimal AP medication regimens, "family management" not only was superior to individual therapy in reducing psychotic relapse but was associated with reduced neuroleptic dosage and fewer deficit symptoms of schizophrenia. This approach emphasized the enhancement of problem-solving and communication skills in both the patient and his or her family/caregivers; family management is *not* a psychodynamically based, "exploratory" form of psychotherapy. Although studies of psychotherapy for schizophrenia have many methodological shortcomings, Harnett (1988) concludes that there is little evidence supporting the utility of *individual psychodynamically oriented therapy* in schizophrenia. On the other hand, Liberman et al. (1986) have shown that *social skills training* improves social adjustment and decreases relapse rates in schizophrenia.

Q. Is it useful to add a conventional neuroleptic to clozapine in patients who do not respond to clozapine alone?

A. In theory, the addition of a classic D_2 receptor blocker might interfere with the relatively benign extrapyramidal side effect profile of clozapine (which has a high ratio of 5-HT_2 to D_2 receptor blockade). However, some limited clinical experience suggests that the addition of a conventional neuroleptic (such as haloperidol) to ongoing clozapine therapy may enhance efficacy, particularly in patients who cannot tolerate high doses of clozapine (Goff and Baldessarini 1995). Thus, a patient maintained on 250 mg/day clozapine might benefit from the addition of 1–2 mg haloperidol or thiothixene, without developing significant extrapyramidal side effects. Theoretically, concomitant use of two APs could increase the risk of agranulocytosis, but the increment above that associated with clozapine alone is probably small.

Q. What about combining clozapine and risperidone in patients refractory to one or the other alone?

A. There are only limited data on the use of this combination, but anecdotal reports suggest that it may be useful in refractory patients (Tyson et al. 1995). One patient with schizoaffective illness, treated with a combination of clozapine 300 mg bid and risperidone 1 mg bid, showed an increase in his clozapine plasma levels from 344 ng/mL to 598 ng/mL. However, this was not associated with any adverse events and actually led to an improvement in the patient's illness (Tyson et al. 1995). Nevertheless, the potential for interaction—probably via competition for the CYP2D6 enzyme system—warrants caution because high plasma levels of clozapine may (in theory) be associated with greater risk of seizures or other side effects. In my experience, risperidone may be safely combined with clozapine in extremely refractory psychotic patients who do not respond to either agent alone; however, blood pressure needs to be monitored closely given the risk of additive hypotensive effects, and the doses of risperidone should be kept low (0.5–3 mg/day).

Q. How useful are anticonvulsants as potentiators of APs in patients with schizophrenia?

A. Although anticonvulsants alone rarely benefit schizophrenic patients, they may be of use in persistently psychotic patients who show prominent positive symptoms, aggressive-impulsive behaviors ("episodic dyscontrol"), or EEG abnormalities (P. F. Buckley and Meltzer 1995). Okuma et al. (1989) found that carbamazepine was more effective than placebo (48% versus 30% response, respectively) when added to ongoing neuroleptic treatment of schizophrenic and schizoaffective patients, particularly for symptoms of excitement, suspiciousness, and poor cooperation. However, some patients with psychosis may worsen with the addition of carbamazepine to a neuroleptic, possibly because of carbamazepine's reduction of plasma neuroleptic levels (Arana et al. 1986). In a retrospective study, Hayes (1989) found that 11 of 14 schizoaffective patients improved with valproate; however, some of these patients also had received lithium.

Q. How useful are benzodiazepines in the treatment of schizophrenia?

A. Janicak et al. (1993) summarize the use of benzodiazepines as either sole or adjunctive agents in psychotic patients, with effects ranging "from deterioration, to no change in most patients, to striking improvement in a rare patient" (pp. 152–153). Benzodiazepines may ameliorate superimposed anxiety, auditory hallucinations, and perhaps negative symptoms in a few schizophrenic patients; however, sedation, ataxia, cognitive impairment, and behavioral disinhibition may occur (Janicak et al. 1993). A number of benzodiazepines (lorazepam, clonazepam, diazepam) have proved useful in catatonic patients, including some with catatonic schizophrenia (Martenyi et al. 1989). Generally, these results have been obtained using IM or IV benzodiazepines, although some studies point to continued benefit when the patient is maintained on oral benzodiazepines (Martenyi et al. 1989). (Keep in mind that catatonia is a symptom, not a diagnosis, and that treatment must be directed at the underlying pathology.) Benzodiazepines also may be helpful in the management of acute psychotic states and may reduce the need for higher doses of neuroleptics in agitated psychotic patients (Tueth et al. 1995).

∎ Use in Special Populations

Q. What are the AP agents and doses of choice in treating patients with seizure disorders?

A. Probably all APs decrease seizure threshold (i.e., make seizures more probable) to some degree, with low-potency agents, such as loxapine and clozapine, having greater effects than high-potency agents, such as haloperidol and molindone (Dubovsky 1994). With clozapine, major motor seizures are induced in 1%–2% of patients at doses below 300 mg/day, 2%–4% at doses above 300 mg/day, and 4%–6% at doses above 600 mg/day (Meltzer 1995); these findings contrast with a prevalence of about 0.1% with conventional neuroleptics and risperidone. A history of epilepsy or "organic brain impairment" is a risk factor for AP-induced seizures (P. F. Buckley and Meltzer 1995). Decreasing the clozapine dose and/or adding valproate is usually sufficient to manage seizures in these patients. (It is also important that the patient avoid epileptogenic agents such as caffeine or theophylline in high doses.) With other APs, using the lowest effective dose, and perhaps checking the plasma level, may help reduce the likelihood of seizures. Thus, with haloperidol, one might begin treatment at 4 mg/day and aim for a plasma level of about 5 ng/mL—parameters that are probably applicable to *most* patients being treated with haloperidol.

Q. How dangerous are APs in pregnancy, and what are the APs of choice in this situation?

A. In general, all psychotropic medications should be avoided during at least the first trimester of pregnancy, if possible. However, the risks of untreated psychosis (e.g., command auditory hallucinations to "stab the baby") must be weighed against the relatively rare teratogenic effects of these medications (Stowe and Nemeroff 1995). A number of studies have shown no increase in malformations after first-trimester exposure to APs, although a few have found an increase in nonspecific congenital anomalies after exposure to phenothiazines. APs also can cause anticholinergic side effects in the fetus (constipation, urinary retention) and may increase the risk of jaundice in premature infants. A mild, transient syndrome of neonatal hypertonia, tremor, and poor motor maturity can be seen after neuroleptic use in late pregnancy. There is little evidence of behavioral toxicity or impaired IQ in infants born to mothers taking APs during pregnancy (Stowe and Nemeroff 1995). Some data suggest that haloperidol or *piperazine-type* phenothiazines are less teratogenic than *aliphatic* phenothiazines, whereas other data do not point to such an advantage. Fetal tachyarrhythmias may be more likely with maternal use of low-potency (hence, more anticholinergic) APs. To prevent fetal sedation and muscle spasms/tremors, some clinicians recommend tapering off the AP a week or two in advance of the expected delivery date. Because APs are variably excreted in breast milk, breast-feeding is best avoided if the mother remains on an AP (McElhatton 1992).

Q. What about the risks of clozapine and risperidone in pregnancy and the postpartum period?

A. Little is known about the effects on, or risks to, the developing fetus as a result of maternal exposure to these agents during pregnancy (Altshuler et al. 1996). The manufacturer of risperidone notes that there are no well-controlled studies in pregnant women (Physicians' Desk Reference 1996), although one report of agenesis of the corpus callosum is cited in an infant exposed to risperidone in utero; obviously, causal connections are hard to establish in such cases. It is also not known whether risperidone is excreted in breast milk, although animal studies suggest that it is. With respect to clozapine, data from animal studies suggest that clozapine has a low risk of causing teratogenesis, but no adequate studies in pregnant women have been done as of yet. Waldman and Safferman (1993) note at least 15 cases of normal births following maternal exposure to clozapine, but such numbers are far too small to provide meaningful data. There is evidence (Barnas et al. 1994) that clozapine enters the fetal circulation in significant amounts, both in utero and as a consequence of breast-feeding, leading to sedation and "floppy baby syndrome." The authors suggest that clozapine dosage be kept low in the days that precede delivery. However, as Altshuler et al. (1996) note, there are substantial risks to the mother and baby if the former has a psychotic relapse; thus, in general, there are few good reasons to discontinue or interrupt clozapine treatment during pregnancy.

Q. How do pharmacokinetic and pharmacodynamic factors interact when APs are used in the elderly?

A. In general, the volume of distribution of APs is increased and their metabolism slowed in the elderly. These actions would be expected to yield a longer time to reach steady state, longer time for drug elimination ("washout"), and prolongation of both therapeutic and toxic effects (Dubovsky 1994). In a study of haloperidol pharmacokinetics, Kelly et al. (1993) found no statistically significant differences in younger versus older patients; however, the older subjects (mean age = 72 years) showed significantly greater decreases in *cognitive function* following IV haloperidol administration. This finding suggests important *pharmacodynamic* mechanisms in aging, perhaps involving increased neuronal sensitivity or decreased dopaminergic transmission in the elderly (Dubovsky 1994). On the other hand, a recent study of serum haloperidol levels in older psychotic patients (Lacro et al. 1996) found that the *ratio of haloperidol level to dose* was higher in elderly patients with Alzheimer's disease than in younger subjects with schizophrenia, suggesting a reduction in haloperidol clearance with age. This finding would be consistent with others in studies of perphenazine, thiothixene, and other neuroleptics (Lacro et al. 1996). The elderly are also more sensitive to anticholinergic effects of APs, including central effects (confusion, delirium).

Q. What concerns are paramount when prescribing risperidone or clozapine in the elderly?

A. There has been only limited experience with these two drugs in elderly populations. Although early results are encouraging, special problems may arise in the elderly (Naimark et al. 1995). Thus, the weekly blood drawings with clozapine may lead to bruising or cellulitis from an infected phlebotomy site, and tachycardia, hypotension, and cardiac conduction abnormalities are not uncommon in elderly patients. Clozapine's anticholinergic side effects may cause urinary retention, fecal impaction, exacerbation of narrow-angle glaucoma, and confusional states in the elderly. Respiratory arrest when clozapine is combined with benzodiazepines may be more likely in elderly patients, although data are lacking on this question. Clozapine dosage should start around 6.25 mg/day in the elderly, with increments of 6.25 mg as tolerated every 3–4 days. Although published data are limited, one study (Madhusoodanan et al. 1995) of risperidone in 11 elderly patients (ages 61–79 years) with various types of psychoses showed this agent to be useful. In doses of 0.5–3 mg/day, risperidone reduced both positive and negative symptoms of psychoses and was associated with reduced EPS and TD in four patients. However, two patients with preexisting heart disease had severe dizziness and hypotension. Risperidone may be associated with a greater incidence of EPS in the elderly than in younger patients (Naimark et al. 1995) and can cause significant hypotension even in therapeutic doses. Special care should be taken when elderly patients are coprescribed antihypertensive agents or drugs that inhibit the CYP2D6 system (such as fluoxetine and paroxetine). Dosage of risperidone in the elderly should begin at no higher than 0.5 mg/day and should be increased slowly as tolerated to around 2–3 mg/day. Despite these caveats, accumulating data suggest that low-dose risperidone may be effective in treating behavioral disturbances in dementia patients (C. A. Pearlman, personal communication, February 1997). A recent open-label study also found risperidone generally well tolerated in elderly schizophrenic patients (Berman et al. 1996).

Q. How do APs compare with buspirone in the treatment of agitated dementia patients?

A. A recent double-blind study (Cantillon et al. 1996) compared buspirone 15 mg/day with haloperidol 1.5 mg/day in a population of 26 nursing home residents with Alzheimer's disease and agitation. Physical tension and motor activity de-

creased to a greater extent in buspirone-treated patients. Although this study is preliminary (e.g., no placebo group was
included), the results certainly suggest that in nonpsychotic
dementia patients with motor agitation, buspirone is worth
trying before initiating a trial of an AP. (Patients with psychotic features were excluded from the study by Cantillon et
al [1996].) In some cases, combined use of an AP and buspirone may be warranted in agitated dementia patients.

Q. What special considerations exist when prescribing APs
for children and adolescents?

A. The main indication for using APs in children is childhood schizophrenia. This disorder is now regarded as essentially the same disorder as that which occurs in adults but
with more severe symptoms and a more chronic course
(Nakane and Rapoport 1995). Unfortunately, there are few
well-designed studies of AP use in this younger population.
Using APs in children and adolescents is further complicated
by resistance to medication and both over- and undermedi-
cation (Dulcan et al. 1995). Although children metabolize APs
more rapidly than adults, they also may require lower
plasma levels for efficacy (Dulcan et al. 1995). The usual dose
range of haloperidol in children is about 0.5–16 mg/day
(0.02–0.2 mg/kg/day). Loxapine in doses of 10–200 mg/day
also was found effective in one study of adolescents with
schizophrenia (Pool et al. 1976). Notwithstanding these dosage guidelines, the best advice is to begin with a very low
dose and to increase it gradually—generally no more than
once or twice a week (Janicak et al. 1993). Older adolescents
with schizophrenia may require AP doses comparable to
those of adults, whereas younger adolescents may require
doses that fall between those used for children and those
used for adults. Some data suggest that adolescent boys are
more susceptible to acute dystonic reactions than are older
patients and are less responsive to anticholinergics, such as

benztropine; thus, reducing AP dosage is the preferred strategy (M. Campbell et al. 1985). It is not yet clear which class of AP is safest and most efficacious in children and adolescents. Preliminary data suggest that both clozapine and risperidone may be effective (Frazier et al. 1994; Grcevich et al. 1995; Nakane and Rapoport 1995), but randomized, controlled trials are needed. The average dosage of clozapine used in an open-label study of 11 adolescents with severe, chronic schizophrenia (Frazier et al. 1994) was 370.5 mg/day (by the end of 6 weeks). By week 6 of treatment, there was an overall 58% improvement in the CGI score. Tachycardia and sedation were the main limiting side effects. However, other data (Freedman et al. 1994; Rapoport 1994; Remschmidt et al. 1994) have raised concerns about potential toxicity in adolescents treated with clozapine (e.g., leukopenia without agranulocytosis, electrocardiogram abnormalities, and a high incidence of EEG abnormalities).

∎ Vignettes and Puzzlers

Q. A 34-year-old woman complains, "I hear this voice telling me I ran someone over in my car." The patient experiences this voice as "probably my own thoughts." She does not perceive two or more voices discussing her in derogatory terms, command auditory hallucinations, ideas of people "reading" her mind, ideas of influence/reference, or paranoid ideation. There are no history of psychological or physical trauma and no history of olfactory hallucinations, amnesic periods, déjà vu, or altered level of consciousness. However, the patient does stop her car periodically along the highway "just to make sure that I haven't killed anybody." She says, "I probably didn't run over anybody, but if I don't stop to check, I just feel like I'm going crazy." The patient has no history of psychiatric hospitalizations. However, she has been in individual psychotherapy for several years because of "strange experiences" she has had most of her life (e.g., "feeling like my soul sometimes leaves my body" or "feeling like there's somebody in the room with me when I'm alone at night"). She also expresses, "I think I may have ESP . . . I can usually tell what people are thinking before they even know what it is." Are APs indicated in this case?

A. There is no simple answer to this question, but the initial approach in this case probably does not include the use of APs (Pies 1984). Most of the clinical symptoms in this case suggest an obsessional disorder with at least partially intact "reality testing," although there are certainly some schizo-typal personality features that complicate this assessment. That the patient experiences the voices as probably her *own thoughts,* rather than an external voice being "broadcast" to her, supports the argument against a psychotic process. Furthermore, there is no delusional elaboration surrounding the voice (e.g., "I think someone must have put a radio transmitter into my car"). Probably, treatment should begin with an SSRI or clomipramine (Goodman et al. 1992). If the patient does not respond to several such trials (especially after attempts to potentiate with buspirone or lithium), a small amount of pimozide or haloperidol might be tried. (Risperidone has had mixed results in the treatment of patients with OCD.) Pimozide has been beneficial in treating patients with OCD and comorbid tic disorder or schizotypal features (see Goodman et al. 1992 and Table 2–1). Of course, the risk of TD must be carefully discussed when APs are used in the treatment of OCD patients.

Q. A 25-year-old man with chronic schizophrenia was taking oral haloperidol 10 mg/day and then converted to haloperidol decanoate. The patient also was taking benztropine 1 mg/day. The formula **monthly IM depot dose = 10–15 times daily oral dose** was followed, and the patient's dosage was tapered down to 5 mg/day, and then an injection of haloperidol decanoate 100 mg IM was given. The oral haloperidol and benztropine were then discontinued. Four days later, the patient was seen in clinic and noted to be significantly more psychotic. Reasoning that the initial IM dose may not have been sufficient, the resident in the emergency room administered an additional 50 mg haloperidol decanoate IM. Two days later, the patient returned to the emergency room with severe torticollis and tongue protrusion. What is the *pharmacokinetic* explanation for this adverse event, and what should have been the initial corrective action?

A. Haloperidol decanoate reaches a peak concentration in the plasma at around day 6, then slowly declines (McNeil Pharmaceutical, package insert, 1987). It has an apparent $t\frac{1}{2}$ of about 3 weeks and reaches steady state in about 3 months (about four to five $t\frac{1}{2}$s). In this case, the second IM injection was producing *rising plasma levels* just as the initial injection was peaking, probably accounting for the severe EPS. (Discontinuing the benztropine probably created a *pharmacodynamic* factor predisposing the patient to EPS [i.e., increased central cholinergic activity].) There seems to be no appreciable *pharmacokinetic* interaction between benztropine and haloperidol (Goff et al. 1991). It would have been wiser to add a small amount of daily oral haloperidol to the patient's regimen (e.g., 2–4 mg po qd) to help until the haloperidol decanoate reached higher plasma levels and produced its pharmacodynamic effect on dopamine receptors in the brain. A significant drop from baseline in total BPRS (Overall and Gorham 1962), clearly detectable by week 4 of haloperidol decanoate treatment (Simpson 1988), correlated with clinical improvement. Another intervention in this case would have been the continuation of an anticholinergic agent on a prophylactic basis, particularly in a young male patient.

Q. A 63-year-old man receiving clozapine 300 mg bid underwent a right hemicolectomy for adenocarcinoma. His clozapine was held on the day before the surgery and on the day of the operation, then restarted at 100 mg/day with increases up to 300 mg/day by day 4. On postoperative day 5, the patient had normal bowel sounds and was able to tolerate a regular diet. By day 6, he complained of "gas pains" and some abdominal tenderness. He showed some abdominal distention and had one bout of vomiting. No bowel sounds were heard on auscultation. He also was noted to have significant orthostatic hypotension and dizziness on standing. What is the diagnosis and etiology?

A. Any drug with significant anticholinergic effects can cause constipation, fecal impaction, and even functional bowel obstruction (paralytic ileus), as in this case. *Abdominal surgery* also may be associated with ileus, but in this case, the relatively delayed onset suggests that clozapine's strong anticholinergic effects were a contributing factor (Erickson and Morris 1995). It is important, in such cases, to avoid premature restoration of full-dose regimens of highly anticholinergic medications. Furthermore, the patient's orthostatic hypotension and dizziness were probably related to the rapid dosage escalation of clozapine *after a 48-hour hiatus.* Although sensitivity to the "restart effects" of clozapine is quite variable, orthostasis and even respiratory arrest have been attributed to high restart doses of clozapine; thus, it is recommended that if there is a hiatus of 2 days or more, dosing be restarted at 12.5 mg once or twice daily.

Q. A 23-year-old patient with schizophrenia is on a stable regimen of clozapine 450 mg/day when she has a grand mal seizure. Her psychosis had been under control for more than 5 months, and two attempts to reduce the clozapine dose have led to worsening of psychosis. Because of a previous allergic reaction to valproate, the patient is started on phenytoin 100 mg tid. Her plasma phenytoin level after 1 week is 12 μg/mL (therapeutic = 10–20 μg/mL). Two weeks later, the patient complains of "the devil's voice rocketing through my brain" and isolates herself in her room. She is oriented to day and date and shows no gross neurological impairment. What is the most likely explanation of this deterioration?

A. Phenytoin may significantly decrease clozapine levels, resulting in decreased clinical efficacy (Ciraulo et al. 1994). Phenytoin toxicity is another possibility, and a follow-up phenytoin level would be indicated; however, in the absence of mental confusion, ataxia, slurred speech, and other signs of toxicity, phenytoin toxicity seems unlikely.

Q. A 25-year-old woman with schizophrenia and apparent comorbid OCD was being treated with clozapine 300 mg/day. Although this dosage ameliorated her psychotic symptoms and was well tolerated, she continued to show extreme obsessive-compulsive behaviors, such as counting backward from 100 every time she needed to leave her bed and arranging her food in a highly idiosyncratic manner before eating it. There did not appear to be specific delusional content behind these behaviors. Because fluvoxamine (Luvox) has been FDA-labeled for the treatment of OCD, the patient's psychiatrist began treatment with fluvoxamine 50 mg bid, which was increased over the subsequent week to 100 mg bid. The patient complained of extreme lethargy, hypersalivation, dizziness, and confusion. What is the explanation?

A. Case reports of markedly elevated clozapine levels during fluvoxamine therapy have now been reported. This elevation of clozapine levels may be mediated through fluvoxamine's strong inhibition of the CYP1A2 system, which is at least partly involved in clozapine's metabolism (in addition to CYP2D6). This combination must be used with great caution and with careful monitoring of clinical status. Clozapine blood levels (before and after fluvoxamine) may also help guide treatment (Nemeroff et al. 1995–1996).

Q. A 23-year-old man with chronic undifferentiated schizo-phrenia complains of a "creepy feeling" in his legs and ap-pears to shift from foot to foot. He has not had a full response to adequate doses or trials of conventional neuroleptics (fluphenazine, haloperidol, thioridazine, loxapine, trifluo-perazine) or risperidone. A trial on clozapine led to some im-provement, but the patient developed severe leukopenia requiring discontinuation of the clozapine. Currently, he complains of auditory hallucinations of a threatening nature and the belief that "the storm troopers are out to get me." He has been aggressive and irritable on the inpatient unit and has required restraints three times in the past 2 weeks. His current regimen is thiothixene 15 mg/day, with evidence of good compliance and CNS penetration (e.g., mild cogwheel-ing at the wrist); benztropine 1 mg bid; and lorazepam 1 mg bid. What is the most *parsimonious* potentiation strategy at this point?

A. Adding a β-blocker may be the most efficient means of treating the patient's evident akathisia, aggressiveness, and *possibly* his refractory psychosis. Wirshing et al. (1995) note that most, but not all, controlled studies have found im-provement in acute schizophrenia when propranolol has been used as an adjunctive agent. Doses have been quite high, ranging from 400 to 2,000 mg/day. Propranolol can ele-vate levels of some APs (e.g., thioridazine), and some clini-cians have suggested that β-blockers ameliorate psychosis through this pharmacokinetic mechanism. However, it is possible that both peripheral and centrally acting β-blockers have *primary* effects on aggression (Yudofsky et al. 1987) and psychosis, perhaps via pharmacodynamic effects of some kind. β-Blockers are relatively contraindicated in patients with obstructive lung disease, diabetes mellitus, or hyperthy-roidism. Care also must be exercised when β-blockers are used with other agents that may slow cardiac conduction or induce hypotension. Indeed, combining propranolol with chlorpromazine may lead to increased risk of hypotension, probably due to mutual inhibition of hepatic metabolism. Although one study failed to demonstrate that propranolol raises haloperidol levels (Greendyke and Kanter 1987), hypotension has been reported with this combination (Ratey and MacNaughton 1995). Another option would be a change from thiothixene to mesoridazine, a somewhat atypical AP with a low incidence of akathisia (Osser and Patterson 1996b).

Q. An 82-year-old woman with a history of dementia with psychosis is admitted to the inpatient psychiatric unit from a local nursing home. The patient has been observed to be confused and belligerent during the past 2 weeks beyond her usual baseline. Because of moderate EPS, her medications were recently changed from haloperidol 2 mg bid and benztropine 1 mg qd to thioridazine 150 mg qd and benztropine 1 mg qd. She also takes dicyclomine (Bentyl) 40 mg qid for irritable bowel syndrome. What is the most likely cause of the patient's recent change in mental status?

A. The change in mental status is probably due to central anticholinergic toxicity (Pies 1994a). Cholinergic projections from the nucleus basalis of Meynert to the cerebral cortex have been linked to the pathophysiology of Alzheimer's disease, in which acetylcholine is generally deficient. Cholinergic dysfunction also may be important in many instances of delirium. Thus, this patient may have been at risk for central anticholinergic toxicity even at baseline. The change from 2 mg/day haloperidol to 150 mg/day thioridazine was not a change to an equivalent dose. The correct conversion would have been to approximately 80–100 mg/day thioridazine (Shader 1994a). Because thioridazine is substantially more anticholinergic than haloperidol, even at equivalent doses, the change in AP markedly increased the patient's anticholinergic burden. The benztropine and dicyclomine also have substantial anticholinergic properties and probably contributed to the patient's confusional state.

References

Adams F: Emergency intravenous sedation of the delirious, medically ill patient. J Clin Psychiatry 49 (suppl):22–27, 1988

Altshuler LL, Cohen L, Szuba MP, et al: Pharmacologic management of psychiatric illness during pregnancy: dilemmas and guidelines. Am J Psychiatry 153:592–606, 1996

American Psychiatric Association: Diagnostic and Statistical Manual of Mental Disorders, 3rd Edition. Washington, DC, American Psychiatric Association, 1980

Arana GW, Goff DC, Friedman H, et al: Does carbamazepine-induced reduction of plasma haloperidol levels worsen psychotic symptoms? Am J Psychiatry 143:650–651, 1986

Ayd FJ: Lexicon of Psychiatry, Neurology, and the Neurosciences. Baltimore, MD, Williams & Wilkins, 1995

Baker RW, Chengappa KN, Baird JW, et al: Emergence of obsessive-compulsive symptoms during treatment with clozapine. J Clin Psychiatry 53:439–442, 1992

Barnas C, Bergant A, Hummer M, et al: Clozapine concentrations in maternal and fetal plasma, amniotic fluid, and breast milk. Am J Psychiatry 151:945, 1994

Berman I, Sapers BL, Chang HHJ, et al: Treatment of obsessive-compulsive symptoms in schizophrenic patients with clomipramine. J Clin Psychopharmacol 15:206–210, 1995

Berman I, Merson A, Rachov-Pavlov J, et al: Risperidone in elderly schizophrenic patients. American Journal of Geriatric Psychiatry 4:173–179, 1996

Borison RL, Diamond BI, Pathiragja A, et al: Clinical overview of risperidone, in Novel Antipsychotic Drugs. Edited by Meltzer HY. New York, Raven, 1992, pp 223–239

Bourgeois JA, Klein M: Risperidone and fluoxetine in the treatment of pedophilia with comorbid dysthymia (letter). J Clin Psychopharmacol 16:257–258, 1996

Breier A, Wolkowitz OM, Doran AR, et al: Neuroleptic responsivity of negative and positive symptoms in schizophrenia. Am J Psychiatry 144:1549–1555, 1987

Buckley NA, Whyte IM, Dawson AH: Cardiotoxicity more common in thioridazine overdose than with other neuroleptics. Clinical Toxicology 33:199–204, 1995

Buckley PF, Meltzer HY: Treatment of schizophrenia, in The American Psychiatric Press Textbook of Psychopharmacology. Edited by Schatzberg AF, Nemeroff CB. Washington, DC, American Psychiatric Press, 1995, pp 615–639

Campbell A, Baldessarini RJ: Prolonged pharmacologic activity of neuroleptics (letter). Arch Gen Psychiatry 42:637, 1985

Campbell M, Green WH, Deutsch SI (eds): Child and Adolescent Psychopharmacology. Beverly Hills, CA, Sage, 1985

Cantillon M, Brunswick R, Molina D, et al: A double-blind trial for agitation in a nursing home population with Alzheimer's disease. American Journal of Geriatric Psychiatry 4:263–267, 1996

Casey DE: Antipsychotic drug therapy and extrapyramidal symptoms: past, present, and future. Syllabus material from the Eighth Annual U.S. Psychiatric and Mental Health Congress, New York City, November 17, 1995

Casey DE: Side effect profiles of new antipsychotic agents. J Clin Psychiatry 57 (suppl 11):40–45, 1996

Castillo E, Rubin RT, Holsboer-Trachsler E: Clinical differentiation between lethal catatonia and neuroleptic malignant syndrome. Am J Psychiatry 146:324–328, 1989

Chin AC, Shaw KA, Ciaranello RD: Molecular neurobiology, in The American Psychiatric Press Textbook of Psychopharmacology. Edited by Schatzberg AF, Nemeroff CB. Washington, DC, American Psychiatric Press, 1995, pp 35–36

Ciraulo DA, Shader RI, Greenblatt DJ, et al: Drug Interactions in Psychiatry. Baltimore, MD, Williams & Wilkins, 1989, pp 88–126

Ciraulo DA, Shader RI, Greenblatt DJ: Drug interactions in psychopharmacology, in Manual of Psychiatric Therapeutics, 2nd Edition. Edited by Shader RI. Boston, Little, Brown, 1994, pp 143–158

Cole JO, Goldberg SC, Klerman GL: Phenothiazine treatment in acute schizophrenia. Arch Gen Psychiatry 10:246–261, 1964

Cornelius JR, Soloff PH, Perel JM, et al: A preliminary trial of fluoxetine in refractory borderline patients. J Clin Psychopharmacol 11:116–120, 1991

Cornelius JR, Soloff PH, Perel JM, et al: Continuation pharmacotherapy of borderline personality disorder with haloperidol and phenelzine. Am J Psychiatry 150:1843–1848, 1993

Cowdry RW: Psychopharmacology of borderline personality disorder: a review. J Clin Psychiatry 48 (suppl):15–22, 1987

Csernansky JG, Newcomer JG: Maintenance drug treatment for schizophrenia, in Psychopharmacology: The Fourth Generation of Progress. Edited by Bloom FE, Kupfer DJ. New York, Raven, 1995, pp 1267–1275

DeVane CL: Pharmacogenetics and drug metabolism of newer antidepressant agents. J Clin Psychiatry 55 (suppl):38–45, 1994

Drug Facts and Comparisons. St. Louis, MO, Facts and Comparisons, 1995

Dubovsky SL: Geriatric neuropsychopharmacology, in The American Psychiatric Press Textbook of Geriatric Neuropsychiatry. Edited by Coffey CE, Cummings JL. Washington, DC, American Psychiatric Press, 1994, pp 596–631

Dulcan MK, Bregman JD, Weller EB: Treatment of childhood and adolescent disorders, in The American Psychiatric Press Textbook of Psychopharmacology. Edited by Schatzberg AF, Nemeroff CB. Washington, DC, American Psychiatric Press, 1995, pp 669–706

Dwight MM, Keck PE, Stanton SP, et al: Antidepressant activity and mania associated with risperidone treatment of schizoaffective disorder. Lancet 344:554–555, 1994

Ellison JM, Adler D: A strategy for the pharmacotherapy of personality disorders, in Treating Personality Disorders. Edited by Adler D. San Francisco, CA, Jossey-Bass, 1990, pp 43–64

Emes C, Millson R: Risperidone-induced priapism (letter). Can J Psychiatry 39:315–316, 1994

Ereshefsky L: Pharmacokinetics and drug interactions: update for new antipsychotics. J Clin Psychiatry 57 (suppl 11):12–15, 1996

Erickson B, Morris D: Clozapine-associated postoperative ileus: case report and review of the literature (letter). Arch Gen Psychiatry 52:508–509, 1995

Falloon IRH, Boyd JL, McGill CW, et al: Family management in the prevention of morbidity of schizophrenia. Arch Gen Psychiatry 42:887–896, 1985

Farde L, Wiesel F-A, Halldin C, et al: Central D_2-dopamine receptor occupancy in schizophrenic patients treated with antipsychotic drugs. Arch Gen Psychiatry 45:71–76, 1988

Fink M: Response to "Neuroleptic malignant-like syndrome due to cyclobenzaprine?" J Clin Psychopharmacol 16:97–98, 1996

Fink M, Bush G, Francis A: Catatonia: a treatable disorder, occasionally recognized. Directions in Psychiatry 13:1–7, 1993

Frankenburg F, Zanarini MC: Clozapine treatment of borderline patients: a preliminary study. Compr Psychiatry 34:402–405, 1993

Frazier JA, Gordon CT, McKenna K, et al: An open trial of clozapine in 11 adolescents with childhood-onset schizophrenia. J Am Acad Child Adolesc Psychiatry 33:658–663, 1994

Freedman JE, Wirshing WC, Russel AT, et al: Absence status seizures during successful long-term clozapine treatment of an adolescent with schizophrenia. Journal of Child and Adolescent Psychopharmacology 4:53–62, 1994

Freudenreich O, McEvoy JP: How much Haldol D does Larry really need? (letter) J Clin Psychiatry 56:331–332, 1995

Friedman H, Greenblatt DJ: Rational therapeutic drug monitoring. JAMA 256:2227–2233,1986

Gelenberg AJ: Clozapine for adolescents? Biological Therapies in Psychiatry Newsletter 17:37–38, 1994

Gelenberg AJ: Bipolar patients. J Clin Psychiatry (October monogr ser) 13:28–29, 1995a

Gelenberg AJ: Risperidone for psychosis of Parkinson's syndrome and Lewy body dementia. Biological Therapies in Psychiatry Newsletter 18:43–44, 1995b

Gelenberg AJ: Fatal risperidone overdose. Biological Therapies in Psychiatry Newsletter 19:34–35, 1996

Goff DC, Baldessarini RJ: Antipsychotics, in Drug Interactions in Psychiatry, 2nd Edition. Edited by Ciraulo DA, Shader RI, Greenblatt DJ, et al. Baltimore, MD, Williams & Wilkins, 1995, pp 129–174

Goff DC, Arana GW, Greenblatt DJ, et al: The effect of benztropine on haloperidol-induced dystonia, clinical efficacy, and pharmacokinetics: a prospective, double-blind trial. J Clin Psychopharmacol 11:106–108, 1991

Goldberg SC, Schulz SC, Schulz PM, et al: Borderline and schizotypal personality disorders treated with low-dose thiothixene versus placebo. Arch Gen Psychiatry 43:680–690, 1986

Goldmann MB, Janecek HM: Adjunctive fluoxetine improves global function in chronic schizophrenia. J Neuropsychiatry Clin Neurosci 2:429–431, 1990

Goodman WK, McDougle CJ, Price LH: Pharmacotherapy of obsessive compulsive disorder. J Clin Psychiatry 53 (suppl):29–37, 1992

Grcevich SJ, Findling RL, Schulz SC, et al: Risperidone in the treatment of children and adolescents with psychotic illness: a retrospective review. Poster presented at the annual meeting of the American Psychiatric Association, Miami, FL, May 20–25, 1995

Green A, Schildkraut J: Should clozapine be a first-line treatment for schizophrenia? the rationale for a double-blind clinical trial in first-episode patients. Harvard Review of Psychiatry 3:1–9, 1995

Greendyke RM, Kanter DR: Plasma propranolol levels and their effect on plasma thioridazine and haloperidol concentrations. J Clin Psychopharmacol 7:178–182, 1987

Guy W: ECDEU Assessment Manual for Psychopharmacology, Revised (DHEW Publ No 76-338). Rockville, MD, U.S. Department of Health, Education and Welfare, 1976

Harnett DS: Psychotherapy and psychopharmacology, in Handbook of Clinical Psychopharmacology. Edited by Tupin JP, Shader R, Harnett DS. Northvale, NJ, Jason Aronson, 1988, pp 401–424

Hayes SG: Long-term use of valproate in primary psychiatric disorders. J Clin Psychiatry 50 (suppl):35–39, 1989

Hegarty JD: Antipsychotic drug withdrawal. Current Approaches to Psychoses 5:1–4, 1996

Hiemke C, Weigmann H, Harter S, et al: Elevated levels of clozapine in serum after addition of fluvoxamine. J Clin Psychopharmacol 14:279–281, 1994

Hirschowitz J, Casper R, Garver DL, et al: Lithium response in good prognosis schizophrenia. Am J Psychiatry 137:916–920, 1980

Hogarty GE, McEvoy JP, Ulrich RF, et al: Pharmacotherapy of impaired affect in recovering schizophrenic patients. Arch Gen Psychiatry 52:29–41, 1995

Honer WG, MacEwan GW, Kopala L, et al: A clinical study of clozapine treatment and predictors of response in a Canadian sample. Can J Psychiatry 40:208–211, 1995

Janicak PG, Davis JM, Preskorn SH, et al: Principles and Practice of Psychopharmacotherapy. Baltimore, MD, Williams & Wilkins, 1993

Jeanblanc W, Davis YB: Risperidone for treating dementia-associated aggression (letter). Am J Psychiatry 152:1239, 1995

Jenkins SC, Hansen MR: A Pocket Reference for Psychiatrists, 2nd Edition. Washington, DC, American Psychiatric Press, 1995

Jibson MD, Tandon R: A summary of research findings on the new antipsychotic drugs. Directions in Psychiatry 16:1–7, 1996

Kaplan HI, Sadock BJ, Grebb JA (eds): Synopsis of Psychiatry, 7th Edition. Baltimore, MD, Williams & Wilkins, 1994

Keck PE, McElroy SL: The new antipsychotics and their therapeutic potential. Psychiatric Annals 27:320–331, 1997

Keck PE, Wilson DR, Strakowski SM, et al: Clinical predictors of acute risperidone response in schizophrenia, schizoaffective disorder, and psychotic mood disorders. J Clin Psychiatry 56:466–470, 1995

Keith SJ, Schooler NR: Treatment of schizophreniform disorder, in Treatment of Psychiatric Disorders. Edited by Karasu TB. Washington, DC, American Psychiatric Association, 1989, pp 1656–1665

Kelly JF, Berardki A, Raffaele K, et al: Intravenous haloperidol causes greater memory impairment in old compared to young healthy subjects. Paper presented at the annual meeting of the American Geriatric Society, New Orleans, LA, November 1993

Koller WC, Megaffin BB: Parkinson's disease and parkinsonism, in The American Psychiatric Press Textbook of Geriatric Neuropsychiatry. Edited by Coffey CE, Cummings JL. Washington, DC, American Psychiatric Press, 1994, pp 433–456

Lacro JP, Kuczenski R, Roznoski M, et al: Serum haloperidol levels in older psychotic patients. American Journal of Geriatric Psychiatry 4:229–236, 1996

Lee HS, Kwon KY, Alphs LD, et al: Effect of clozapine on psychogenic polydipsia in chronic schizophrenia. J Clin Psychopharmacol 11:222–223, 1991

Leipzig RM, Mendelowitz A: Adverse psychotropic drug-drug interactions, in Adverse Effects of Psychotropic Drugs. Edited by Kane JM, Lieberman JA. New York, Guilford, 1992, pp 13–76

Levinson DF, Simpson GM, Singh H, et al: Fluphenazine dose, clinical response, and extrapyramidal symptoms during acute treatment. Arch Gen Psychiatry 47:761–768, 1990

Liberman RP, Mueser RP, Mueser KT, et al: Social skills training for schizophrenic individuals at risk for relapse. Am J Psychiatry 143:523–526, 1986

Lieberman JA, Safferman AZ, Pollack S, et al: Clinical effects of clozapine and chronic schizophrenia: response to treatment and predictors of outcome. Am J Psychiatry 151:1744–1752, 1994

Lindenmayer J-P, Apergi F-S: The relationship between clozapine plasma levels and clinical response. Psychiatric Annals 26:406–412, 1996

Madhusoodanan S, Brenner R, Araujo L, et al: Efficacy of risperidone treatment for psychoses associated with schizophrenia, schizoaffective disorder, bipolar disorder, or senile dementia in 11 geriatric patients: a case series. J Clin Psychiatry 56:514–518, 1995

Manschreck TC: Delusional disorder. Current Approaches to Psychoses 5:7–9, 1996

Marsden CD, Jenner P: The pathophysiology of extrapyramidal side-effects of neuroleptic drugs. Psychol Med 10:55–72, 1980

Martenyi F, Harangozo J, Laszlo M: Clonazepam for the treatment of catatonic schizophrenia (letter). Am J Psychiatry 146:1230, 1989

McCarthy RH, Terkelsen KG: Esophageal dysfunction in two patients after clozapine treatment (letter). J Clin Psychopharmacol 14:281–283, 1994

McDougle CJ, Goodman WK, Price LH, et al: Neuroleptic addition in fluvoxamine-refractory obsessive-compulsive disorder. Am J Psychiatry 147:652–654, 1990

McDougle CJ, Fleischmann RL, Epperson CN, et al: Risperidone addition in fluvoxamine-refractory obsessive-compulsive disorder: three cases. J Clin Psychiatry 56:526–528, 1995

McElhatton PR: The use of phenothiazines during pregnancy and lactation. Reprod Toxicol 6:475–490, 1992

McEvoy JP, VanderZwaag C, McGee M, et al: A double-blind randomized trial comparing clozapine treatment within three distinct serum level ranges in patients with refractory schizophrenia (abstract). Paper presented at the winter schizophrenia meeting, Crans, Switzerland, March 1996

McGlashan TH: Schizophrenia: psychosocial treatments and the role of psychosocial factors in its etiology and pathogenesis, in Psychiatry Update: American Psychiatric Association Annual Review, Vol 5. Edited by Frances AJ, Hales RE. Washington, DC, American Psychiatric Press, 1986, pp 96–111

Meltzer HY: Atypical antipsychotic drugs, in Psychopharmacology: The Fourth Generation of Progress. Edited by Bloom FE, Kupfer DJ. New York, Raven, 1995, pp 1277–1286

Meltzer HY: Predictors of response to clozapine. Psychiatric Annals 26:385–389, 1996

Meltzer HY, Matsubara S, Lee JC: Classification of typical and atypical drugs on the basis of dopamine D_1, D_2 and serotonin2 pKi values. J Pharmacol Exp Ther 251:238–246, 1989

Naimark D, Harris J, Jeste DV: Use of atypical neuroleptics in the elderly. Geriatric Psychiatry News 1:12–13, 1995

Nakane Y, Rapoport J: Childhood-onset schizophrenia. Current Approaches to Psychoses 4:1–4, 1995

Nemeroff CB, Devane CL, Pollack BG: Summary and review of antidepressants and the cytochrome P450 system. Progress Notes, Fall/Winter 1995–1996, pp 38–40

Okuma T, Yamashita I, Takahashi R, et al: A double-blind study of adjunctive carbamazepine versus placebo on excited states of schizophrenic and schizoaffective disorders. Acta Psychiatr Scand 80:250–259, 1989

Osser DN: A systematic approach to pharmacotherapy in patients with neuroleptic-resistant psychosis. Hospital and Community Psychiatry 40:921–926, 1989

Osser DN, Patterson RD: Pharmacotherapy of schizophrenia, I: acute treatment, in Handbook for the Treatment of the Seriously Mentally Ill. Edited by Soreff SM. Seattle, WA, Hogrefe & Huber, 1996a, pp 91–119

Osser DN, Patterson RD: Pharmacotherapy of schizophrenia, II: an algorithm for neuroleptic-resistant patients, in Handbook for the Treatment of the Seriously Mentally Ill. Edited by Soreff SM. Seattle, WA, Hogrefe & Huber, 1996b, pp 121–155

Overall JE, Gorham DR: The Brief Psychiatric Rating Scale. Psychol Rep 10:799–812, 1962

Ovsiew F: Bedside neuropsychiatry: eliciting the clinical phenomena of neuropsychiatric illness, in The American Psychiatric Press Textbook of Neuropsychiatry, 2nd Edition. Edited by Yudofsky SC, Hales RE. Washington, DC, American Psychiatric Press, 1992, pp 99–101

Owens MJ, Risch SC: Atypical antipsychotics, in The American Psychiatric Press Textbook of Psychopharmacology. Edited by Schatzberg AF, Nemeroff CB. Washington, DC, American Psychiatric Press, 1995, pp 263–280

Pearlman CA: Neuroleptic malignant syndrome: a review of the literature. J Clin Psychopharmacol 6:257–273, 1986

Pearlman CA: Clozapine, nocturnal sialorrhea, and choking (letter). J Clin Psychopharmacol 14:283, 1994

Petersdorf RG: Hypothermia and hyperthermia, in Harrison's Principles of Internal Medicine, 12th Edition. Edited by Wilson JD, Braunwald E, Isselbacher KJ, et al. New York, McGraw-Hill, 1991, pp 2194–2200

Peterson BS: Natural history, pathophysiology, and treatment of Tourette's syndrome. J Clin Psychiatry 13 (monogr ser):17–19, 1995

Phillips KA: Body dysmorphic disorder: the distress of imagined ugliness. Am J Psychiatry 148:1138–1149, 1991

Physicians' Desk Reference, 50th Edition. Montvale, NJ, Medical Economics, 1996

Pickar D: Serotonin and dopamine abnormalities in schizophrenia. J Clin Psychiatry 12 (monogr ser):10–16, 1994

Pickar D: Relative receptor affinities of selected antipsychotic compounds. Psychiatric Times (suppl), November 1995, p 2

Pies R: Distinguishing obsessional from psychotic phenomena. J Clin Psychopharmacol 6:345–347, 1984

Pies R: Beware this fate. Psychiatric Times, November 1994a, pp 40–41

Pies R: Clinical Manual of Psychiatric Diagnosis and Treatment. Washington, DC, American Psychiatric Press, 1994b, pp 466–469

Pies R, Popli AP: Self-injurious behavior: pathophysiology and implications for treatment. J Clin Psychiatry 56:580–588, 1995

Pool D, Bloom W, Mielke DH, et al: A controlled evaluation of Loxitane in seventy-five adolescent schizophrenia patients. Curr Ther Res Clin Exp 19:99–104, 1976

Rapoport JL: Clozapine and child psychiatry. Journal of Child and Adolescent Psychopharmacology 4:1–3, 1994

Raskind MA: Treatment of Alzheimer's disease and other dementias, in The American Psychiatric Press Textbook of Psychopharmacology. Edited by Schatzberg AF, Nemeroff CB. Washington, DC, American Psychiatric Press, 1995, pp 657–667

Ratey JJ, MacNaughton KL: β-Blockers, in Drug Interactions in Psychiatry, 2nd Edition. Edited by Ciraulo DA, Shader RI, Greenblatt DJ, et al. Baltimore, MD, Williams & Wilkins, 1995, pp 311–355

Remschmidt H, Schulz E, Martin M: An open trial of clozapine in thirty-six adolescents with schizophrenia. Journal of Child and Adolescent Psychopharmacology 4:31–41, 1994

Richelson E: Preclinical pharmacology of neuroleptics: focus on new generation compounds. J Clin Psychiatry 57 (suppl 11):4–11, 1996

Rosebush P, Stuart T: A prospective analysis of 24 episodes of neuroleptic malignant syndrome. Am J Psychiatry 146:717–725, 1989

Roth M: Delusional (paranoid) disorders, in Treatment of Psychiatric Disorders. Edited by Karasu TB. Washington, DC, American Psychiatric Association, 1989, pp 1609–1648

Sachdev P, Loneragan C: Intravenous benztropine and propranolol challenges in acute neuroleptic-induced akathisia. Clin Neuropharmacol 16:324–331, 1993

Sachdev P, Kruk J, Kneebone M, et al: Clozapine-induced neuroleptic malignant syndrome: review and report of new cases. J Clin Psychopharmacol 15:365–370, 1995

Salzman C, Satlin A, Burrows AB: Geriatric psychopharmacology, in The American Psychiatric Press Textbook of Psychopharmacology. Edited by Schatzberg AF, Nemeroff CB. Washington, DC, American Psychiatric Press, 1995, pp 803–821

Schaffer CB, Schaffer LC: The use of risperidone in the treatment of bipolar disorder (letter). J Clin Psychiatry 57:136, 1996

Schexnayder LW, Hirschowitz J, Sautter FJ, et al: Predictors of response to lithium in patients with psychoses. Am J Psychiatry 152:1511–1513, 1995

Seeman P: Dopamine receptor sequences: therapeutic levels of neuroleptics occupy D_2 receptors, clozapine occupies D_4. Neuropsychopharmacology 7:261–284, 1992

Seeman P: Dopamine receptors: clinical correlates, in Psychopharmacology: The Fourth Generation of Progress. Edited by Bloom FE, Kupfer DJ. New York, Raven, 1995, pp 295–302

Segraves RT: Sexual dysfunction complicating the treatment of depression. J Clin Psychiatry 10 (monogr ser):75–79, 1992

Shader RI: Approaches to the treatment of schizophrenia, in Manual of Psychiatric Therapeutics, 2nd Edition. Edited by Shader RI. Boston, MA, Little, Brown, 1994a, pp 311–336

Shader RI: Dissociative, somatoform, and paranoid disorders, in Manual of Psychiatric Therapeutics, 2nd Edition. Edited by Shader RI. Boston, MA, Little, Brown, 1994b, pp 15–23

Simpson GM: Postmarketing evaluation of haloperidol decanoate injection: efficacy, safety, and dosing considerations. J Clin Psychiatry 1:1–8, 1988

Small JG, Hirsch SR, Arvanitis LA, et al: Quetiapine in patients with schizophrenia. Arch Gen Psychiatry 54:549–557, 1997

Soloff RH, George A, Nathan R, et al: Progress in pharmacotherapy of borderline disorders: a double-blind study of amitriptyline, haloperidol, and placebo. Arch Gen Psychiatry 43:691–697, 1986

Spears NM, Leadbetter RA, Shutty MS: Clozapine treatment in polydipsia and intermittent hyponatremia. J Clin Psychiatry 57:123–128, 1996

Spitzer RL, Gibson M, Endicott J: Global Assessment Scale. New York, New York State Department of Mental Hygiene, 1973

Springfield AC, Bodiford E: An overdose of risperidone. J Anal Toxicol 20:202–203, 1996

Stanilla JK, Simpson GM: Drugs to treat extrapyramidal side effects, in The American Psychiatric Press Textbook of Psychopharmacology. Edited by Schatzberg AF, Nemeroff CB. Washington, DC, American Psychiatric Press, 1995, pp 281–299

Sternbach H: The serotonin syndrome. Am J Psychiatry 148:705–713, 1991

Stowe ZN, Nemeroff CB: Psychopharmacology during pregnancy and lactation, in The American Psychiatric Press Textbook of Psychopharmacology. Edited by Schatzberg AF, Nemeroff CB. Washington, DC, American Psychiatric Press, 1995, pp 823–837

Suppes T, McElroy SL, Gilbert J, et al: Clozapine in the treatment of dysphoric mania. Biol Psychiatry 32:270–280, 1992

Theoharides TC, Harris RS, Weckstein D: Neuroleptic malignant-like syndrome due to cyclobenzaprine? J Clin Psychopharmacol 15:79–81, 1995

Thompson JW Jr, Ware MR, Blashfield RK: Psychotropic medication and priapism: a comprehensive review. J Clin Psychiatry 51:430–433, 1990

Tsang MW, Shader RI, Greenblatt DJ: Metabolism of haloperidol: clinical implications and unanswered questions (editorial). J Clin Psychopharmacol 14:159–161, 1994

Tueth MJ, DeVane CL, Evans DL: Treatment of psychiatric emergencies, in The American Psychiatric Press Textbook of Psychopharmacology. Edited by Schatzberg AF, Nemeroff CB. Washington, DC, American Psychiatric Press, 1995, pp 769–781

Tyson SC, DeVane CL, Risch SC: Pharmacokinetic interaction between risperidone and clozapine (letter). Am J Psychiatry 152:1401–1402, 1995

VanderZwaag C, McGee M, McEvoy JP, et al: Response of patients with treatment-refractory schizophrenia to clozapine within three serum level ranges. Am J Psychiatry 153:1579–1584, 1996

van Kammen DP, McEvoy JP, Targum SD, et al: A randomized, controlled, dose-ranging trial of sertindole in patients with schizophrenia. Psychiatric Times, August 1996, pp 7–13

Van Putten T, Marder SR, Mintz J: A controlled dose comparison of haloperidol in newly admitted schizophrenic patients. Arch Gen Psychiatry 47:754–758, 1990a

Van Putten T, Marder SR, Wirshing W, et al: Neuroleptic plasma levels in treatment-resistant schizophrenic patients, in The Neuroleptic-Nonresponsive Patient: Characterization and Treatment. Edited by Angrist B, Schulz SC. Washington, DC, American Psychiatric Press, 1990b, pp 69–85

Velamoor VR, Swamy GN, Parmar RS, et al: Management of suspected neuroleptic syndrome. Can J Psychiatry 40:545–550, 1995

Viguera AC, Baldessarini RJ, Hegarty JM, et al: Clinical risk following abrupt and gradual withdrawal of maintenance neuroleptic treatment. Arch Gen Psychiatry 54:49–55, 1997

Waldman MD, Safferman AZ: Pregnancy and clozapine (letter). Am J Psychiatry 150:168–169, 1993

Warner JP, Barnes TRE, Henry JA: Electrocardiographic changes in patients receiving neuroleptic medication. Acta Psychiatr Scand 93:311–313, 1996

Webster P, Wijeratne C: Risperidone-induced neuroleptic malignant syndrome (letter). Lancet 344:1228–1229, 1994

Wirshing WC, Marder SR, Van Putten T, et al: Acute treatment of schizophrenia, in Psychopharmacology: The Fourth Generation of Progress. Edited by Bloom FE, Kupfer DJ. New York, Raven, 1995, pp 1259–1266

Young CR, Bostic JQ, McDanald CL: Clozapine and refractory obsessive-compulsive disorder: a case report. J Clin Psychopharmacol 14:209–210, 1994

Yudofsky SC, Silver JM, Schneider SE: Pharmacologic treatment of aggression. Psychiatric Annals 17:397–406, 1987

Zarate CA, Tohen M, Baldessarini RJ: Clozapine in severe mood disorders. J Clin Psychiatry 56:411–417, 1995

CHAPTER 3

Anxiolytics and Sedative-Hypnotics

Overview

▊ Drug Class

Anxiolytics and hypnotics include a variety of pharmacological agents, but the benzodiazepines (BZDs) are by far the most frequently used. Although the BZDs are sometimes classified by chemical structure, their clinical properties are more closely related to pharmacokinetic factors. However, triazolo-BZDs may have some qualitatively different properties from nontriazolo-BZDs. Other anxiolytics and hypnotics include some antihistamines, β-blockers, and the azapirone anxiolytic buspirone. Barbiturates and meprobamate are rarely used in clinical psychiatry. Clonidine is occasionally used to treat various forms of anxiety or agitation.

▊ Indications

The BZD anxiolytics and hypnotics are used primarily in the treatment of generalized anxiety disorder (GAD) and panic disorder and in the short-term treatment of stress-related insomnia. However, the BZDs have found increasing use as adjunctive agents in the treatment of mania and acute psychosis; in such cases, the BZDs are usually combined with mood stabilizers and antipsychotics, respectively. The BZDs are also the agents of choice in the treatment of alcohol withdrawal and may be useful for various kinds of extrapyramidal symptoms, nocturnal myoclonus, and night terrors. There is less-convincing evidence for the role of BZDs in the adjunctive treatment of obsessive-compulsive disorder (OCD), social phobic disorder, avoidant personality disorder, posttraumatic stress disorder (PTSD), and depression. There is controversy as to the efficacy and safety of long-term BZD use for chronic insomnia. The non-BZD anxiolytic buspirone is useful in the treatment of GAD but not of panic disorder. Buspirone also can be useful as an adjunctive agent in the treatment of OCD, dementia-related agitation, sexual dysfunction, and—in higher doses (> 50 mg/day)—depression.

▋ Mechanisms of Action

BZDs appear to bind to the α subunit of the γ-aminobutyric acid (GABA) receptor. There, BZDs increase the affinity of the receptor for GABA, an inhibitory neurotransmitter that leads to increased chloride ion conductance, which hyperpolarizes the neuron and leads to decreased excitability. The mechanism of the azapirone anxiolytic, buspirone, is completely different, involving variable effects at serotonin (5-HT) receptors. Buspirone may have dose-dependent antidepressant effects.

▋ Pharmacokinetics

The BZDs may be divided into three main groups—long-, intermediate-, and short-acting—based on their elimination half-lives ($t\frac{1}{2}$s). Most of the *longer-acting* agents share a common active intermediate, *desmethyldiazepam*, which has an elimination $t\frac{1}{2}$ exceeding *60 hours* (and generally longer in the elderly). Long-acting BZDs undergo oxidative metabolism, which is sensitive to alterations in hepatic function. Three of the *intermediate-acting* BZDs—*lorazepam, oxazepam,* and *temazepam*—require only *glucuronidation* and are relatively unaffected by alterations in hepatic function. *Estazolam* (used as a hypnotic agent) and *alprazolam* are intermediate-duration BZDs; both undergo oxidative metabolism but have no active metabolites of significant duration. Another intermediate-acting agent, *clonazepam*, undergoes *nitroreduction* as its primary metabolic step. *Triazolam*, which has a $t\frac{1}{2}$ of about only 3 hours, is the only *short-acting* BZD in general clinical use. (*Midazolam*, which has a $t\frac{1}{2}$ of about 2 hours, is used primarily as a presurgical sedative.) BZDs are metabolized primarily via the cytochrome P450 (CYP) 3A4 and 2C19 systems.

■ Main Side Effects

The side effects of BZDs are primarily extensions of their sedative properties. Although generally well tolerated, BZDs can produce drowsiness, fatigue, weakness, light-headedness, ataxia, respiratory suppression, and falls. Confusion, psychomotor impairment, amnesia, depression, and paradoxical excitation are also seen. Some predisposed individuals can become psychologically and/or physically dependent on BZDs. Significant withdrawal effects may be seen if BZDs are suddenly discontinued, and "rebound insomnia" may be seen with sudden discontinuation of short-acting (and to some degree intermediate-acting) BZDs. Buspirone is generally well tolerated, although it occasionally can produce dizziness, gastrointestinal (GI) disturbance, or headache. The antihistamines may produce memory impairment or confusion in susceptible individuals.

■ Drug-Drug Interactions

BZDs are generally safe in combination with most other medications. However, a variety of drugs may increase the plasma levels and/or toxicity of oxidatively metabolized BZDs (e.g., cimetidine, ketoconazole, metoprolol, valproate, fluoxetine, and erythromycin). Nefazodone may increase plasma levels of triazolo-BZDs. In contrast, rifampin and phenytoin may decrease the clinical effects of some BZDs, probably via induction of hepatic metabolism. Ranitidine and various antacids may reduce or delay oral absorption of BZDs. The coadministration of BZDs and anticholinergic agents may lead to greater cognitive impairment than administration of either drug class alone. The combination of BZDs with clozapine has led to severe sedation and/or cardiorespiratory suppression in some individuals. BZDs may increase the neurotoxicity of alcohol, narcotics, and other central nervous system (CNS) depressants. Although BZDs by themselves have little toxicity in overdose, they may be lethal when combined with alcohol or other CNS depressants. Finally, alprazolam, and perhaps diazepam, may lead to increased digoxin levels. Buspirone is generally well tolerated in combination with most other drugs, although adverse interactions may occur in combination with monoamine oxidase inhibitors (MAOIs) or other agents with serotonergic properties.

▋ Potentiating Maneuvers

Some reports suggest that BZDs may be potentiated by the addition of buspirone (e.g., in the treatment of GAD). β-Blockers also may be used in combination with BZDs, although hypotension may result. BZDs are often used in combination with antidepressants, but their effect on depression per se is equivocal (e.g., sometimes BZDs may worsen preexisting depression). BZDs are useful in potentiating the effects of antimanic and antipsychotic agents and may reduce the dosage of antipsychotic medication needed for management of acute psychosis.

▋ Use in Special Populations

The use of BZDs during the first trimester of pregnancy is associated with cleft lip or palate and possibly with impaired intrauterine growth. However, the absolute risk of such problems appears small. Infants exposed to BZDs either in the last trimester or at the time of parturition may show muscular hypotonicity, failure to feed, impaired temperature regulation, apnea, and low Apgar scores. There are insufficient data in humans to determine the risks of buspirone during pregnancy.

In elderly and medically ill populations, the use of BZDs may be associated with cognitive impairment, falls and hip fractures, behavioral disinhibition or confusion (particularly in dementia patients), reduced hepatic metabolism, drug-drug interactions, and hangover effects from long-acting hypnotic agents. Buspirone is relatively well tolerated in the elderly and medically ill.

Tables

▌ Drug Class

Table 3–1. Commonly used benzodiazepine anxiolytics

Agent/brand	Tablet/capsule strengths (mg)	Usual daily adult dose (mg)
Alprazolam (Xanax)	0.25, 0.5, 1, 2	0.75–4 (up to 10 mg for panic disorder)
Chlordiazepoxide (Librium)	5, 10, 25	15–100
Clonazepam (Klonopin)	0.5, 1, 2	0.5–4
Clorazepate (Tranxene)	3.75, 7.5, 15 (11.25, 22.5 single-dose tablets)	15–60
Diazepam (Valium)	2, 5, 10 (15 mg sustained release)	4–40
Halazepam (Paxipam)	20, 40	60–160
Lorazepam (Ativan)	0.5, 1, 2	2–6
Oxazepam (Serax)	10, 15, 30	30–120
Prazepam (Centrax)	5, 10, 20	20–60

Sources.   Data from Drug Facts and Comparisons 1995; Shader and Greenblatt 1994a.

Table 3–2. Benzodiazepine hypnotics

Agent	Tablet/capsule strengths (mg)	Usual daily adult dose (mg)
Estazolam (ProSom)	1, 2	1–2
Flurazepam (Dalmane)	15, 30	15–30
Quazepam (Doral)	7.5, 15	7.5–15
Temazepam (Restoril)	7.5, 15, 30	15–30
Triazolam (Halcion)	0.125, 0.25	0.125–0.5[a]

[a]Do not exceed 0.25 mg in elderly (see also Tables 3–12 and 3–16).

Table 3–3. Nonbenzodiazepine anxiolytics and hypnotics

Agent	Comments
Antihistamines (diphenhydramine, hydroxyzine)	Not as well studied as anxiolytics or hypnotics; anticholinergic effects can be sedating but may cause cognitive impairment in elderly/dementia patients; may lose effectiveness after a few weeks; occasionally useful as short-term anxiolytics in agitated psychotic patients and may ameliorate extrapyramidal symptoms
Barbiturates	Effective anxiolytics but too prone to abuse and lethality (in overdose) to be useful in most cases
Buspirone	Azapirone that acts as a 5-HT agonist at the presynaptic $5-HT_{1A}$ receptor but as a *partial agonist* at postsynaptic $5-HT_{1A}$ receptors; causes downregulation of $5-HT_2$ receptors (similar to antidepressants); has anxiolytic and (in high doses) antidepressant properties; useful in generalized anxiety disorder, perhaps social phobia, agitated dementia patients, aggressive/self-injurious mentally retarded patients; does not impair psychomotor performance; has little if any abuse potential and is relatively safe in overdose; not useful for panic disorder, BZD withdrawal
Meprobamate	Structurally, does not resemble BZDs or other psychoactive drugs; has muscle relaxant and anxiolytic properties; may bind to BZD-GABA-Cl⁻ ionophore and competitively inhibit BZD binding; may also potentiate adenosine; has significant abuse liability, and withdrawal from high doses resembles barbiturate withdrawal; rarely used in clinical practice, but if BZDs and alternative agents fail, meprobamate could be considered

Zolpidem

Marketed as hypnotic agent (5–10 mg hs); binds to BZD type 1 receptors with very low affinity for other receptor subtypes; little effect on sleep architecture; has no muscle relaxant, anxiolytic, or anticonvulsant properties (unlike BZDs); generally well tolerated and effective in inducing and maintaining sleep in adults, with minimal residual cognitive effects in the morning; some reports of tolerance, withdrawal symptoms, amnesic psychotic reactions, and hallucinatory phenomena (the last occurring at therapeutic doses)

Note. 5-HT = serotonin; BZD = benzodiazepine; GABA = γ-aminobutyric acid; Cl⁻ = chloride ion.
Sources. Ayd 1995; Cole and Yonkers 1995; Pies 1995a.

Table 3–4. Off-label uses for clonidine and β-blockers for anxiety and agitation in selected disorders

Agent	Off-label uses
β-Blockers	Akathisia
	Aggressive-impulsive behaviors following brain damage
	Performance anxiety
	Tremor (essential, drug related)
	Adjunct to BZDs in alcohol withdrawal
	?Generalized anxiety disorder
	?Panic disorder, agoraphobia
	?Adjunctive agent in narcotic/BZD withdrawal
	?Management of cocaine intoxication
	?Adjunctive agent in treatment of schizophrenia
	?Adjunctive agent in mania
Clonidine	Attention-deficit/hyperactivity disorder
	Opioid detoxification
	Nicotine dependence
	?Posttraumatic stress disorder (augmenting agent)
	Tourette's syndrome
	?Panic disorder
	?Augmenting agent for obsessive-compulsive disorder
	?Generalized anxiety disorder
	?Refractory mania
	?Tricyclic-induced sweating

Note. BZDs = benzodiazepines; ? = data base is limited or contradictory.
Sources.   Ayd 1995; Cornish et al. 1995; Dulcan et al. 1995; Pies and Parks 1996; Yudofsky et al. 1995

Table 3–5. Dosage of selected benzodiazepines roughly equivalent (anxiolytic-hypnotic effect) to 5 mg diazepam

Agent	Equivalent dose (mg)
Alprazolam (Xanax)	0.5
Chlordiazepoxide (Librium)	10
Clonazepam (Klonopin)	0.25
Clorazepate (Tranxene)	7.5
Estazolam (ProSom)	2
Flurazepam (Dalmane)	15
Halazepam (Paxipam)	20
Lorazepam (Ativan)	1
Oxazepam (Serax)	15
Prazepam (Centrax)	10
Quazepam (Doral)	15
Temazepam (Restoril)	15
Triazolam (Halcion)	0.25

Source. Data from Jenkins and Hansen 1995.

Table 3–6.   Comparative expense of selected benzodiazepines

Agent (daily dosage in low therapeutic range)	Approximate monthly cost
Alprazolam (1 mg/day)	$11
Chlordiazepoxide (not sustained release) (30 mg/day)	$11
Clonazepam (0.5 mg/day)	$29
Diazepam (not sustained release) (10 mg/day)	$8
Estazolam (1 mg qhs)	$39
Flurazepam (15 mg qhs)	$15
Lorazepam (2 mg/day)	$8
Oxazepam (30 mg/day)	$14
Temazepam (15 mg qhs)	$8

Source.   Data from a suburban Boston pharmacy, March 1997.

▌ Indications

Table 3–7. Indications for benzodiazepines

Indication	Data base/comments
Generalized anxiety disorder	BZDs are primary pharmacological treatment for generalized anxiety disorder; virtually all BZDs are more effective than placebo during short-term, outpatient treatment; controlled studies fail to demonstrate superiority of one BZD over another; choice of agent depends heavily on side effect profile, patient-specific factors, medical issues
Panic disorder	Most data derived from studies of alprazolam, showing efficacy significantly greater than placebo in reducing frequency, severity of panic attacks; alprazolam is FDA-approved for treatment of panic disorder, but other BZDs, including clonazepam, diazepam, and lorazepam, may have comparable efficacy; clonazepam may provide better "coverage" of panic disorder, with less breakthrough of symptoms, perhaps fewer dependency, withdrawal problems than with alprazolam; in general, BZDs are now used as second-line treatments for panic disorder, with SSRIs as first line (as well as cognitive-behavior therapy)
Obsessive-compulsive disorder	Clonazepam may be modestly effective in obsessive-compulsive disorder, based on a few case reports
Social phobic disorder	In small, uncontrolled studies, alprazolam and clonazepam have been effective in social phobic disorder

(continued)

Table 3–7.   Indications for benzodiazepines *(continued)*

Indication	Data base/comments
Avoidant personality disorder	Little systematic investigation of medication for "pure" avoidant personality disorder (comorbidity/overlap with social phobia is high); one study found alprazolam helpful in reducing many symptoms of avoidant personality disorder in a small sample ($n = 14$) of social phobic patients
Posttraumatic stress disorder	Few systematic trials of BZDs; a small retrospective study ($n = 20$) showed that alprazolam (0.5–6 mg/day) reduced many PTSD symptoms in 16 cases, but *disinhibited behavior* was seen in 4 patients; a placebo-controlled study of alprazolam showed modest improvement in anxiety and in subjective sense of well-being, but no significant improvement in core PTSD symptoms of intrusion and avoidance; because substance abuse is common in PTSD, BZDs should be used conservatively in this population
Insomnia	Nearly all BZDs are effective short-term (1–4 weeks) hypnotics; use in long term is controversial, and problems with dependency, withdrawal must be considered; use of long-acting BZDs, such as flurazepam, usually not optimal for most patients with insomnia because of hangover effects; very short acting agents (such as triazolam) may lead to breakthrough insomnia/early awakening; triazolam also associated with higher-than-average cognitive impairment; some clinicians recommend use of BZDs every second or third night in cases of chronic insomnia, to reduce tolerance

(continued)

Table 3–7. Indications for benzodiazepines *(continued)*

Indication	Data base/comments
Mania	Both lorazepam and clonazepam have been found useful as antimanic agents and may reduce need for adjunctive neuroleptics during initiation of mood stabilizers; some evidence that lorazepam may work more rapidly than clonazepam during first 2 weeks of acute mania
Depression	With the exception of alprazolam, and possibly clonazepam, there is little evidence that BZDs have antidepressant properties; some data indicate that BZDs (including clonazepam) can worsen depression, but during initiation of treatment with "stimulating" antidepressants (e.g., fluoxetine, desipramine, bupropion), a brief period of adjunctive BZD use may be warranted, particularly as an at-bedtime dose
Acute psychosis	Short-term use of BZDs, either po or IM, can reduce the need for neuroleptics in the management of acute psychosis, particularly when accompanied by agitated or catatonic features; BZDs may be useful for agitated PCP-induced psychosis; haloperidol and lorazepam may be combined in same syringe for IM treatment of severe/psychotic agitation
Akathisia/ dyskinesia	Clonazepam, diazepam, lorazepam all reported useful in small, open, short-term studies of neuroleptic-induced akathisia, parkinsonism, TD; little controlled data in large populations; in open studies of TD, about 58% of patients improved with BZDs; in double-blind studies, the rate is 43%
Nocturnal myoclonus	BZDs reduce periodic leg movements of sleep; preliminary data suggest BZDs (clonazepam) also may be helpful in REM sleep behavioral disorder

(continued)

Table 3–7.   Indications for benzodiazepines *(continued)*

Indication	Data base/comments
Night terrors/other sleep disorders	Because they suppress delta (stages 3 and 4) sleep, BZDs are useful for night terrors; there is risk of worsening sleep apnea, so this should be ruled out before using BZDs
Substance withdrawal	BZDs are the treatment of choice for alcohol withdrawal; duration of clinical action after single oral dose is not related to elimination half-life of BZD but to its distribution in lipid compartments (CNS and outside CNS); repeated doses of diazepam, for example, may be necessary in initial treatment of DTs; note poor IM absorption of all commonly prescribed BZDs except lorazepam

Note.   BZDs = benzodiazepines; FDA = Food and Drug Administration; SSRIs = selective serotonin reuptake inhibitors; PTSD = posttraumatic stress disorder; IM = intramuscular; PCP = phencyclidine; TD = tardive dyskinesia; REM = rapid eye movement; CNS = central nervous system; DTs = delirium tremens.

Sources.   Data from Ballenger 1995; Braun et al. 1990; Cornish et al. 1995; Davidson et al. 1991; Feldmann 1987; Gardos and Cole 1995; Hewlett et al. 1990; Janicak et al. 1993; Pagel 1996; Reich et al. 1989; Shader and Greenblatt 1994a, 1994b; Stanilla and Simpson 1995; Taylor 1995.

▊ Mechanisms of Action

Table 3–8.   Effect of various agents on $GABA_A$ receptors

Agent	Effect on receptor
Alcohol	Weakly augments GABA-activated Cl⁻ ion conductance but also inhibits NMDA receptor–mediated depolarization
Barbiturates	Augment receptor affinity for GABA (like BZDs) but also *directly* increase channel opening, even in absence of GABA; dual mechanism may account for greater toxicity of barbiturates versus BZDs
Benzodiazepines	Bind to α subunit; increase the affinity of the receptor for GABA, an inhibitory neurotransmitter that leads to increased Cl⁻ ion conductance, hyperpolarizing the neuron and leading to decreased excitability; BZDs have no direct effect on Cl channel opening
Buspirone	No effect on GABA-BZD complex
Zolpidem	Appears to interact with same binding site as BZDs, since effects of zolpidem can be prevented by flumazenil (BZD receptor antagonist)

Note.   GABA = γ-aminobutyric acid; Cl⁻ = chloride;
NMDA = *N*-methyl-D-aspartate; BZDs = benzodiazepines.
Sources.   Kaplan et al. 1995; Paul 1995.

▌ Pharmacokinetics

Table 3–9. Orally administered benzodiazepine
pharmacokinetics: anxiolytics

Agent	Onset of peak action (hrs)	Effective elimination $t\frac{1}{2}$ (hrs)[a]	Active metabolites
Alprazolam	1.5	12–15	No
Chlordiaze-poxide	2	> 50	Yes
Clonazepam	1.5	18–50	No
Clorazepate	1.5	> 50	Yes
Diazepam	1.3	> 50	Yes
Halazepam	2.5	> 50	Yes
Lorazepam	1.3	12–15	No
Oxazepam	3	12–15	No
Prazepam	5	> 50	Yes

Note.   Onset of peak action after oral dosing varies from patient to patient,
and the above data are based on my experience, as well as on published
data pertaining to peak blood levels. $t\frac{1}{2}$ = half-life.
[a]Includes effects of long-acting metabolites, usually *desmethyldiazepam.*
Elimination $t\frac{1}{2}$ may vary with age and hepatic function, with elderly
patients usually showing longer elimination $t\frac{1}{2}$.
Sources.   Data from Ballenger 1995; Drug Facts and Comparisons 1995;
Physicians' Desk Reference 1996; Shader and Greenblatt 1994b.

Table 3–10. Benzodiazepine pharmacokinetics: hypnotics

Agent	Onset of peak action (hrs)	Effective elimination $t\frac{1}{2}$ (hrs)[a]	Active metabolites
Estazolam (ProSom)	2	10–24	No
Flurazepam (Dalmane)	0.5–2	> 50	Yes
Quazepam (Doral)	2	> 50	Yes
Temazepam (Restoril)	1–2	7–12	No
Triazolam (Halcion)	0.5–2	2–5	No

Note. Onset of peak action varies from patient to patient, and the above data are based on my experience, as well as on published data pertaining to peak blood levels. $t\frac{1}{2}$ = half-life.
[a]Includes effects of long-acting active metabolites (e.g., desalkylflurazepam and desalkyl-2-oxoquazepam).
Sources. Data from Ballenger 1995; Drug Facts and Comparisons 1995; Physicians' Desk Reference 1996; Shader and Greenblatt 1994a.

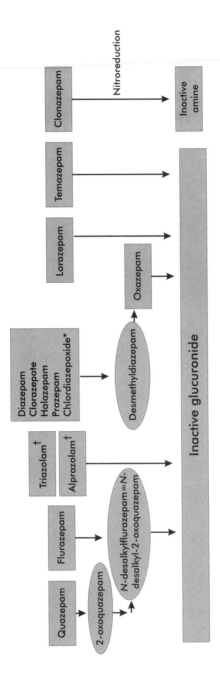

Figure 3–1. Simplified metabolic pathways. *Intermediates include desmethylchlordiazepoxide and demoxepam. †Very transient active metabolites (little clinical importance).

▌Main Side Effects

Table 3–11. Frequency of benzodiazepine and buspirone side effects (average for various benzodiazepines)

Side effect	Benzodiazepines (%)	Buspirone (%)
Hypotension	4.7	< 1
Hypertension	0	< 1
Dizziness	3.4	13.6
Fainting	3.1	< 1
Tachycardia	7.7	1.3
Palpitations	7.7	1
Bradycardia	< 1	< 1
Dyspnea	< 1	< 1
Chest pain	—	1.5
Dry mouth/throat	12.6	5.3
Salivation	4.2	< 1
Nausea, vomiting	7.4	10.8
Diarrhea	7	2.5
Constipation	7.1	1.3
Weight gain	2.7	—
Sexual dysfunction	11	1
Blurry vision	10.6	2
Weakness, fatigue	17.7	7.6
Clumsiness	20	—
Headache	9.1	10.6
Ataxia, incoordination	17.6	2.5

(continued)

Table 3–11. Frequency of benzodiazepine and buspirone side effects (average for various benzodiazepines) *(continued)*

Side effect	Benzodiazepines (%)	Buspirone (%)
Confusion/ disorientation	6.9	1.4
Insomnia	6.4	6.7
Unusual dreams	—	5.5
Hallucinations	5.5	< 1
Paradoxical anxiety, nervousness	4.1	5
Irritability, hostility	5.5	2
Depression	8.3	1.4

Note. — = no data available.
Source. Data from Maxmen 1991.

Table 3–12. Benzodiazepine side effects and management

Side effect	Comments/management
Drowsiness, fatigue, weakness	At fixed dose of BZD, sedation usually subsides after about a week as anxiolytic action emerges; dosage reduction and administration mostly at bedtime may reduce the problem
Light-headedness, ataxia, falls	Some, but not all, studies show BZDs linked with risk of falls and hip fractures in elderly; although some studies suggest less risk of falls with short-acting BZDs, other data suggest that risk of falls/hip fractures is related to *rate of dosage increase and total dose;* reduce dosage; educate patients regarding rising slowly from bed
Slurred speech, double vision	Dosage reduction
Confusion, psychomotor impairment	Visual-spatial ability, coordination, sustained attention may be impaired and may affect driving skills (although no conclusive evidence linking BZDs with automobile accidents); patients often not aware of decreased ability until stopping the BZD; dysfunction is synergistic with use of alcohol; elderly may be especially susceptible to cognitive decrements; some cognitive dysfunction may diminish with time/chronic dosing; use minimal effective dose, avoid sudden dosage increases; some patients may benefit from a small amount of caffeine

(continued)

Table 3–12.   Benzodiazepine side effects and
management *(continued)*

Side effect	Comments/management
Memory impairment, anterograde amnesia	All BZDs can cause memory impairment to some degree; triazolam probably has somewhat greater risk of causing dose-related amnesic and cognitive symptoms than do other BZD hypnotics; BZD-related confusion/amnesia may be misdiagnosed as dementia in elderly; triazolam may be especially likely to cause memory impairment in the elderly; avoid triazolam dose > 0.125 mg in the elderly
Depression	When depression occurs after onset of panic disorder, BZDs may be useful for both anxiety and depression; with exception of alprazolam, BZDs generally lack antidepressant properties and may cause or exacerbate depression in some patients
Paradoxical stimulation/ disinhibition	Can manifest as irritability, increased anxiety, aggression, euphoria, psychosis; tends to occur in patients with underlying brain damage, dementia, also in some borderline personality disorder patients; may be more likely with alprazolam based on anecdotal reports, but not all data support this association

(continued)

Table 3–12. Benzodiazepine side effects and management *(continued)*

Side effect	Comments/management
Respiratory suppression	Flurazepam and probably all BZDs may exacerbate sleep apnea; chlordiazepoxide and probably all BZDs can exacerbate breathing difficulties in patients with chronic lung disease; reports of respiratory suppression/arrest when BZDs combined with clozapine (see also Table 3–13); avoid BZDs if possible in patients with sleep-related breathing problems; avoid high doses of BZDs in other patients at risk; increase dose slowly; SSRIs, buspirone may be good alternatives in anxious patients at risk for respiratory suppression
Miscellaneous (GI complaints, dry mouth, urinary hesitancy)	Dosage reduction; administration with food may reduce GI complaints (also may slow rate of absorption); urinary hesitancy may respond to bethanechol
Discontinuation/ withdrawal syndromes	Withdrawal of BZDs may lead to continuum of symptoms, ranging from restlessness, headaches, insomnia, hyperacusis to (rarely) severe depression, myoclonus, involuntary movements, delirium, and seizures; likelihood of withdrawal reaction probably related to duration of BZD use and daily dosage, possibly related to use of short-acting BZDs; alprazolam, perhaps other triazolo-BZDs, may be especially hard to discontinue; key management strategy is very slow taper of BZDs over weeks to months; "coverage" of triazolo-BZD may not be complete with nontriazolo (e.g., "covering" a patient withdrawing from alprazolam by using clonazepam)

Note. BZD = benzodiazepine; SSRIs = selective serotonin reuptake inhibitors; GI = gastrointestinal.
Sources. Ballenger 1995; Creelman et al. 1989; Herings et al. 1995; Janicak et al. 1993; Jenkins and Hansen 1995; Pies 1992; Smoller 1996; Woods et al. 1995.

∎ Drug-Drug Interactions

Table 3–13.   Benzodiazepine drug-drug interactions

Index drug (added to BZD)	Clinical effect/other interactions
Cimetidine, isoniazid, disulfiram, oral contraceptives, ketoconazole, metoprolol, propranolol, valproate, propoxyphene, erythromycin, omeprazole	Potential for increased toxicity of diazepam, chlordiazepoxide, other BZDs that undergo *oxidative* hepatic metabolism, due to inhibition of BZD metabolism; dosage adjustment of BZD may be necessary; ketoconazole-type agents affect mainly triazolo-BZD metabolism (alprazolam, triazolam, midazolam); metoprolol, propranolol may inhibit metabolism of demethylated BZDs (e.g., diazepam) but do not interfere with metabolism of alprazolam, lorazepam, oxazepam, and (probably) temazepam
Oral contraceptives	Some (but not all) data suggest that OCs can *increase* clearance rate/reduce levels of BZDs that undergo *glucuronidation* (lorazepam, oxazepam); in contrast, OCs *decrease* clearance of diazepam and other BZDs undergoing *oxidative* metabolism; diazepam plus an OC may increase psychomotor/cognitive impairment; lorazepam dose might need upward adjustment with OCs, whereas diazepam dose might need downward adjustment; alprazolam clearance probably not affected by OCs
Rifampin, phenytoin, carbamazepine	Decreased clinical effect of BZDs, due to induction of hepatic metabolism (e.g., phenytoin may increase oxazepam clearance, decrease levels)

(continued)

Table 3–13. Benzodiazepine drug-drug interactions *(continued)*

Index drug (added to BZD)	Clinical effect/other interactions
Ranitidine	May reduce GI absorption of diazepam but does not impair oxidative or conjugative metabolism of diazepam, lorazepam (as may cimetidine)
Antacids, anticholinergics	Suspension-type antacids (e.g., magnesium/aluminum hydroxide) may alter *rate* but usually not *extent* of GI absorption; delay in oral absorption and/or onset of effect of BZDs possible, but this is probably most relevant after single-dose (rather than chronic) treatment; biodegradation of clorazepate (prodrug) to active desmethyldiazepam may be delayed with antacids
Anticholinergics	Coadministration may produce more cognitive impairment than with either drug alone, particularly in the elderly
Digoxin	Alprazolam, and perhaps diazepam, may lead to increased digoxin levels (could lead to toxicity)
Alcohol, narcotics, other CNS depressants	Increased CNS sedation, toxicity
Tricyclic antidepressants	Increased imipramine and desipramine (but not nortriptyline) levels with concomitant alprazolam administration; amitriptyline may increase psychomotor effects of BZDs

(continued)

Table 3–13.   Benzodiazepine drug-drug interactions *(continued)*

Index drug (added to BZD)	Clinical effect/other interactions
SSRIs	*Fluoxetine* and *fluvoxamine* may reduce clearance of some oxidatively metabolized BZDs, including diazepam and alprazolam, leading to increased BZD levels/effects; fluoxetine does not appear to affect metabolism of glucuronidated BZDs (lorazepam, oxazepam), triazolam, or clonazepam; data not yet available for sertraline, paroxetine, but metabolite of sertraline would be expected to affect CYP3A4 (which metabolizes triazolo-BZDs)
Nefazodone	Increased levels of triazolo-BZDs (e.g., alprazolam elimination half-life may double)
Antipsychotics/ clozapine	BZDs may act synergistically with clozapine to cause severe sedation, hypotension, respiratory depression (may be related to dose of BZD)
L-Dopa	Possibly decreased effect of L-dopa when BZDs coadministered

Note. BZD = benzodiazepine; OCs = oral contraceptives; GI = gastrointestinal; CNS = central nervous system; SSRIs = selective serotonin reuptake inhibitors; CYP = cytochrome P450.
Sources. Abernethy et al. 1982, 1984; Ayd 1995; Cobb et al. 1991; Drug Facts and Comparisons 1995; Ellinwood et al. 1984; Pies and Weinberg 1990; Preskorn 1996; Salzman et al. 1986; Sands et al. 1995.

▌Potentiating Maneuvers

Table 3–14. Agents used in combination with benzodiazepines for augmentation of effect

Agent combined with BZD	Rationale/comment
Anticholinergic/anti-parkinsonian agents	BZDs may augment antiparkinsonian effect of benztropine, similar agents, in treatment of neuroleptic-induced tremor, muscle rigidity, akathisia (*Note:* Anticholinergics may slow BZD absorption)
Antidepressants	BZDs may provide early relief of agitation, insomnia in patients with depression or panic disorder before primary (coadministered antidepressant) treatment has become effective; some patients may become more depressed with continued use of BZDs
Antipsychotics	BZDs (e.g., lorazepam) may augment effect of haloperidol in acute psychosis; BZDs also may be of help for catatonic features
Buspirone	Buspirone may augment anxiolytic effect of BZDs in panic disorder; may facilitate discontinuation of BZDs
Mood stabilizers	Clonazepam, lorazepam potentiate antimanic effect of valproate, lithium

Note. BZD = benzodiazepine.
Sources. Cole and Yonkers 1995; Coplan and Gorman 1990; Fawcett 1990; Gastfriend and Rosenbaum 1989; Lenox and Manji 1995; Tueth et al. 1995.

▌Use in Special Populations

Table 3–15.   Potential concerns of benzodiazepine use during pregnancy

Potential problem	Comments/management
Cleft lip and palate	Recent evidence suggests small absolute risk from BZD exposure during first trimester (< 1%) but higher than in general population (0.06%); informed consent, discussion with mother and obstetrician are indicated; if possible, minimize/avoid BZD use during first trimester
Impaired intrauterine growth and various dysmorphic birth defects	Data mostly derived from one group (Laegreid et al. 1992); informed consent, discussion with mother and obstetrician are indicated; if possible, minimize/avoid use during first trimester
Condition resembling fetal alcohol syndrome	As yet unconfirmed
Increased duration of labor	Consult with obstetrician in advance of expected delivery date
Withdrawal symptoms in neonate	May be manifest as tremulousness, hypertonicity, irritability, hyperactivity, disturbed sleep, tremors, in neonate; avoid high doses of short-acting BZDs; do not discontinue BZDs suddenly during pregnancy but rather taper slowly as delivery approaches

(continued)

Table 3–15. Potential concerns of benzodiazepine use during pregnancy *(continued)*

Potential problem	Comments/management
Appearance of BZDs in breast milk	Mothers should avoid nursing while taking BZDs if possible or use lowest effective dose; amount of BZD in breast milk appears to be very small percentage of maternal dose and is unlikely to pose a threat to the nursing infant

Note. BZD = benzodiazepine.
Sources. Data from Altshuler et al. 1996; Ayd 1995; Laegreid et al. 1992; Pies 1995b; Stowe and Nemeroff 1995.

Table 3–16.   Risks of benzodiazepine use in elderly and/or dementia patients

Risk/problem	Management
Cognitive dysfunction/ amnesia	Use lowest-effective dose; intermediate-duration agents with no active metabolites may be preferable; if triazolam is used, avoid dose > 0.125 mg; reassess rationale for long-term BZD use periodically
Falls, hip fractures	Use lowest-effective dose; avoid sudden increases in dose; instruct patient to rise slowly; check blood pressure supine and standing after dose increases; reassess rationale for long-term BZD use periodically; ?avoid long-acting BZDs (conflicting data)
Behavioral disinhibition	Avoid BZDs for most agitated dementia patients (most likely to become disinhibited or confused); if BZD must be used, prescribe lowest-effective dose for limited duration; ?avoid alprazolam (data are weak but clinical experience suggests caution)
Reduced hepatic metabolism	Use intermediate-duration agents that do not undergo oxidative metabolism (e.g., oxazepam, lorazepam, temazepam)
Drug-drug interactions	Be aware of metabolic route of coprescribed agents and avoid those that specifically inhibit CYP2C19 and/or CYP3A4 (see "Questions and Answers," "Drug-Drug Interactions")

Hangover effect from hypnotic	Avoid long-acting agents (e.g., flurazepam, any BZD with desmethyldiazepam metabolite) when treating simple insomnia (without daytime anxiety); reassess rationale for long-term BZD use periodically

Note. ? = conflicting data; BZD = benzodiazepine; CYP = cytochrome P450.
Source. Data from Dubovsky 1994.

Questions and Answers

▌ Drug Class

Q. What is the main factor determining the choice of one BZD versus another for any given indication?

A. Because all the BZDs are probably equal in efficacy for their principal indications, the choice of agent is dictated mainly by pharmacokinetic considerations (Arana and Hyman 1991). The onset of action, distribution in body compartments, metabolic pathway, and elimination $t\frac{1}{2}$ are more important factors than the specific chemical structure of the BZD (see Table 3–9). The triazolo-BZDs may be a partial exception to this in that their chemical structure may confer somewhat atypical properties (e.g., high-potency and antidepressant effects [the latter having been demonstrated in some studies of alprazolam]). This qualitative difference between triazolo- and nontriazolo-BZDs also may make it difficult to "cover" a patient withdrawing from alprazolam by using another (nontriazolo-) BZD, such as clonazepam. Some patients will continue to complain of withdrawal symptoms as they are tapered off alprazolam, despite equipotent doses of clonazepam or other long-acting BZDs. Another factor in choosing a BZD is the potential for interaction with other medications (see "Drug-Drug Interactions"). Triazolo-BZDs are metabolized mainly by CYP3A4. With the release of two new antidepressants that inhibit the CYP 3A4 system—nefazodone and fluvoxamine—use of triazolo-BZDs may be problematic in patients taking these new agents. Thus, choice of BZD is influenced by a variety of pharmacokinetic (and to some degree pharmacodynamic) factors.

Q. Can BZDs be administered sublingually?

A. Lorazepam, alprazolam, and triazolam are well absorbed sublingually. Although the time to peak plasma levels is only modestly reduced for sublingual versus oral alprazolam (about 1.2 versus 1.7 hours, respectively [Scavone et al. 1987]), the sublingual route may be preferable in acutely anxious patients who cannot swallow pills, or have a full stomach, which would slow absorption (Arana and Hyman 1991). Dry mouth may interfere with the sublingual route.

Q. Are the BZDs ever used intravenously (IV) in psychiatry?

A. The IV route is rarely used, except for preoperative sedation and in treating seizures; however, IV diazepam, lorazepam, or midazolam may be used to treat neuroleptic-induced laryngeal dystonia, if anticholinergics fail (Arana and Hyman 1991). Occasionally, IV midazolam may be used in the treatment of severe alcohol withdrawal (Ciraulo et al. 1994). The IV route carries a substantial risk of respiratory suppression or arrest and should not be attempted without adequate medical support.

■ Indications

Q. How effective are BZDs in the psychic versus the somatic aspects of GAD, and how long do these effects last?

A. Most studies of two commonly used BZDs—chlordiazepoxide and diazepam—have found evidence of global effectiveness in GAD or similar conditions when compared with placebo; however, few such studies have distinguished psychic versus somatic aspects of relief (Hollister et al. 1993). In a recent study of diazepam, Pourmotabbed et al. (1996) found that *somatic* symptoms of GAD are more responsive to diazepam than are psychic symptoms. However, superiority of diazepam over placebo was seen only for the first 3 *weeks*, after which time the *placebo group* continued to improve.

Pourmotabbed et al. (1996) suggest that diazepam be used to treat symptoms of GAD for only a few weeks; however, their results do not indicate that diazepam is *ineffective* for GAD after the first 3 weeks, and I have seen some patients with GAD who appear to benefit from—and indeed require—longer use of BZDs. One study of diazepam noted that the improvement obtained by the 6th week was sustained when medication was continued for 22 weeks (Rickels et al. 1983).

Q. How do the indications for BZDs differ from those for buspirone?

A. Buspirone—an azapirone anxiolytic that does not interact with brain BZD receptors—differs from BZDs in its pharmacodynamic profile (Janicak et al. 1993). First, its clinical effect takes several weeks to accrue, so buspirone is not useful in treating an acute episode of anxiety. Second, buspirone is not useful when taken on a prn basis, in contrast to BZDs (for some patients). Third, buspirone has not been shown effective for panic attacks or panic disorder. Neither is buspirone capable of covering BZD withdrawal symptoms. Finally, buspirone—in doses greater than 50 mg/day—has demonstrable antidepressant properties, based on double-blind studies (Rickels et al. 1990). In contrast—with the exception of alprazolam and possibly clonazepam—BZDs have minimal antidepressant activity and may sometimes be associated with treatment-emergent depression (Janicak et al. 1993; Tesar 1990). Buspirone may be useful for patients with generalized anxiety who cannot tolerate respiratory suppression or sedation.

Q. Besides insomnia, are there any other indications for the use of zolpidem (Ambien)?

A. There are no other indications that have been well documented. However, Jackson et al. (1996) recently reported the successful use of low-dose zolpidem (2.5 mg/day) for the management of agitation in two elderly dementia patients. This interesting observation must be tempered by several reports of cognitive side effects with zolpidem at therapeutic doses (Pies 1995a).

Q. How effective are BZDs in the treatment of OCD?

A. There are few controlled studies bearing on this question, but clinical experience has not generally supported use of the BZDs for this disorder. However, Hewlett et al. (1990) reported on three patients who met DSM-III-R (American Psychiatric Association 1987) criteria for OCD and who responded well to clonazepam (3–5 mg/day) over a 1-year period. One patient showed a reduction in obsessions and compulsions that was equal to or greater than that seen with clomipramine treatment and also experienced improvement in depressive symptoms. The authors note that clonazepam does have complex effects on 5-HT metabolism. In my experience with OCD, clonazepam sometimes may be a useful adjunct in combination with a selective serotonin reuptake inhibitor (SSRI).

Q. How are BZDs employed in the treatment of acute psychosis or severe agitation in the emergency setting?

A. Most experience has been gained with lorazepam, which is the only conventional BZD (excluding midazolam) that is reliably absorbed via the intramuscular (IM) route. For the agitated, psychotic patient, lorazepam 1–2 mg po or IM may be given alone, every ½–2 hours, up to 6–12 mg over a 24-hour period. Lorazepam is often coprescribed with variable amounts of an antipsychotic. Alternatively, lorazepam (2–4 mg) may be *combined in the same syringe* with haloperidol (2.5–5 mg) and administered every 1–2 hours, up to five times or so in a 24-hour period. The disadvantage of such a "cocktail" is that adverse reactions (including allergic ones) are difficult to sort out (i.e., which agent was responsible?). On the other hand, some data suggest that this combination may be superior to either agent alone in the acute care setting (Garza-Trevino et al. 1989). Keep in mind that elderly patients may experience hypotension from IM lorazepam and that some patients with underlying brain damage may become disinhibited with BZD administration.

Q. Are BZDs useful in the long-term management of schizophrenia?

A. Because BZDs appear to inhibit dopamine neurotransmission and decrease presynaptic dopamine release, there is some theoretical justification for their use in schizophrenia (Wolkowitz and Pickar 1991). Of 16 double-blind studies assessing adjunctive use of BZDs in schizophrenia, 7 reported positive results, but 4 reported mixed or transiently positive results. The overall response rate in such patients is about 40% (Ayd 1995; Wolkowitz and Pickar 1991). Wolkowitz and Pickar (1991) have noted "rapid (within 1–2 weeks) and occasionally striking improvements in social relatedness, affability, spontaneity, humor, and interest in family and social life in some benzodiazepine-treated patients" (p. 720). However, some patients appear to lose therapeutic response within a few weeks. BZDs may be useful in ameliorating neuroleptic-induced extrapyramidal effects, which may secondarily improve psychotic features. Patients with high initial anxiety, psychosis, or motor disturbance may be most likely to respond to adjunctive BZDs (Wolkowitz and Pickar 1991).

Q. Are BZDs indicated in the *long-term* treatment of chronic insomnia?

A. Opinion differs on this issue, with most experts counseling that BZDs are indicated primarily for the *short-term* treatment of insomnia (Janicak et al. 1993). This advice seems prudent, in general, because there are few studies showing hypnotic efficacy of BZDs beyond 12 weeks (Janicak et al. 1993) and because of the risks of cognitive impairment, tolerance, withdrawal, and exacerbation of sleep-related breathing disorders. On the other hand, as Hollister et al. (1993) cogently stated, "the labeling of benzodiazepine hypnotic drugs typically recommends that prescriptions should not exceed 1 month. Such statements have been widely interpreted as reflecting evidence that the drugs lose efficacy after these periods of time. *In fact, they reflect only that there have simply not been enough studies of long-term efficacy from which to draw definitive conclusions*" (p. 138S, italics added). Moreover, some sleep laboratory data have documented continued benefits for up to 6 months after the start of regular BZD use (Hollister et al. 1993). A recent study spanning 12 years found that long-term nightly treatment of sleep disorders with BZDs was effective and did not lead to dosage escalation or drug abuse in the vast majority of patients (Schenck and Mahowald 1996). In summary, the issue of long-term BZD hypnotic therapy has not been settled. In my experience, there is a small subgroup of patients with mixed anxiety and depression whose chronic insomnia does respond well to low doses of BZDs over a period of months to years, with no evidence of tolerance, abuse, or cognitive impairment. (Almost always, the BZD is an adjunct to ongoing antidepressant therapy.) Nevertheless, prudence would dictate use of alternative regimens whenever possible. Trazodone or (in selected cases) small amounts of doxepin may be useful for chronic, intractable insomnia not amenable to behavioral methods. Other clinicians suggest that if BZDs are used chronically for insomnia without complicating anxiety, the patient should try to take the hypnotic every second or third night. To my knowledge, however, this method has not been compared with every-night dosing in a controlled study.

Q. What BZDs are employed in the treatment of periodic leg movements of sleep?

A. Although most BZDs could be used for periodic leg movements of sleep, clonazepam (1 mg hs) is probably the most commonly used agent for this purpose because of its intermediate $t\frac{1}{2}$, allowing coverage of periodic leg movements of sleep for 6–8 hours (Nofzinger and Reynolds 1996). However, as with all BZDs, adaptation to or tolerance of the effects of clonazepam may develop, and BZDs must be used cautiously when a patient has obstructive sleep apnea (Nofzinger and Reynolds 1996) (see discussion on "Main Side Effects" that follows).

Q. What is the role of BZDs in the management of bipolar disorder?

A. BZDs may be useful as adjunctive agents in the management of acute mania (Chouinard 1987; McElroy and Keck 1995). Thus, in one controlled study comparing lorazepam with haloperidol as adjuncts to lithium in acute mania, the two treatments were comparable (Lenox et al. 1992). Typically, clonazepam 0.5–2 mg q 2–6 hours is used until the patient is calm or sedated. The maximum daily dose is usually less than 6 mg/day (Sachs 1996), although higher doses (more than 12 mg/day) may be employed. One study (Bradwejn et al. 1990) found lorazepam superior to clonazepam during the first 2 weeks of treatment, but these differences may diminish with time. After 2–3 weeks, and usually after the primary mood-stabilizing agents have achieved control of the mania, the BZD can often be tapered and discontinued. However, some bipolar patients—particularly those with comorbid anxiety disorders—may benefit from longer-term BZD treatment. Contraindications for BZD maintenance would include a history of BZD-induced behavioral dyscontrol/paradoxical response or substance abuse (Sachs 1996).

Although one study found neurotoxicity when clonazepam was combined with lithium (Koczerginski et al. 1989), the patients also were taking neuroleptics, which may have contributed to this problem (Sarid-Segal et al. 1995).

Q. What about the use of BZDs in the *depressed* phase of bipolar illness?

A. Anxiety may intensify dysphoria and insomnia during bipolar depression, and loss of sleep is a risk factor for the "switch" into mania. Therefore, brief periods of BZD use may be warranted in depressed bipolar patients with anxiety and/or insomnia (Sachs 1996). Because alprazolam occasionally may induce mania, use of lorazepam or clonazepam is probably preferable. Although one study of clonazepam (1.5–6 mg/day) showed that it improved depression in bipolar depressed patients (Kishimoto et al. 1988), the evidence that clonazepam has significant antidepressant properties is weak. BZDs also may be associated with treatment-emergent depression in patients with some anxiety disorders (Janicak et al. 1993; Tesar 1990). Thus, the use of BZDs for bipolar depression must be monitored and limited carefully.

Q. Are BZDs effective in the treatment of unipolar depression?

A. In a review of 20 controlled studies of BZDs in patients with depressive disorders, Schatzberg and Cole (1978) concluded that although anxiety and insomnia may be significantly relieved, BZDs do not have significant impact on core depressive symptoms (e.g., psychomotor retardation, diurnal mood variation). There was little evidence for efficacy in severe depression unless prominent anxiety also was present (Janicak et al. 1993). Some data suggest that BZDs may aggravate depression and/or suicidality (Klerman 1986). Alprazolam, however, is an exception, and one study showed alprazolam had antidepressant properties equal to those of imipramine (Feighner 1982). Another study (Jonas and Hearron 1996) of alprazolam in patients with major depression compared its effects on suicidality with both placebo and various "active comparator" medications (including several tricyclics). Alprazolam-treated patients showed greater improvement in suicidality than did placebo-treated patients, although somewhat less than patients treated with active comparator drugs. The authors interpreted the results to indicate that "although alprazolam may have efficacy in mild-to-moderate depression, standard antidepressants are more effective in severe depression" (Jonas and Hearron 1996, p. 211).

Q. Are there any appropriate indications for barbiturates in modern clinical psychiatry?

A. In my opinion, there are rarely any good reasons to use barbiturates in preference to safer agents, such as BZDs. Amobarbital (50–100 mg IM) is sometimes used in emergency settings to control agitation; however, laryngospasm and respiratory depression may occur, and IM lorazepam may be just as effective (Kaplan et al. 1995). Some chronically anxious patients who have serious adverse side effects to BZDs and buspirone may be candidates for barbiturates (Kaplan et al. 1995), but my preference is to attempt treatment with valproate, trazodone, or a sedating tricyclic (e.g., doxepin 25 mg hs). Amobarbital has been used, historically, for diagnostic purposes (Amytal interview), but both clinical and medicolegal considerations make this use problematic (e.g., the *Ramona* case, in California, has cast suspicion on the amobarbital interview because of fears of "implanted memories"). Finally, although barbiturates may be useful in activating some "catatonic" patients, IM lorazepam may be just as effective and is considerably safer.

Q. What about the use of chloral hydrate for insomnia?

A. Chloral hydrate (500–1,000 mg hs) occasionally may be indicated in the *short-term* treatment (two to three nights) of insomnia if BZDs are not effective. However, the lethal dose of chloral hydrate is only 5–10 times the "therapeutic" dose, giving this drug a very narrow therapeutic index. Moreover, symptoms of intoxication, dependence, and withdrawal may be associated with chloral hydrate, and tolerance develops after only 2 weeks of treatment (Kaplan et al. 1995). GI side effects are also common (e.g., gastritis and gastric ulceration).

Q. What is *guanfacine,* and what are its indications in psychiatry?

A. Guanfacine is an α_2-adrenergic agonist, similar to clonidine in its reduction of autonomic arousal. Guanfacine also suppresses REM sleep. It has been used in lieu of clonidine in the treatment of attention-deficit/hyperactivity disorder and in one case of PTSD-related nightmares (Horrigan and Barnhill 1996). Because it has a longer elimination $t\frac{1}{2}$ than clonidine, guanfacine may have some advantages in various disorders of autonomic arousal or REM sleep. Controlled studies are needed to establish the indications, benefits, and risks of guanfacine.

■ Mechanisms of Action

Q. Baclofen, like BZDs, is also active at GABA receptors. Does baclofen have anxiolytic properties?

A. Baclofen is active at $GABA_B$ receptors, whose activation results in an increase in potassium channel conductance and hyperpolarization of the neuron. Baclofen is not active at $GABA_A$ receptors (the site of action of BZDs) and seems to have primarily antispasmodic properties (Paul 1995). However, baclofen does have sedative properties and can lead to somnolence, tolerance, and respiratory depression (Drug Facts and Comparisons 1995).

Q. Do BZDs have effects on other neurotransmitters besides GABA?

A. In animal studies, BZDs have been shown to decrease nigrostriatal dopamine release and turnover, to block stress-induced activation in cortical dopamine turnover, and to augment the chronic decreases in dopamine turnover seen with neuroleptics (Wolkowitz and Pickar 1991). It also has been hypothesized that the antipanic properties of BZDs relate to their inhibitory effects on noradrenergic function in the locus ceruleus (Charney and Heninger 1985). Clonazepam, perhaps more so than other BZDs, may have significant effects on 5-HT (Kishimoto et al. 1988).

Q. What is buspirone's mechanism of action, and how does this relate to its clinical use?

A. Buspirone has no effect on the GABA-BZD receptor complex; rather, it is an agonist or partial agonist at the 5-HT$_{1A}$ receptor. Buspirone also may have activity at the 5-HT$_2$ and D$_2$ receptors, but the clinical significance of these effects is not clear (Kaplan et al. 1995). Buspirone's action at the 5-HT$_{1A}$ receptor is complex, depending on whether the receptor is pre- or postsynaptic. It appears that buspirone acts as a 5-HT agonist at presynaptic 5-HT$_{1A}$ receptors but as a *partial agonist* at postsynaptic 5-HT$_{1A}$ receptors. This pharmacodynamic flexibility may permit buspirone to act as either an anxiolytic or an antidepressant, depending on the concentration of ambient serotonin (Eison 1990; Pies 1993). In anxiety states, buspirone's net effect may be to reduce serotonergic function in some brain regions, via effects on the (presynaptic) 5-HT$_{1A}$ autoreceptor; however, in depressive conditions characterized by *low ambient levels of 5-HT,* buspirone (in doses of 50 mg/day or more) may enhance serotonergic function by acting as a substitute for endogenous 5-HT (Eison 1990; Pies 1993; Rickels et al. 1990).

Q. How does zolpidem (Ambien) work?

A. Zolpidem is a non-BZD that interacts with the GABA-BZD receptor. Its binding site may be the same as that of the BZDs, because zolpidem's effects can be reversed via administration of the BZD antagonist, flumazenil (Kaplan et al. 1995). Zolpidem is thought to bind preferentially to the BZD_1 receptor (Ayd 1995), which in theory may reduce the risk of cognitive side effects; however, excessive use of zolpidem can produce cognitive and perceptual disturbance (Pies 1995a).

▌ Pharmacokinetics

Q. What issues arise regarding absorption (GI, IM) of BZDs?

A. With the exception of clorazepate, all BZDs are absorbed unchanged from the GI tract. Clorazepate is converted in the GI tract to desmethyldiazepam, and this conversion requires an acidic medium. Thus, concomitant administration of antacids may impair absorption of clorazepate, at least acutely (see the discussion on "Drug-Drug Interactions" that follows). The BZDs differ in their rates of absorption from the GI tract (e.g., lorazepam is rapidly absorbed, whereas oxazepam is slowly absorbed). The rate of absorption largely determines onset of clinical action after oral dosing, but other factors are involved (see the next question). Oral absorption may be affected by the presence of food (e.g., patients who take a BZD with a snack at bedtime may experience a slower onset of hypnotic activity than if the same drug had been taken several hours after a meal [Janicak et al. 1993]). Loraze-

pam is the only commonly used BZD that is well absorbed
IM; thus, IM administration of other BZDs (e.g., for the treatment of delirium tremens) is unlikely to be reliable. Midazolam, which also is well absorbed IM, is a BZD usually used as
a preanesthetic agent (e.g., prior to surgical procedures) and
in some emergency situations where rapid sedation is de-
sired.

Q. What is the relationship between how lipophilic a BZD is
and its onset of clinical action?

A. More lipophilic compounds would cross the blood-brain
barrier more rapidly than less lipophilic ones and, in principle, have a more rapid onset of action (Greenblatt 1991). This
onset of action has been demonstrated with IV-administered
BZDs, such as the highly lipophilic diazepam (which has an
almost immediate onset) and the less lipophilic lorazepam
(which has a more delayed onset). However, after oral dosage, the rate-limiting step in onset of clinical action is the
drug's rate of absorption from the GI tract (Greenblatt 1991).

Q. What are the specific metabolic pathways for BZD metabolism?

A. Three BZDs—*lorazepam, oxazepam,* and *temazepam*—require only *glucuronidation* and are relatively unaffected by alterations in hepatic function, as in cirrhosis. Most of the other
BZDs—including *diazepam, chlordiazepoxide, flurazepam,* and
the *triazolo-BZDs*—undergo *oxidative metabolism* (phase I reaction). *Clonazepam* undergoes *nitroreduction* as its primary
metabolic step, which is also sensitive to alterations in hepatic function (Sands et al. 1995). Most phase I oxidative metabolism is mediated by the cytochrome P450 system; in the
case of BZDs, the CYP3A4 and CYP2C19 systems appear to
be primarily involved. Thus, the triazolo-BZDs—*alprazolam,
midazolam,* and *triazolam*—are metabolized via CYP3A4. Di-

azepam has a complex route of demethylation, involving both CYP2C19 and CYP3A4 (Sands et al. 1995).

Q. What is "single-dose kinetics," and in what clinical situations when BZDs are used is this important?

A. Single-dose kinetics refers to the distribution and accumulation of a drug after a single oral or parenteral dose. Single-dose kinetics with respect to BZDs is governed mainly by the distribution of the agent in particular body compartments (e.g., blood, CNS lipids, or lipid stores outside the CNS). The elimination $t\frac{1}{2}$ of a BZD becomes important only after *repeated* dosing. Single-dose kinetics applies in situations such as a single night's treatment of insomnia or jet lag, emergency treatment of alcohol withdrawal, status epilepticus, preoperative sedation, and induction of anesthesia (Arana and Hyman 1991; Greenblatt 1991). (See the discussion on "Drug-Drug Interactions" that follows [antacid-BZD interaction].)

∎ Main Side Effects

Q. What are the most common BZD side effects and their frequency?

A. BZD side effects tend to be extensions of their sedative properties (e.g., drowsiness or light-headedness). Using lorazepam as a prototypical agent, one might expect the following common side effect frequency: sedation (15.9%), dizziness (6.9%), weakness (4.2%), and unsteadiness (3.4%) (Physicians' Desk Reference 1996). For alprazolam, a triazolo-BZD, the *placebo-adjusted* rate of side effects is as follows: drowsiness (19.4%), hypotension (2.5%), increased salivation (1.8%), dry mouth (1.4%), light-headedness (1.5%), and dizziness (1%). It is important to note that some side effects actually occur more frequently in the placebo group than in the BZD group; thus, side effects reported *less frequently* in the alprazolam group ($n = 565$) than in the placebo group ($n = 505$) include depression, headache, confusion, insomnia, nervousness, constipation, diarrhea, tachycardia, rigidity, and tremor (Physicians' Desk Reference 1996). With the hypnotic agent, quazepam, placebo-adjusted side effects were as follows: daytime drowsiness (8.7%), headache (2.3%), and fatigue (1.9%) (Physicians' Desk Reference 1996). (See also Table 3–11.)

Q. What effects do BZDs have on memory, and do these differ among agents?

A. All BZDs may cause varying degrees of memory impairment. If we divide memory into several components—*acquisition, retention, consolidation,* and *retrieval*—it is clear that BZDs impair memory at the level of consolidation (i.e., when data are transferred from short- to long-term memory [American Psychiatric Association 1990]). Thus, a person who has taken a BZD will recall something told to him or her after 1–2 minutes but will be unable to recall this information after 15–20 minutes. Anterograde amnesia associated with BZDs (difficulty in learning material presented after drug administration) may be seen even after a single oral dose of a BZD and is not correlated with degree of psychomotor impairment and sedation (Roache and Griffiths 1985). Some data suggest that high-potency, short $t\frac{1}{2}$ BZDs (e.g., triazolam) impair memory *more* than comparable therapeutic doses of low-potency, short $t\frac{1}{2}$ agents (e.g., oxazepam) (American Psychiatric Association 1990; Scharf et al. 1987). It should be borne in mind, however, that even over-the-counter sedative-hypnotics—mainly antihistamines—also can impair memory, probably via their anticholinergic effects. (Elderly or dementia patients may show persistent cognitive deficits in some cases [Pies 1992].)

Q. Isn't the hypnotic agent quazepam (Doral), which acts selectively on BZD_1 receptors, less likely to affect memory and cognitive function than are other nonselective BZDs?

A. It has been hypothesized that BZD_1 receptors in the brain are primarily involved in sleep induction, whereas BZD_2 receptors are thought to affect cognitive, memory, and motor functions (Ayd 1995). Quazepam has preferential affinity for BZD_1 receptors and may be less likely to affect memory than other BZDs (Wamsley and Hunt 1991). However, quazepam has two metabolites—2-oxoquazepam (OQ) and N-desalkyl-2-oxoquazepam (DOQ). The latter is *chemically identical* to desalkylflurazepam, the major metabolite of flurazepam (Dalmane), a BZD that may produce carryover sedation in some patients. DOQ is *not* selective for the BZD_1 receptor (Ayd 1995). Nevertheless, at least one study (Dement 1991) found that quazepam at doses of 15 mg or 30 mg produced less daytime somnolence and fewer psychomotor performance decrements than did flurazepam (15 mg or 30 mg hs).

Q. What is the abuse liability of BZDs?

A. This question is almost always a source of controversy among mental health professionals, depending on their philosophy and background (Pies 1991). Clinicians with a "12-step" orientation sometimes take the view that BZDs are widely abused and discourage their long-term use. Certainly, this concern is warranted with respect to individuals with either a personal or family history of alcohol/substance abuse. Actual BZD abuse seems to occur primarily in persons who abuse other drugs (Schweizer et al. 1995). Compared with other drugs of abuse, the reinforcing properties of BZDs appear to be fairly low in nonaddict populations. There is some evidence suggesting that diazepam—and perhaps alprazolam and lorazepam—is more likely to be abused than other BZDs in at-risk populations (Griffiths and Wolf 1990;

Schweizer et al. 1995). For example, anecdotal data suggest that alprazolam is the preferred agent for self-medication of cocaine "crashes" (C. A. Pearlman, personal communication, February 1997). In contrast, oxazepam, halazepam, and possibly chlordiazepoxide have a relatively low abuse potential (Griffiths and Wolf 1990). Keep in mind that *abuse liability* as determined by clinical studies of euphoria and interviews with addicted individuals is not necessarily related to *actual rates of abuse.* The latter term has to do with overall availability of a drug, its cost on the street, and other factors. Thus, although lorazepam and alprazolam constitute a small percentage of illicit drug traffic, they may still have a high abuse potential for a given individual (Griffiths and Wolf 1990). The bottom line is that BZDs should be used very conservatively, if at all, in patients with known histories of substance abuse and/or dependence and only when other alternatives (such as a sedating antidepressant) have been exhausted.

Q. What is the abuse liability of BZDs in relatives of substance/alcohol abusers?

A. Several studies now indicate that subjective response to alprazolam and diazepam differs in subjects who have first-degree relatives with alcoholism versus subjects who do not. Thus, Ciraulo et al. (1996) have found that both the sons and daughters of alcoholic individuals have "positive mood responses" to alprazolam more often than control subjects, despite similar alprazolam plasma levels. Ciraulo et al. (1996) conclude that these data are consistent with greater risk of alprazolam (and possibly ethanol) abuse in the siblings of alcoholic patients, although the siblings did not have alcohol abuse or dependence.

Q. Do the BZDs differ in their tendency to produce discontinuation/withdrawal syndromes?

A. Although controlled research studies are lacking, The American Psychiatric Association Task Force Report *Benzodiazepine Dependence, Toxicity, and Abuse* (1990) noted that "anecdotal reports and clinical experience . . . have increasingly noted severe discontinuance with the high-potency, short half-life benzodiazepines alprazolam, lorazepam, and triazolam . . . there have also been suggestions that high-potency, short half-life benzodiazepines have been associated with a higher incidence of seizures following abrupt withdrawal" (p. 30). Thus, discontinuation should be very gradual with these agents.

Q. What are the main symptoms of BZD withdrawal, and how are they managed?

A. Discontinuation of BZDs may result in *recurrence* or *relapse* symptoms (return of the original symptoms for which BZDs were prescribed), *rebound* symptoms (symptoms such as anxiety or insomnia that are *more intense* than at baseline), and true *withdrawal* symptoms (probably representing the reaction of the CNS to loss of GABA) (Jenkins and Hansen 1995; Shader and Greenblatt 1994a). These three types of symptoms often can be difficult to distinguish in a given patient. However, a study of diazepam discontinuation (Pourmotabbed et al. 1996) found that discontinuation of clinical doses produced *rebound anxiety* rather than physical withdrawal symptoms in women with GAD. Most of these rebound symptoms (anxiety, insomnia, GI symptoms) were mild and transient. Withdrawal symptoms can include anxiety, agitation, tachycardia, palpitations, anorexia, blurred vision, muscle cramps, insomnia, nightmares, hyperacusis (increased sensitivity to noise), and seizures (Ayd 1995; Jenkins and Hansen 1995). Although various non-BZD agents have been used to manage BZD withdrawal (e.g., phenobarbital, carbamazepine), the best approach is to avoid the syndrome in the first place by very slow tapering of

BZDs—particularly short-acting agents (Shader and Greenblatt 1994a). One approach is the "quarter per week" method, in which the daily dose of alprazolam, for example, is reduced by 25% once per week. Thus, a patient taking 4 mg/day alprazolam would reduce the daily dose to 3 mg in week 1, 2 mg in week 2, 1 mg in week 3, then discontinue it completely (Shader and Greenblatt 1994a). However, this discontinuation in week 4 may be too abrupt for many patients, and the last 0.5–1 mg of alprazolam may be particularly difficult to discontinue. Thus, extending the tapering schedule to 6–8 weeks, with very small decrements, may be necessary (Shader and Greenblatt 1994a).

Q. If tolerance develops in a patient with periodic leg movements of sleep who has been treated successfully with a BZD (e.g., clonazepam), what is the best management strategy?

A. Tolerance to clonazepam has been reported to develop over a period of about 6 months (Nofzinger and Reynolds 1996). An increase in clonazepam dose (e.g., from 1 to 1.5 mg hs) could be tried, but tolerance may occur fairly rapidly on this higher dose. The use of L-dopa/carbidopa (25-mg/100-mg strength, with upward titration as appropriate) may be a good alternative for periodic leg movements of sleep and "restless leg syndrome" (Nofzinger and Reynolds 1996). An alternative is a 1-month "clonazepam holiday" every 6 months to prevent occurrence of tolerance in the first place (C. A. Pearlman, personal communication, February 1997). Of course, sudden discontinuation of any BZD should be avoided.

▌ Drug-Drug Interactions

Q. What are the most common and serious drug-drug interactions involving BZDs?

A. The most common and serious drug-drug interactions occur with alcohol and other sedative-hypnotics (American Psychiatric Association 1990), often producing severe CNS toxicity and/or respiratory suppression. BZDs also augment the euphoric effects of opiates. Finally, the sedating effects of BZDs may mask the early warning signs of tricyclic antidepressant toxicity (Beresford et al. 1981; Sands et al. 1995).

Q. Is there a clinically significant decrement in the effectiveness of BZDs when antacids are taken simultaneously?

A. With the exception of single-dose treatment, the basic answer is no. Although antacids may slow the *rate* of BZD absorption, the *completeness* of absorption and resultant steady-state concentration are not affected. However, because slowed absorption may affect subjective antianxiety effects, use of a BZD with an antacid may be undesirable if the patient requires rapid onset of anxiolytic action. It is also possible that somewhat lower plasma levels (due to slowed absorption) may decrease efficacy in some patients (Creelman et al. 1989).

Q. What is the effect of taking BZDs with food?

A. As with the use of antacids, food delays absorption of BZDs without diminishing completeness of absorption (area under the curve when one plots plasma level of the drug versus time). When rapid anxiolysis is necessary, BZDs should be taken on an empty stomach (Creelman et al. 1989).

Q. How important is protein-binding displacement (e.g., by warfarin-type anticoagulants) when treating a patient with BZDs?

A. Although heparin can cause a rapid rise in the free fraction of diazepam, this rise is probably transient and rapidly compensated for by increased exposure of the BZD to hepatic metabolism. Thus, such interactions are unlikely to be of enduring clinical significance (Ayd 1995; Sands et al. 1995).

Q. What are the risks of combining BZDs and clozapine?

A. Severe sedation, delirium, and respiratory arrest have been reported with the combination of BZDs and clozapine (Ayd 1995), although such extreme reactions appear to be rare. Indeed, Meltzer (1995) notes that "reliable evidence for a negative interaction between clozapine and benzodiazepines is very slight" (p. 1280) and further notes that "benzodiazepines are sometimes useful in diminishing anxiety when initiating clozapine treatment"(p. 1280). Adverse reactions seem to occur within 1–2 days of starting high doses of clozapine in patients taking long-acting BZDs (Ayd 1995; Grohmann et al. 1989). In my experience, initiation of low-dose benzodiazepine treatment (e.g., 0.25–0.5 mg clonazepam or the equivalent) is usually tolerated in otherwise healthy patients taking moderate doses of clozapine (250–400 mg/day). However, vital signs should be monitored for the first week or so of treatment, and the rationale for using BZDs (as well as known risks) should be documented clearly in the medical record.

Q. Which antidepressants are best to avoid when prescribing concomitant BZDs?

A. As previously mentioned, the CYP3A4 and CYP2C19 systems appear to be primarily involved in BZD metabolism. The triazolo-BZDs—alprazolam, midazolam, and triazolam—as well as clonazepam are metabolized via CYP3A4. Diazepam has a complex route of demethylation, involving both CYP2C19 and CYP3A4 (Sands et al. 1995). Thus, antidepressants that are *strong* inhibitors of CYP3A4 (e.g., nefazodone) or CYP2C19 (e.g., fluvoxamine) should be used with caution when BZDs are coadministered (Preskorn 1996; Shader et al. 1996). Keep in mind, however, that norfluoxetine (the active metabolite of fluoxetine), sertraline and its metabolite desmethylsertraline, and fluvoxamine can all have *moderate* degrees of inhibition on CYP3A4 (Shader et al. 1996). In contrast, venlafaxine appears to have little effect on CYP3A4 or CYP2C9 (Shader et al. 1996); its effects on CYP2C19 are not yet known. Finally, keep in mind that increased imipramine and desipramine (but not nortriptyline) levels may be seen with concomitant alprazolam administration. Amitriptyline may increase psychomotor effects of BZDs (Sands et al. 1995).

Q. What about specific SSRIs interacting with BZDs?

A. It appears from in vivo studies that fluoxetine and fluvoxamine are likely to *increase* diazepam and alprazolam levels. Fluoxetine can elevate levels of both these BZDs 25%–50%, whereas fluvoxamine can lead to increases of these BZDs from 100%–300% (Preskorn 1996). Comparable in vivo studies have not yet been carried out with sertraline and paroxetine (Preskorn 1996).

Q. What drug-drug interactions can occur with buspirone?

A. Buspirone and MAOI combinations (according to the manufacturer of buspirone) may lead to hypertension; thus, a 2-week washout should follow discontinuation of an MAOI before initiating buspirone. Buspirone has been implicated in cases of serotonin syndrome (see Chapter 1). Buspirone also may result in increased haloperidol levels (Kaplan et al. 1995).

Q. What is the preferred method of switching someone from a BZD to buspirone?

A. Because buspirone is not cross-reactive with BZDs, BZD withdrawal symptoms may occur during the switch unless the BZD is slowly tapered. Most clinicians would add buspirone to the BZD regimen, stabilize the dose of buspirone, then gradually taper the BZD (Arana and Hyman 1991; Schatzberg and Cole 1991). Remember that some patients who have taken BZDs for many years may not experience much subjective relief from buspirone and will require several months to be weaned from the BZD. Other patients may need to be maintained indefinitely on a small BZD dose in combination with buspirone.

▮ Potentiating Maneuvers

Q. Is it useful to combine buspirone with a BZD in cases of GAD or panic disorder?

A. Some small-sample reports suggest improvement when buspirone is added to a BZD (Cole and Yonkers 1995; Udelman and Udelman 1990). Thus, although buspirone does *not* block BZD withdrawal symptoms, it may reduce anxiety in patients undergoing withdrawal from alprazolam (Udelman and Udelman 1990). Gastfriend and Rosenbaum (1989) also described four patients with panic disorder, incompletely controlled on BZDs, who had reduced *generalized* and *anticipatory anxiety* after the addition of buspirone.

Q. Can BZDs be used to potentiate the primary effects of mood stabilizers and antidepressants?

A. BZDs are routinely used in combination with mood stabilizers in the treatment of manic patients, and BZD hypnotic agents are often recommended for insomniac bipolar patients taking lithium (Lenox and Manji 1995). BZDs are important adjunctive agents in the management of acute mania (see Chapter 4). The issue of BZDs in depression is less clear.

Fawcett (1990) has found that in patients with major depression and severe anxiety, "aggressive treatment with a benzodiazepine anxiolytic is indicated for immediate relief of anxiety" (p. 42) because antidepressants may take 3–6 weeks to reach peak effectiveness. Fawcett (1990) further states, "the rapid action of benzodiazepines in relieving symptoms of anxiety increases the likelihood that the patient will continue therapy long enough to feel the effects of the antidepressant. As the antidepressant becomes fully effective, benzodiazepine therapy may be discontinued in slowly tapered doses" (p. 42). Similarly, in patients with comorbid panic disorder and depressive symptoms, Coplan and Gorman (1990) note that relief of panic is usually more rapid (1–2 weeks) with the concomitant use of a high-potency BZD and an antidepressant as compared with an antidepressant alone (4–6 weeks). On the other hand, several BZDs may have pharmacokinetic interactions with antidepressants such as fluoxetine and nefazodone (see previous discussion on "Drug-Drug Interactions" [specific SSRIs that interact with BZDs] and Table 3–13), and BZDs may sometimes worsen depression or increase antidepressant side effects. Thus, I prefer to begin treatment of the anxious, depressed patient with a *single agent* possessing both anxiolytic/hypnotic and antidepressant properties, if possible. Nefazodone appears to be a good candidate in this respect (Zajecka 1995). Use of an SSRI may sometimes necessitate use of a BZD at bedtime, but, ideally, BZD use should be tapered and discontinued within the first few weeks of treatment. The patient should also understand at the outset that the BZD is a temporary measure.

Q. Do BZDs potentiate the effects of antipsychotic agents?

A. BZDs as either sole or adjunctive agents in psychotic patients may ameliorate superimposed anxiety, auditory hallucinations, and perhaps negative symptoms in a few schizophrenic patients; however, sedation, ataxia, and cognitive impairment may occur (Janicak et al. 1993). A number of BZDs (lorazepam, clonazepam, diazepam) have proved useful in catatonic patients, including some with catatonic schizophrenia (Martenyi et al. 1989; see also Chapter 2). BZD augmentation of neuroleptics may help control agitation during exacerbations of schizophrenia (Tueth et al. 1995); however, some psychotic patients may experience increased arousal or aggression when treated with BZDs (Arana et al. 1986; Janicak et al. 1993).

∎ Use in Special Populations

Q. What are the teratogenic and behavioral risks to the fetus during exposure to BZDs in utero? What about buspirone?

A. In the 1970s and 1980s, diazepam (Valium) was found to be associated with cleft lip and palate in the fetus, and other BZDs were suspected of this association. One Swedish group (Laegreid et al. 1992) has linked maternal use of BZDs during pregnancy with both impaired intrauterine growth and various dysmorphic birth defects. A recent review (Altshuler et al. 1996) concluded that the available data "indicate a positive association between first-trimester in utero exposure to benzodiazepines and a specific anomaly, oral cleft" (p. 598). Diazepam may double the risk of oral cleft, whereas alprazolam may increase the risk by more than 11-fold. However, most available data suggest that BZDs do not markedly increase the *absolute risk* of cleft palate or other congenital abnormalities in exposed fetuses. Thus, the baseline risk of cleft palate is about 6 in 10,000. With alprazolam exposure during the first trimester, the risk may rise to 7 in 1,000—still less than 1 in 100 (Altshuler et al. 1996). The teratogenicity of lorazepam (Ativan) is less clear. Clonazepam (Klonopin) has not been evaluated for teratogenesis in controlled studies of human subjects; however, based on animal data, clonazepam seems to have low teratogenic potential (Altshuler et al. 1996). The presence of alcohol and other substance abuse in pregnant women using BZDs complicates interpretation of the data. Infants exposed to BZDs either in the last trimester or at the time of parturition may show muscular hypotonicity, failure to feed, impaired temperature regulation, apnea, and low Apgar scores. The data on "behavioral teratogenicity" and developmental delay are inconclusive (Altshuler et al. 1996). There is also some evidence that BZDs may increase duration of labor and lead to prolonged withdrawal symptoms in the neonate when mothers have been maintained on these agents throughout pregnancy. Withdrawal effects may be more likely when high doses of short-acting BZDs have been used. BZDs should not be stopped suddenly during pregnancy but rather tapered slowly as delivery approaches (Stowe and Nemeroff 1995).

The non-BZD anxiolytic buspirone (BuSpar) has been shown to increase the number of stillbirths in rats when given in high doses; however, there are insufficient data in humans to determine the risks of buspirone during pregnancy.

Q. Given the above risks, are BZDs contraindicated during pregnancy?

A. There is no absolute contraindication; rather, the modest risks of BZD exposure must be weighed against the severity of the patient's condition, the risks of no medication, and the risks of alternative medications. For example, inadequately treated panic attacks may themselves pose a risk to the fetus (Cohen et al. 1989). Tricyclic antidepressants or fluoxetine (and perhaps other SSRIs) may be reasonable alternatives to BZDs for the treatment of panic disorder during pregnancy (see Chapter 1). Cognitive-behavior therapy also may be helpful in a variety of anxiety disorders and may reduce the need for psychotropics during pregnancy (Altshuler et al. 1996).

Q. What are the risks of breast-feeding when the nursing mother is taking a BZD?

A. Although there is evidence that several BZDs (e.g., diazepam, lorazepam, oxazepam) are excreted into breast milk, the actual levels of BZDs detected in breast milk seem to be fairly low and the consequent risk to the infant seems to be quite small (McElhatton 1994; Pons et al. 1994). Lorazepam seems to have minimal accumulation in the fetus, and the percentage of the maternal dose of lorazepam to which a nursing infant is exposed is roughly 2.2% (Summerfield and Nielsen 1985). Thus, use of low-dose lorazepam in the nursing mother—particularly on a prn or short-term basis—is probably safe for the infant. The excretion of buspirone into human breast milk has not been adequately studied.

Q. What are the risks of falls and fractures in elderly patients treated with BZDs?

A. BZD use seems to increase the risk of falls among elderly patients from one and a half to three times over baseline, with a 60% increase in risk of femur fracture (Gelenberg 1996; Herings et al. 1995). There is some controversy as to whether these effects are more likely with *long-acting* BZDs. Although such risk was found in some studies (e.g., Ray et al. 1989), Herings et al. (1995) found that short $t_{1/2}$ BZDs were actually associated with a slightly *greater* risk for falls and fractures than long-acting agents. Risk was increased further when short- and long-acting agents were used together. *Sudden increases* in BZD dose, and total dose, were more important in predicting falls than the pharmacokinetics of the agent.

Q. What are the risks of respiratory suppression when using BZDs in patients with chronic lung or other respiratory problems? Are other agents preferable for treating anxiety in these populations?

A. Although early reports suggested that BZDs may actually improve dyspnea in patients with chronic obstructive pulmonary disease (COPD), other reports have shown that BZDs may depress respiration and worsen carbon dioxide (CO_2) retention in these populations (Smoller 1996). In general, BZDs should be used conservatively in patients with COPD, with shorter-acting agents preferable. Preliminary data from Smoller (1996) suggest that sertraline has a beneficial effect on dyspnea and overall well-being in COPD patients and is effective for treatment of panic attacks. (There also is some evidence that serotonergic agents may block panic attacks by decreasing CO_2 sensitivity [Klein 1993].) Although buspirone is not effective for panic attacks, it may be useful in COPD patients with generalized anxiety and does not reduce ventilatory drive (Garner et al. 1989; Smoller 1996).

Vignettes and Puzzlers

Q. Lorazepam has an elimination $t_{1/2}$ of about 10 hours. Diazepam has an elimination $t_{1/2}$ exceeding 50 hours, if the effects of its metabolite desmethyldiazepam are included. An acutely psychotic patient in the emergency room is given 1 mg lorazepam orally, becomes less agitated, and remains so for about 4 hours. Another acutely psychotic, agitated patient is given an equipotent dose of oral diazepam (5 mg), becomes less agitated, but remains so for only 2 hours. Given the elimination $t_{1/2}$s of these agents, how do you account for these findings?

A. Clinical effects after single doses of BZDs are not related to elimination $t_{1/2}$s but to the lipophilicity and volume of distribution of the agent (see previous discussion on "Pharmacokinetics" [relationship between how lipophilic a BZD is and onset of clinical action]). Diazepam, which is highly lipophilic, rapidly crosses the blood-brain barrier and produces its clinical effect. However, diazepam is rapidly "sucked" from the CNS lipids into extra-CNS lipids (e.g., in the thighs)—often a very large volume of distribution. This translocation rapidly terminates the *single-dose* effect of diazepam. In contrast, lorazepam is less lipophilic, takes slightly longer to have its clinical effect, but also has a smaller volume of distribution. Lorazepam is thus longer acting than diazepam after a single oral dose (Arana and Hyman 1991; Greenblatt 1993). These factors become less important after chronic dosing, during which diazepam, for example, generates a long-acting, less lipophilic metabolite (desmethyl-diazepam).

Q. A 73-year-old woman living in a nursing home had been successfully treated for major depression with 300 mg/day nefazodone. Her one residual symptom was significant initial insomnia, for which her physician added triazolam 0.25 mg hs. When the patient awakened at 3 A.M.—two nights after initiation of the triazolam—the nursing staff reported that she was "totally out of it," disoriented to place and date, as well as ataxic and dysarthric. What is the likely explanation?

A. Nefazodone is an inhibitor of the CYP3A4 system, which metabolizes the triazolo-BZDs. It is likely that the nefazodone raised plasma levels of the triazolam, which is itself associated with confusional states in older patients. There also may have been pharmacodynamic synergism between the nefazodone (which can cause dose-related cognitive impairment in some elderly patients) and the triazolam (Gelenberg 1995; van Laar et al. 1995).

Q. A 70-year-old man was taking L-dopa and benztropine to control his parkinsonism. Because he complained of acute situational anxiety, 50 mg/day chlordiazepoxide was prescribed. The patient's parkinsonism worsened significantly 2 days later. What is the likely mechanism?

A. Most likely, the GABA agonist effect of BZDs reduces dopaminergic outflow in the basal ganglia, interfering with the effects of L-dopa (Sands et al. 1995; Yosselson-Superstine and Lipman 1982).

Q. A 35-year-old woman with panic disorder had been maintained for 1 year on alprazolam 1 mg po tid. Over the past 3 weeks, the patient had begun to use more alprazolam, on a more frequent basis, to control breakthrough panic attacks. Her psychiatrist decided to switch her to the longer-acting agent, clonazepam, with an initial dose of 0.75 mg bid (one-half the total prescribed dose of alprazolam). After 2 weeks, the patient's panic attacks were well controlled on clonazepam alone. However, she began to complain of increasing depression. Why?

A. Most patients appear to tolerate the alprazolam-to-clonazepam switch quite well (Herman et al. 1987); however, there is some evidence that clonazepam may induce depression more often than alprazolam (Janicak et al. 1993). Thus, Cohen and Rosenbaum (1987) reported that 5.5% of clonazepam-treated patients developed depression versus only 0.7% of patients taking alprazolam. Alprazolam also may have intrinsic antidepressant properties, and for this patient, alprazolam may have been treating an undiagnosed, comorbid depressive disorder.

Q. A 25-year-old man with panic disorder has been stable on 1 mg bid clonazepam. He has a manic episode and is placed on 200 mg tid carbamazepine, with resultant plasma levels of 8 µg/mL (therapeutic = 5–12 µg/mL). The patient's manic symptoms abate after 1 week, but his panic disorder worsens. What is the mechanism?

A. Carbamazepine is a powerful inducer of hepatic metabolism and is known to decrease clonazepam levels by as much as 37% (Creelman et al. 1989). When these drugs are coadministered, some patients may need an upward adjustment of their clonazepam dose.

Q. A patient with chronic alcohol abuse and dependence successfully maintained with 250 mg/day disulfiram complains of "leg muscle spasms" that interfere with his sleep. A polysomnogram confirms the presence of nocturnal myoclonus (periodic leg movements of sleep). A trial on valproate is attempted, but the patient cannot tolerate the GI side effects. Chlordiazepoxide 25 mg hs is prescribed, with good control of the periodic leg movements of sleep on the first and second nights. By the third night, however, the patient complains of feeling "groggy" and "hungover." What is the problem and what is a possible alternative treatment?

A. Disulfiram inhibits metabolism of oxidatively metabolized BZDs (see Table 3–13), leading in this case to increased levels of chlordiazepoxide. Use of short-acting BZDs that undergo glucuronidation (lorazepam, oxazepam) may be a viable option (Creelman et al. 1989; Sands et al. 1995).

▮ References

Abernethy DR, Greenblatt DJ, Divoll M, et al: Impairment of diazepam metabolism by low-dose estrogen-containing oral contraceptive steroids. N Engl J Med 306:791–792, 1982

Abernethy DR, Greenblatt DJ, Eshelman FN, et al: Ranitidine does not impair oxidative or conjugative metabolism: noninteraction with antipyrine, diazepam and lorazepam. Clin Pharmacol Ther 35:188–192, 1984

Altshuler LL, Cohen L, Szuba MP, et al: Pharmacologic management of psychiatric illness during pregnancy: dilemmas and guidelines. Am J Psychiatry 153:592–606, 1996

American Psychiatric Association: Diagnostic and Statistical Manual of Mental Disorders, 3rd Edition, Revised. Washington, DC, American Psychiatric Association, 1987

American Psychiatric Association: Benzodiazepine Dependence, Toxicity, and Abuse: A Task Force Report of the American Psychiatric Association. American Psychiatric Association, Washington, DC, 1990

Arana GW, Hyman SE: Handbook of Psychiatric Drug Therapy, 2nd Edition. Boston, Little, Brown, 1991

Arana GW, Ornsteen ML, Kanter F, et al: The use of benzodiazepines for psychotic disorders: a literature review and preliminary clinical findings. Psychopharmacol Bull 22:77–87, 1986

Ayd FJ: Lexicon of Psychiatry, Neurology, and the Neurosciences. Baltimore, MD, Williams & Wilkins, 1995

Ballenger JC: Benzodiazepines, in The American Psychiatric Press Textbook of Psychopharmacology. Edited by Schatzberg AF, Nemeroff CB. Washington, DC, American Psychiatric Press, 1995, pp 215–230

Beresford TP, Feinsilver DL, Hall RC: Adverse reactions to a benzodiazepine-tricyclic antidepressant compound. J Clin Psychopharmacol 1:392–394, 1981

Bradwejn J, Shriqui C, Koszycki D, et al: Double-blind comparison of the effects of clonazepam and lorazepam in acute mania. J Clin Psychopharmacol 10:403–408, 1990

Braun P, Greenberg D, Dasberg H, et al: Core symptoms of posttraumatic stress disorder unimproved by alprazolam treatment. J Clin Psychiatry 51:236–238, 1990

Charney DS, Heninger GR: Noradrenergic function and the mechanism of action of antianxiety treatment, I: the effect of long-term alprazolam treatment. Arch Gen Psychiatry 42:458–467, 1985

Chouinard G: Clonazepam in the acute and maintenance treatment of bipolar affective disorder. J Clin Psychiatry 48 (suppl 10): 29–36, 1987

Ciraulo DA, Shader RI, Ciraulo AM, et al: Alcoholism and its treatment, in Manual of Psychiatric Therapeutics, 2nd Edition. Edited by Shader RI. Boston, Little, Brown, 1994, pp 181–210

Ciraulo DA, Sarid-Segal O, Knapp C, et al: Liability to alprazolam abuse in daughters of alcoholics. Am J Psychiatry 153:956–958, 1996

Cobb CD, Anderson CB, Seidel D: Possible interaction between clozapine and lorazepam. Am J Psychiatry 148:1606–1607, 1991

Cohen LS, Rosenbaum JF: Clonazepam: new uses and potential problems. J Clin Psychiatry 48 (suppl 10):50–55, 1987

Cohen LS, Rosenbaum J, Heller VL: Panic attack-associated placental abruption: a case report. J Clin Psychiatry 50:266–267, 1989

Cole JO, Yonkers KA: Nonbenzodiazepine anxiolytics, in The American Psychiatric Press Textbook of Psychopharmacology. Edited by Schatzberg AF, Nemeroff CB. Washington, DC, American Psychiatric Press, 1995, pp 231–244

Coplan JD, Gorman JM: Treatment of anxiety disorder in patients with mood disorders. J Clin Psychiatry 51 (suppl):9–13, 1990

Cornish JW, McNicholas LF, O'Brien CP: Treatment of substance-related disorders, in The American Psychiatric Press Textbook of Psychopharmacology. Edited by Schatzberg AF, Nemeroff CB. Washington, DC, American Psychiatric Press, 1995, pp 707–724

Creelman W, Sands BF, Ciraulo DA: Benzodiazepines, in Drug Interactions in Psychiatry. Edited by Ciraulo DA, Shader RI, Greenblatt DJ, et al. Baltimore, MD, Williams & Wilkins, 1989, pp 158–180

Davidson JRT, Ford SM, Smith RD, et al: Long-term treatment of social phobia with clonazepam. J Clin Psychiatry 51:16–20, 1991

Dement WC: Objective measurements of daytime sleepiness and performance comparing quazepam with flurazepam in two adult populations using the multiple sleep latency test. J Clin Psychiatry 52 (suppl):31–37, 1991

Drug Facts and Comparisons. St. Louis, MO, Facts and Comparisons, 1995

Dubovsky SL: Geriatric neuropsychopharmacology, in The American Psychiatric Press Textbook of Geriatric Neuropsychiatry. Edited by Coffey CE, Cummings JL. Washington, DC, American Psychiatric Press, 1994, pp 596–631

Dulcan MK, Bregman JD, Weller EB, et al: Treatment of childhood and adolescent disorders, in The American Psychiatric Press Textbook of Psychopharmacology. Edited by Schatzberg AF, Nemeroff CB. Washington, DC, American Psychiatric Press, 1995, pp 669–706

Eison MS: Serotonin: a common neurobiologic substrate in anxiety and depression. J Clin Psychopharmacol 10 (suppl):26–30, 1990

Ellinwood EH, Easter ME, Linoilla M, et al: Effects of oral contraceptives on diazepam-induced psychomotor impairment. Clin Pharmacol Ther 35:360–366, 1984

Fawcett J: Targeting treatment in patients with mixed symptoms of anxiety and depression. J Clin Psychiatry 51 (suppl):40–43, 1990

Feighner JP: Benzodiazepines as antidepressants: a triazolobenzo-diazepine used to treat depression, in Modern Problems of Pharmacopsychiatry, Vol 18. Edited by Ban TA, Hollender MH. Basel, Switzerland, S Karger, 1982, pp 196–212

Feldmann TB: Alprazolam in the treatment of post-traumatic stress disorder. J Clin Psychiatry 48:216–217, 1987

Gardos G, Cole JO: The treatment of tardive dyskinesia, in Psycho-pharmacology: The Fourth Generation of Progress. Edited by Bloom FE, Kupfer DJ. New York, Raven, 1995, pp 1503–1511

Garner SJ, Eldridge FL, Wagner PG, et al: Buspirone, an anxiolytic drug that stimulates respiration. American Review of Respiratory Disease 139:946–950, 1989

Garza-Trevino ES, Hollister LE, Overall JE, et al: Efficacy of combinations of intramuscular antipsychotics and sedative-hypnotics for control of psychotic agitation. Am J Psychiatry 146:1598–1601, 1989

Gastfriend DR, Rosenbaum JF: Adjunctive buspirone in benzodiazepine treatment of four patients with panic disorder. Am J Psychiatry 146:914–916, 1989

Gelenberg A: The P450 family. Biological Therapies in Psychiatry Newsletter 18:29–31, 1995

Gelenberg A: Benzodiazepine use and hip fractures in the elderly. Biological Therapies in Psychiatry Newsletter 19:3, 1996

Greenblatt DJ: Benzodiazepine hypnotics: sorting the pharmacokinetic facts. J Clin Psychiatry 52 (suppl):4–10, 1991

Greenblatt DJ: Basic pharmacokinetic principles and their application to psychotropic drugs. J Clin Psychiatry 54 (suppl):8–13, 1993

Griffiths RR, Wolf B: Relative abuse liability of different benzodiazepines in drug abusers. J Clin Psychopharmacol 10:237–243, 1990

Grohmann R, Ruther E, Sassim N, et al: Adverse effects of clozapine. Psychopharmacology 99 (suppl):101–104, 1989

Herings RMC, Stricker BHC, de Boer A, et al: Benzodiazepines and the risk of falling leading to femur fractures: dosage more important than elimination half-life. Arch Intern Med 155:1801–1807, 1995

Herman JB, Rosenbaum JF, Brotman AW: The alprazolam to clonazepam switch for the treatment of panic disorder. J Clin Psychopharmacol 7:175–178, 1987

Hewlett WA, Vinogradov S, Agras WS: Clonazepam treatment of obsessions and compulsions. J Clin Psychiatry 51:158–161, 1990

Hollister LE, Muller-Oerlinghausen, Rickels K, et al: Clinical uses of benzodiazepines. J Clin Psychopharmacol 13 (suppl 1):1–169, 1993

Horrigan JP, Barnhill LJ: The suppression of nightmares with guanfacine (letter). J Clin Psychiatry 57:371, 1996

Jackson CW, Pitner JK, Mintzer JE: Zolpidem for the treatment of agitation in elderly demented patients (letter). J Clin Psychiatry 57:372–373, 1996

Janicak PG, Davis JM, Preskorn SH, et al: Principles and Practice of Psychopharmacotherapy. Baltimore, MD, Williams & Wilkins, 1993

Jenkins SC, Hansen MR: A Pocket Reference for Psychiatrists, 2nd Edition. Washington, DC, American Psychiatric Press, 1995

Jonas JM, Hearron AE: Alprazolam and suicidal ideation: a meta-analysis of controlled trials in the treatment of depression. J Clin Psychopharmacol 16:208–211, 1996

Kaplan HI, Sadock BJ, Grebb JA (eds): Synopsis of Psychiatry, 7th Edition. Baltimore, MD, Williams & Wilkins, 1994

Kishimoto A, Kamata K, Sugihara T, et al: Treatment of depression with clonazepam. Acta Psychiatr Scand 77:81–86, 1988

Klein DF: False suffocation alarms, spontaneous panics, and related conditions: an integrative hypothesis. Arch Gen Psychiatry 50:306–317, 1993

Klerman GL: The use of benzodiazepines in the treatment of depression. International Drug Therapy Newsletter 21:37–38, 1986

Koczerginski D, Kennedy SH, Swinson RP: Clonazepam and lithium: a toxic combination in treatment of mania? Int Clin Psychopharmacol 4:195–199, 1989

Laegreid L, Hagberg G, Lundberg A: The effect of benzodiazepines on the fetus and the newborn. Neuropediatrics 23:18–23, 1992

Lenox RH, Manji HK: Lithium, in The American Psychiatric Press Textbook of Psychopharmacology. Edited by Schatzberg AF, Nemeroff CB. Washington, DC, American Psychiatric Press, 1995, pp 303–349

Lenox RH, Newhouse PA, Creelman WL, et al: Adjunctive treatment of manic agitation with lorazepam versus haloperidol: a double blind study. J Clin Psychiatry 53:47–52, 1992

Martenyi F, Harangozo J, Laszlo M: Clonazepam for the treatment of catatonic schizophrenia (letter). Am J Psychiatry 146:1230, 1989

Maxmen JS: Psychotropic Drugs: Fast Facts. New York, WW Norton, 1991

McElhatton PR: The effects of benzodiazepine use during pregnancy and lactation. Reprod Toxicol 8:461–475, 1994

McElroy SL, Keck PE: Antiepileptic drugs, in The American Psychiatric Press Textbook of Psychopharmacology. Edited by Schatzberg AF, Nemeroff CB. Washington, DC, American Psychiatric Press, 1995, pp 351–375

Meltzer HY: Atypical antipsychotic drugs, in Psychopharmacology: The Fourth Generation of Progress. Edited by Bloom FE, Kupfer DJ. New York, Raven, 1995, pp 1277–1286

Nofzinger EA, Reynolds CF: Sleep impairment and daytime drowsiness in later life. Am J Psychiatry 153:941–943, 1996

Pagel JF: Disease, psychoactive medication, and sleep states. Primary Psychiatry 1:47–51, 1996

Paul SM: GABA and glycine, in Psychopharmacology: The Fourth Generation of Progress. Edited by Bloom FE, Kupfer DJ. New York, Raven, 1995, pp 87–94

Physicians' Desk Reference, 50th Edition. Montvale, NJ, Medical Economics, 1996

Pies R: Benzodiazepine abuse: how real, how serious? Psychiatric Times 8:13–14, 1991

Pies R: Halcion: is a balanced view possible? Psychiatric Times 8:28–30, 1992

Pies R: The azapirones: broad-spectrum psychotropics? Psychiatric Times 9:30–31, 1993

Pies R: Dose-related sensory distortions with zolpidem (letter). J Clin Psychiatry 66:35–36, 1995a

Pies R: Psychotropic medication during pregnancy and postpartum. Clinical Advances in the Treatment of Psychiatric Disorders 9:4–7, 1995b

Pies R, Parks A: Beta blockers in neuropsychiatry: an update. Horizon Physician Quarterly 2:1–10, 1996

Pies R, Weinberg AD: Quick Reference Guide to Geriatric Psychopharmacology. Branford, CT, American Medical Publishing, 1990

Pons G, Rey E, Matheson I: Excretion of psychoactive drugs into breast milk: pharmacokinetic principles and recommendations. Clin Pharmacokinet 27:270–289, 1994

Pourmotabbed T, McLeod DR, Hoehn-Saric R, et al: Treatment, discontinuation, and psychomotor effects of diazepam in women with generalized anxiety disorder. J Clin Psychopharmacol 16:202–207, 1996

Preskorn SH: Clinical Pharmacology of Selective Serotonin Reuptake Inhibitors. Caddo, OK, Professional Communications, 1996

Ray WA, Griffin MR, Downey M: Benzodiazepines of long and short elimination half-life and the risk of hip fracture. JAMA 262:3303–3307, 1989

Reich J, Noyes R, Yates W: Alprazolam treatment of avoidant personality traits in social phobic patients. J Clin Psychiatry 50:91–95, 1989

Rickels K, Case WG, Downing RW, et al: Long-term diazepam therapy and clinical outcome. JAMA 250:767–771, 1983

Rickels K, Amsterdam J, Clary C, et al: Buspirone in depressed outpatients: a controlled study. Psychopharmacol Bull 26:163–167, 1990

Roache JD, Griffiths RR: Comparison of triazolam and pentobarbital: performance impairment, subjective effects, and abuse liability. J Pharmacol Exp Ther 234:120–133, 1985

Sachs GS: Bipolar mood disorder: practical strategies for acute and maintenance phase treatment. J Clin Psychopharmacol 16 (suppl 1):32S–47S, 1996

Salzman C, Green AI, Rodriquez-Villa F, et al: Benzodiazepines combined with neuroleptics for management of severe disruptive behavior. Psychosomatics 27:17–21, 1986

Sands BF, Creelman WL, Ciraulo DA, et al: Benzodiazepines, in Drug Interactions in Psychiatry, 2nd Edition. Edited by Ciraulo DA, Shader RI, Greenblatt DJ, et al. Baltimore, MD, Williams & Wilkins, 1995, pp 214–248

Sarid-Segal O, Creelman WL, Shader RI: Lithium, in Drug Interactions in Psychiatry, 2nd Edition. Edited by Ciraulo DA, Shader RI, Greenblatt DJ, et al. Baltimore, MD, Williams & Wilkins, 1995, pp 175–213

Scavone JM, Greenblatt DJ, Shader RI: Alprazolam kinetics following sublingual and oral administration. J Clin Psychopharmacol 7:332–334, 1987

Scharf MB, Saskin P, Fletcher K: Benzodiazepine-induced amnesia: clinical laboratory findings. J Clin Psychiatry 5 (monogr ser):14–17, 1987

Schatzberg AF, Cole JO: Benzodiazepines in depressive disorders. Arch Gen Psychiatry 24:509–514, 1978

Schatzberg AF, Cole JO: Manual of Clinical Psychopharmacology, 2nd Edition. Washington, DC, American Psychiatric Press, 1991

Schenck C, Mahowald M: Long-term, nightly benzodiazepine treatment of injurious parasomnias and other disorders of disrupted nocturnal sleep in 170 adults. Am J Med 100:333–337, 1996

Schweizer E, Rickels K, Uhlenhuth EH: Issues in the long-term treatment of anxiety disorders, in Psychopharmacology: The Fourth Generation of Progress. Edited by Bloom FE, Kupfer DJ. New York, Raven, 1995, pp 1349–1359

Shader RI, Greenblatt DJ: Approaches to the treatment of anxiety states, in Manual of Psychiatric Therapeutics, 2nd Edition. Edited by Shader RI. Boston, Little, Brown, 1994a, pp 275–298

Shader RI, Greenblatt DJ: Treatment of transient insomnia, in Manual of Psychiatric Therapeutics, 2nd Edition. Edited by Shader RI. Boston, Little, Brown, 1994b, pp 211–216

Shader RI, von Moltke LL, Schmider J, et al: The clinician and drug interactions: an update. J Clin Psychopharmacol 16:197–201, 1996

Smoller JW: Panic-anxiety in patients with respiratory disease. American Society of Clinical Psychopharmacology Progress Notes 7:4–5, 1996

Stanilla JK, Simpson GM: Drugs to treat extrapyramidal side effects, in The American Psychiatric Press Textbook of Psychopharmacology. Edited by Schatzberg AF, Nemeroff CB. Washington, DC, American Psychiatric Press, 1995, pp 281–299

Stowe ZN, Nemeroff CB: Psychopharmacology during pregnancy and lactation, in The American Psychiatric Press Textbook of Psychopharmacology. Edited by Schatzberg AF, Nemeroff CB. Washington, DC, American Psychiatric Press, 1995, pp 823–837

Summerfield RJ, Nielsen MS: Excretion of lorazepam into breast milk. Br J Anaesth 57:1042–1043, 1985

Taylor CB: Treatment of anxiety disorders, in The American Psychiatric Press Textbook of Psychopharmacology. Edited by Schatzberg AF, Nemeroff CB. Washington, DC, American Psychiatric Press, 1995, pp 641–655

Tesar GE: High potency benzodiazepines for short-term management of panic disorder: the U.S. experience. J Clin Psychiatry 51 (suppl):4S–10S, 1990

Tueth MJ, DeVane CL, Evans DL: Treatment of psychiatric emergencies, in The American Psychiatric Press Textbook of Psychopharmacology. Edited by Schatzberg AF, Nemeroff CB. Washington, DC, American Psychiatric Press, 1995, pp 769–781

Udelman HD, Udelman DL: Concurrent use of buspirone in anxious patients during withdrawal from alprazolam therapy. J Clin Psychiatry 51 (suppl):46–50, 1990

van Laar MW, van Willigenburg APP, Volkerts ER: Acute and subchronic effects of nefazodone and imipramine on highway driving, cognitive functions, and daytime sleepiness in healthy adult and elderly subjects. J Clin Psychopharmacol 15:30–40, 1995

Wamsley JK, Hunt MAE: Relative affinity of quazepam for type-1 benzodiazepine receptors in brain. J Clin Psychiatry 52 (suppl):15–20, 1991

Wolkowitz OM, Pickar D: Benzodiazepines in the treatment of schizophrenia: a review and reappraisal. Am J Psychiatry 148: 714–726, 1991

Woods JH, Katz JL, Winger G: Abuse and therapeutic use of benzodiazepines and benzodiazepine-like drugs, in Psychopharmacology: The Fourth Generation of Progress. Edited by Bloom FE, Kupfer DJ. New York, Raven, 1995, pp 1777–1791

Yosselson-Superstine S, Lipman AG: Chlordiazepoxide interaction with levodopa. Ann Intern Med 96:259–260, 1982

Yudofsky SC, Silver JM, Hales RE: Treatment of aggressive disorders, in The American Psychiatric Press Textbook of Psychopharmacology. Edited by Schatzberg AF, Nemeroff CB. Washington, DC, American Psychiatric Press, 1995, pp 735–752

Zajecka JM: Treatment strategies for depression complicated by anxiety disorders. Paper presented at the Eighth Annual U.S. Psychiatric and Mental Health Congress, New York City, November 16, 1995

CHAPTER 4

Mood Stabilizers

Overview

▌ Drug Class

The mood stabilizers class includes *lithium, valproate, carbamazepine,* and a few adjunctive agents that have not been fully validated as "mood stabilizers." In general, when we speak of mood stabilizers, we have in mind certain agents used in the management of bipolar disorder. However, lithium, valproate, and carbamazepine have been found to have many other uses (see the following discussion on "Indications"), not necessarily based on well-designed studies. To qualify as a mood stabilizer, an agent must have some ability to treat both phases of bipolar illness (manic or depressed) while not worsening overall mood stability or cycling when the patient is followed longitudinally. This ability is not an all-or-none phenomenon (e.g., valproate is considered a mood stabilizer even though it is at best a mediocre antidepressant agent and even though it has not yet been demonstrated to have *long-term* prophylactic efficacy in bipolar disorder). (The Food and Drug Administration [FDA] recently permitted the makers of divalproex [Depakote] to list "acute mania" as a labeled indication, which is technically not the equivalent of labeling for "bipolar disorder," although most clinicians are satisfied that divalproex works for bipolar prophylaxis.) Other agents that *may* have mood-stabilizing properties include thyroxine (T_4), calcium channel blockers such as nimodipine and bupropion, and to some degree benzodiazepines such as clonazepam and lorazepam. (These last two are much more useful in the management of acute mania than of depression.) Recent studies also suggest that two anticonvulsants—lamotrigine and gabapentin—may have mood-stabilizing properties.

▌ Indications

The mood stabilizers, as noted, are used in all phases of bipolar illness. Although lithium remains the usual drug of first choice for the prophylaxis of "classic" bipolar disorder, it is rapidly being supplanted by valproate (divalproex [Depakote]) for the treatment of *rapid-cycling* bipolar disorder and *mixed* bipolar states (Bowden 1995a). Indeed, it is increasingly clear that lithium (alone) is not terribly effective in such cases. Carbamazepine has a more ambiguous status, mainly because of its higher side effect profile and potential (although rare) hematological complications. Some data suggest that carbamazepine, like valproate, may be useful for rapidly cycling or mixed states, but the evidence is not as compelling as that for valproate. Both valproate and carbamazepine may have advantages in bipolar patients with electroencephalogram abnormalities. Patients with psoriasis, impaired renal function, and thyroid disorders may be candidates for either valproate or carbamazepine in preference to lithium (Bowden 1995b). The benzodiazepines—particularly lorazepam (Ativan) and clonazepam (Klonopin)—are useful mainly in the adjunctive treatment of acute mania. Limited evidence suggests that clonazepam may have some antidepressant properties and perhaps some prophylactic effects in bipolar patients already maintained on lithium. Benzodiazepines may permit lower doses of antipsychotics during the stabilization of acute mania. In addition to being used in the treatment of bipolar disorder, lithium, valproate, and carbamazepine have been used in the treatment of various excited psychotic states, schizoaffective disorder, and conditions characterized by impulsive aggression or self-injurious behavior. To a more limited degree, these agents have been useful in some cases of posttraumatic stress disorder and borderline personality disorder. Outside of the evidence for their use in bipolar disorder, however, most of the evidence for using lithium, valproate, and carbamazepine is anecdotal or uncontrolled.

■ Mechanisms of Action

The precise mechanism of action for the three main mood stabilizers remains unknown (Table 4–2a). Lithium has numerous actions on neurotransmitters, secondary messengers, and membrane transport mechanisms (the various ion channels and "pumps" that maintain the resting potential across the cell membrane). Effects on dopamine formation, norepinephrine turnover, cholinergic transmission, phosphoinositide turnover, and adenylyl cyclase are but a few of the ways lithium may act on the brain. Valproate, a simple branched-chain carboxylic acid, may have both antiepileptic and antimanic effects via its effects on γ-aminobutyric acid (GABA), the main inhibitory neurotransmitter in the mammalian central nervous system. Valproate also may decrease dopamine turnover, possibly accounting for its modest antipsychotic effects. The correlation between valproate serum concentration and its antimanic effect is poor, but the concentration range usually required for good clinical effect is about 50–135 µg/mL (McElroy and Keck 1995). Carbamazepine—like valproate—has numerous effects on neurotransmitters, including adenosine, norepinephrine, dopamine, and serotonin (5-HT). Its actual mechanism of action in mood stabilization is not known, and it is not clear whether these actions are related to carbamazepine's antiepileptic effects. As with valproate, there is not a good correlation between plasma level and mood stabilization, but clinical response is usually seen within the range of 4–15 µg/mL (McElroy and Keck 1995).

▌Pharmacokinetics

Lithium is virtually the only psychotropic agent in common use that does not undergo hepatic metabolism; rather, it is eliminated almost entirely via the kidneys. Lithium is not protein bound and has an elimination half-life ($t\frac{1}{2}$) of approximately 24 hours, implying that steady-state levels are usually reached after 4–6 days on a fixed dose (Janicak et al. 1993). Peak lithium levels may be reduced via once-daily dosing, which may have beneficial effects on some aspects of treatment (see the following discussion on "Main Side Effects"). Lithium retention and excretion may be affected by sodium (salt) restriction or "loading." Valproate is highly protein-bound, which may have implications for some drug-drug interactions. Valproate metabolism is quite complex, mediated via two hepatic pathways (one mitochondrial, one microsomal). One valproate metabolite appears to be hepatotoxic. Valproate has an elimination $t\frac{1}{2}$ of roughly 12 hours (range of 5–20 hours), which may be altered by drugs that affect mitochondrial and/or microsomal enzymes (McElroy and Keck 1995). Carbamazepine, like valproate, is highly protein-bound. It has erratic absorption, possibly related to slow dissolution rate in the gastrointestinal (GI) tract. Carbamazepine also undergoes complex metabolism, with production of a 10,11-epoxide being of greatest significance for both pharmacological activity and neurotoxicity. At least one portion of carbamazepine's metabolism is thought to go through cytochrome P450 3A4 (CYP3A4) (DeVane 1994), the pathway inhibited by nefazodone, ketoconazole, and other drugs. Carbamazepine's elimination $t\frac{1}{2}$ ranges from 18–55 hours, and autoinduction (induction of its own metabolism) occurs during the first few months of treatment, which may reduce $t\frac{1}{2}$ to 5–26 hours and also reduce plasma levels (McElroy and Keck 1995). Valproate-carbamazepine pharmacokinetic interactions are complex and sometimes clinically troublesome.

∎ Main Side Effects

Lithium commonly produces increased urination with associated thirst and increased water intake (polyuria/polydipsia), mild GI problems (e.g., loose stools), and mild tremor. Most of these side effects may be mitigated by reducing the dosage and/or peak plasma levels. Hypothyroidism may be found in roughly 5%–10% of patients, particularly in women (who also have a higher intrinsic rate of thyroid disease) (Lenox and Manji 1995; Pies 1995b). Cognitive dulling or slowed thinking related to lithium may be a source of poor medication compliance. Frank nephrogenic diabetes insipidus is uncommon with lithium but is seen more frequently than glomerular dysfunction (Lenox and Manji 1995). Valproate generally produces few side effects, with the main exception being dose- or plasma level–related GI disturbance (McElroy and Keck 1995). Some patients may develop weight gain, transient hair loss, or tremor. Alterations in liver function with valproate are usually benign. Teratogenicity, however, is a significant problem with both valproate and carbamazepine. In approximately 40% of patients, carbamazepine may be associated with side effects, including fatigue, gait instability, headache, light-headedness, and rash (Shader 1994). However, carbamazepine may produce less weight gain, hair loss, and tremor than does valproate and less memory impairment than does lithium (Andrews et al. 1990; Mattson et al. 1992). Transient leukopenia occurs in about 10% of carbamazepine-treated patients but is usually benign; the much-feared complication of aplastic anemia is exceedingly rare (about 1 in 125,000). Hyponatremia, altered liver functions, and cardiac conduction abnormalities may sometimes be seen with carbamazepine.

Drug-Drug Interactions

Clinically significant drug-drug interactions with lithium include nonsteroidal anti-inflammatory drugs (NSAIDs) such as ibuprofen, thiazide diuretics, indapamide (a nonthiazide diuretic), and tetracyclines. These drug-drug interactions may lead to increased lithium levels and potential toxicity (Janicak et al. 1993). Theophylline, caffeine, verapamil, and carbonic anhydrase inhibitors all can increase lithium excretion, thus reducing lithium levels. Valproate tends to be a mild *inhibitor* of hepatic oxidative metabolism and thus may increase plasma levels of carbamazepine and its epoxide metabolite, phenobarbital, phenytoin, tricyclics, and to a small degree antipsychotics (McElroy and Keck 1995). Cimetidine, salicylates, and chlorpromazine may decrease valproate clearance, thus raising valproate levels. Fluoxetine (Prozac) also may raise valproate concentrations (Sovner and Davis 1991). As a general rule, carbamazepine tends to be a strong *inducer* of hepatic metabolism, generally reducing levels of other hepatically metabolized drugs. Thus, carbamazepine reduces valproate levels but may *raise* levels of valproate's hepatotoxic metabolite. Carbamazepine significantly reduces levels of haloperidol and probably other antipsychotics, as well as levels of tricyclics, benzodiazepines, warfarin, prednisone, theophylline, and oral contraceptives. Carbamazepine metabolism may be reduced (and carbamazepine increased to potentially toxic levels) by verapamil, diltiazem, erythromycin, valproate, and other agents (McElroy and Keck 1995). In addition to the pharmacokinetic interactions previously discussed, numerous pharmacodynamic interactions may occur between the mood stabilizers and other agents acting on the central nervous system (e.g., a subset of patients taking carbamazepine and lithium or antipsychotics may be prone to neurotoxicity [Fogel 1988]).

▌ Potentiating Maneuvers

In treating refractory bipolar disorder, the three main mood stabilizers—lithium, valproate, and carbamazepine—are often used in various combinations. A valproate-lithium regimen is often used in patients with mixed or rapid-cycling mania who do not respond to valproate alone. Patients who remain refractory may have carbamazepine added to this regimen, although the pharmacokinetic and pharmacodynamic interactions may be problematic. In addition to the three main mood stabilizers, adjunctive antipsychotics, benzodiazepines, and other agents are sometimes necessary, in either the acute or maintenance phases of treatment. Antipsychotics or benzodiazepines play an important adjunctive role during the first week or two of acute mania when lithium or valproate is still reaching therapeutic levels or efficacy (therapeutic levels and efficacy may occur more rapidly with valproate than with lithium [McElroy and Keck 1995]). Lorazepam and clonazepam are often used as adjunctive antimanic agents, with some data suggesting that lorazepam has a more rapid onset (Bradwejn et al. 1990). Thyroid supplementation, calcium channel blockers, β-blockers, and clonidine all have been used as adjunctive treatments for mania or rapid cycling, with generally limited success.

▌ Use in Special Populations

There is reasonably good evidence that lithium use during early pregnancy is associated with the development of cardiac abnormalities, especially *Ebstein's anomaly*, a severe, sometimes fatal malformation involving a downward displacement of the tricuspid valve into the right ventricle. However, the actual likelihood of lithium-related cardiac malformations appears to be lower than previously believed.

Until quite recently, carbamazepine was considered a safe alternative to lithium in treating the pregnant bipolar patient. More recent studies, unfortunately, have linked in utero carbamazepine exposure to higher-than-expected rates of craniofacial defects, developmental delay, and spina bifida (see McElroy and Keck 1995 for review). There is also a 1% rate of spina bifida in infants exposed to the anticonvulsant mood stabilizer valproate (divalproex [Depakote]) (McElroy and Keck 1995). The rate of spina bifida associated with exposure to valproate is clearly much higher than the risk of lithium-induced Ebstein's anomaly, and most clinicians do not advocate substituting valproate for lithium in the pregnant bipolar patient.

Lithium is the mood stabilizer most commonly used in children and adolescents, although few double-blind studies of its efficacy exist for this population. Valproate is also being used more frequently in the adolescent population.

Although all three mood stabilizers have been used in the elderly, there are relatively few well-controlled studies. Lithium may have an increased likelihood of neurotoxicity in elderly and dementia populations and must be used cautiously in patients (such as the elderly) with reduced renal function. Valproate appears to be relatively well tolerated in the elderly, whereas carbamazepine seems to be better tolerated than lithium by elderly patients with brain damage (Dubovsky 1994).

Tables

■ Drug Class

Table 4–1.   Mood stabilizers: preparations and doses

Generic drug	Brand names	Capsules/ tablets (mg)	Usual daily dose (mg)
Carbamaze-pine	Tegretol	100 (chewable), 200 (suspension also available as 100 mg/ 5 mL)	400–800
Divalproex	Depakote	125, 250, 500	500–1,250
	Depakote Sprinkle	125	—
Lithium carbonate	Eskalith, Lithonate, Lithane	150, 300, 600	600–1,500, usually in divided doses
Slow-release lithium carbonate	Lithobid	300	600–1,500, usually as bid dosing
	Eskalith CR	450	450–1,350, usually as bid dosing
Lithium citrate (syrup)	—	8 mEq/5mL	Each 5 mL = 300 mg lithium carbonate

Sources.   Data from Drug Facts and Comparisons 1995; Physicians' Desk Reference 1996.

▌ Indications

Table 4–2. Indications for lithium

Strength of data base	Condition	Comments
Strong	Acute mania	Lithium seems most effective when acute mania is "classic" type, not mixed with depression, dysphoria, irritability (valproate more effective)
	Prophylaxis of bipolar disorder	As many as 50% of bipolar patients show inadequate long-term response to lithium monotherapy; breakthrough depression may be more common than hypomania (?reporting artifact)
Moderate	Depressed phase of bipolar disorder	Lithium may be effective for the majority of depressed bipolar patients but may take 3–4 weeks of treatment; lithium averts risk of rapid cycling from ADs, although some patients may require brief course of ADs
	Potentiation of AD response in unipolar and bipolar depression	Lithium potentiation of tricyclics and probably SSRIs successful in about 50% of cases, often within 1–2 weeks (more likely to help in bipolar than unipolar patients)
	Schizoaffective disorder	Overall response rate of lithium-treated schizoaffective patients is > 70%; schizomanic patients respond better than depressed subtype

(continued)

Table 4–2. Indications for lithium *(continued)*

Strength of data base	Condition	Comments
Moderate *(continued)*	Impulsive aggression	Lithium has antiaggressive effects in wide range of psychiatric patients, including developmentally delayed/mentally retarded patients, prisoners with "rage outbursts," self-injurious patients; patients with underlying brain damage may be prone to lithium toxicity (?use lower doses)
Weak/ question- able	Schizophrenia	Lithium may improve some affective symptoms in schizophrenia but rarely improves "core" features of illness; subset of psychotic patients with absence of negative features and schizophrenia spectrum disorders in family may be lithium responsive
	OCD (adjunct)	In OCD, addition of lithium to primary serotonergic agent appears to produce only a few responders
	BPD	Some BPD patients may show decreased impulsivity with lithium but controlled studies lacking
	Alcoholism	Lithium for alcoholism has had mixed results (three positive, four negative outcome studies)

Note. ? = possibly; ADs = antidepressants; SSRIs = selective serotonin re-uptake inhibitors; OCD = obsessive-compulsive disorder; BPD = border-line personality disorder.
Sources. Hester 1994; Lenox and Manji 1995; Pies and Popli 1995; Rifkin et al. 1972; Schexnayder et al. 1995.

▌ Mechanisms of Action

Table 4–2a.   Mood stabilizer mechanisms of action

Mood stabilizer or putative mood stabilizer	Hypothesized mechanism(s) of action
Lithium	Antimanic activity may relate to reduction of dopaminergic function; antidepressant activity may relate to enhanced serotonergic function. May reduce "excessive signaling" via PI system, at least during mania.
Valproate	May enhance GABA function; decrease dopaminergic function. Does not appear to work via the PI system.
Carbamazepine	Antiseizure activity linked with inactivation of sodium channels and reduction of sodium influx; mood-stabilizing properties may relate to reduction of aspartate and/or glutamate release (excitatory neurotransmitters).
Lamotrigine[a]	Blocks voltage-sensitive sodium channels in presynaptic neuron, thus stabilizing presynaptic neuronal membrane and inhibiting release of glutamate, aspartate. (Unclear if this relates to mood-stabilizing effects.)
Gabapentin[a]	Structurally related to GABA but does not interact with GABA receptors. Inhibits voltage-dependent sodium channels and release of excitatory neurotransmitters. (Unclear if this relates to mood-stabilizing effects.)

Note.   PI = phosphatidylinositol; GABA = γ-aminobutyric acid.
[a]Under active investigation as mood stabilizers or adjunctive agents in bipolar disorder.
Sources.   Lenox and Manji 1995; McElroy and Keck 1995; Stoll and Severus 1996; Sussman 1997.

▌ Pharmacokinetics

Table 4–3. Mood stabilizer pharmacokinetics

Chemical name	$t_{1/2}$[a]	Time to steady state[a]	Metabolism	Active metabolites
Carbamazepine	15–50 hours initially; 8–20 hours chronically	2–4 days initially; after first 2 weeks, autometabolism means more than a month may be required to reach stable level, assuming dose is increased	Hepatic microsomal oxidation (at least in part via CYP3A4)	10,11-epoxide, which may be neurotoxic; $t_{1/2}$ of metabolite is approximately 6.5 hours
Divalproex	6–16 hours	1.5–3.5 days	Hepatic, via two pathways: mitochondrial β oxidation and CYP microsomal metabolism	Several active metabolites, including 2-propyl-4-pentanoic acid, which is hepatotoxic and teratogenic
Lithium	20–27 hours	4–7 days	Renal excretion	—

Note. $t_{1/2}$ = half-life; CYP = cytochrome P450.
[a]Values are only estimates derived from several studies.
Sources. Data from DeVane 1994; Drug Facts and Comparisons 1995; Janicak et al. 1995; McElroy and Keck 1995.

Main Side Effects

Table 4–4.   Lithium side effects

Subjective side effect of lithium	% of patients complaining
Excessive thirst	35.9
Polyuria	30.4
Memory problems	28.2
Tremor	26.6
Weight gain	18.9
Drowsiness/fatigue	12.4
Diarrhea	8.7

Sources.   Lenox and Manji 1995; Goodwin and Jamison 1990.

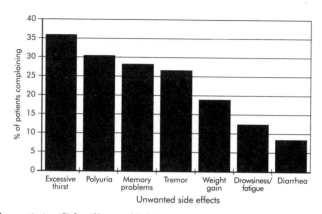

Figure 4–1. Side effects of lithium.

Sources. Lenox and Manji 1995; Goodwin and Jamison 1990 (does not include placebo control data).

Table 4–5. Stages of lithium toxicity

Stage	Lithium level (mEq/L)	Clinical picture
Early toxicity	1.2–1.5	Slight ataxia, dysarthria, lack of coordination
Mild toxicity	1.5–2	Listlessness, nausea, slurring of speech, diarrhea, coarse tremor
Moderate toxicity	2–2.5	Coarse tremor, confusion, delirium, pronounced ataxia
Severe toxicity	2.5–3 or greater	Stupor, spontaneous attacks of hyperextension of extremities, choreoathetosis, seizures, coma

Source. Adapted from Janicak et al. 1993, p. 397.

Table 4–6.   Five most common side effects with carbamazepine

Unwanted side effect	% of patients complaining
Dizziness	35
Drowsiness	29
Nausea	13
Skin reactions	12
Asthenia	11

Source.   Data from Sillanpaa 1981 (based on Ciba-Geigy data on patients taking carbamazepine for neuralgia, epilepsy, and miscellaneous conditions).

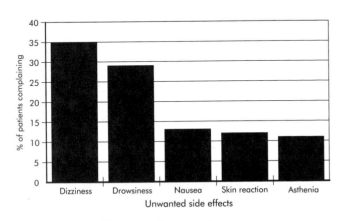

Figure 4–2.   Side effects of carbamazepine.
Source.   Data from Sillanpaa 1981 (based on Ciba-Geigy data on patients taking carbamazepine for neuralgia, epilepsy, and miscellaneous conditions).

Table 4–7. Management of side effects of anticonvulsant mood stabilizers

Agent	Side effect/average reporting (%)[a]	Management
Carbamazepine	Neurological (ataxia, vertigo, diplopia, sedation, blurred vision) (36)	Usually transient; reversible with dosage reduction; may be related to carbamazepine 10,11-epoxide
	Leukopenia (10)	Usually transient, benign granulocytopenia (not related to aplastic anemia); usually resolves spontaneously or with dosage reduction (*Note:* Aplastic anemia seen in about 1 in 575,000 cases)
	Rash (10)	May respond to topical steroids; discontinue carbamazepine if rash accompanied by fever, bleeding, exfoliative skin lesions (Stevens-Johnson syndrome)
	Hyponatremia (17)	If severe, may require discontinuation; tetracyclines may be helpful (e.g., demeclocycline)
	Liver enzyme elevations (10)	Usually benign; dosage reduction helps; monitor clinical status to rule out malaise, vomiting, jaundice; if transaminases are three times normal, or if alkaline phosphatase or bilirubin elevated, hold carbamazepine, consider alternative agent; monitor LFTs periodically

(continued)

Table 4–7.　Management of side effects of anticonvulsant mood stabilizers (*continued*)

Agent	Side effect/average reporting (%)[a]	Management
Carbamazepine (*continued*)	Thyroid dysfunction (8)	Slight decrease in total or free T_4 or elevation of TSH, rarely of clinical significance; may be dose related; thyroid supplement if necessary
	GI (10)	Side effects usually abate after first few weeks of treatment; dosage reduction or multiple dosing schedule may help
Valproate[b] (divalproex)	GI (anorexia, nausea, vomiting, diarrhea) (18)	Side effects related to onset of treatment (may be transient), dose, and plasma level; rarely a significant problem with plasma levels below 90 µg/mL; may be reduced with use of divalproex "sprinkles," addition of H_2 blocker (e.g., famotidine)
	Tremor (5)	Dosage reduction or use of β-blocker
	Hair loss/thinning (6)	Usually transient; may respond to zinc/selenium supplement
	Increased appetite, weight gain (5)	Exercise and fat/sugar reduction occasionally helpful, but side effects may be refractory

Elevated liver functions (20)	Usually benign, dose-related elevation of transaminases; not necessarily associated with hepatic dysfunction; monitor clinical status to rule out malaise, vomiting, jaundice; check alkaline phosphatase and bilirubin; if transaminases are three times normal and/or if alkaline phosphatase or bilirubin elevated, hold valproate, consider alternative agent

Note. LFTs = liver function tests; T_4 = thyroxine; TSH = thyroid-stimulating hormone; GI = gastrointestinal; H_2 = histamine-2.
[a]Figures are not placebo adjusted.
[b]Published data are rare regarding the percentage of side effects due to valproate monotherapy. Percentages represent composite averages from several of the sources, as well as from my clinical experience.
Sources. Data from Calabrese et al. 1992; Janicak et al. 1993; Lenox and Manji 1995; Maxmen 1991; Sillanpaa 1981.

Table 4–8.   Management of lithium side effects

Side effect	Specific symptoms	Management strategy
Gastrointestinal	Nausea, vomiting, anorexia, diarrhea, cramping; common at start of therapy, often transient	Reduce dose and/or slow rate of dose increase early in treatment; give lithium with meals; slow-release preparations can decrease nausea but increase diarrhea; lithium citrate syrup may help GI side effects; if GI toxicity develops late in treatment, rule out toxicity
Renal	Glomerular dysfunction is rare at therapeutic doses; renal tubular effects are fairly common (e.g., polyuria in about 60% of patients on long-term maintenance treatment); NDI in about 10% of cases (> 3 L/day urine output); edema is usually not due to change in renal function and may resolve spontaneously	If creatinine rises abruptly, hold lithium and check creatinine clearance; consider decreasing or discontinuing lithium; some patients may experience less polydipsia/polyuria if most of lithium dose is given at bedtime (reduce total dose by about 20%); some data suggest that every-other-day schedule may be feasible; thiazide diuretics may help with polyuria but can increase lithium levels about 40% (must decrease lithium dose); thiazides also may reduce K⁺; use of amiloride (K⁺–sparing diuretic, 5–10 mg bid) may be preferable for treatment of polyuria and usually does not affect lithium or K⁺

Neurological/cognitive	Neurological side effects may be related to peak plasma levels; include cognitive effects (slowing, memory impairment), lethargy, weakness, postural tremor (7–16 Hz); lithium may increase extrapyramidal side effects in patients taking neuroleptics; rarely, lithium may reactivate NMS, cause pseudotumor cerebri	Reduce dosage or increase interdose interval; for tremor, reduce caffeine, stimulant, tricyclic use; β-blockers (e.g., atenolol 50 mg bid) may help with tremor (must monitor pulse to avert bradycardia); always rule out lithium toxicity with new-onset neurological symptoms; use lower levels in dementia, brain-injured patients, perhaps elderly
Endocrine	Hypothyroidism develops in about 20% of patients treated chronically; possible elevations of parathyroid hormone and serum calcium (rarely)	Check baseline TFTs and follow up every 6 months; if TSH elevated, consider adding T_4; hypothyroidism not a reason to discontinue lithium, but different agent could be considered; baseline calcium, phosphorus with one follow-up after 6 months of lithium may be prudent
Cardiac	T-wave flattening/inversion, S-A node dysfunction; bradycardia; rare ventricular premature contractions	Baseline ECG for patients older than age 50 years or with history of cardiac symptoms, concomitant use of β-blockers or calcium channel blockers; check K^+ if T-wave flattening present (usually not due to low serum K^+); monitor pulse periodically; avoid coprescribing other drugs that cause bradyarrhythmias

(continued)

Table 4–8.   Management of lithium side effects (*continued*)

Side effect	Specific symptoms	Management strategy
Dermatological	Acne, psoriasis, pruritis, hair loss; dermatological side effects not clearly dose related	Antiacne regimens may help; consider change to alternative mood stabilizer; check TFTs if hair loss present (rule out hypothyroidism)
Weight gain	Lithium may have insulin-like effect on carbohydrate metabolism; increased intake of liquids may promote weight gain	Begin weight management program (exercise, avoid sugary drinks; change to carbamazepine may help (weight gain also associated with valproate)

Note.   GI = gastrointestinal; NDI = nephrogenic diabetes insipidus; K^+ = potassium; NMS = neuroleptic malignant syndrome; TFTs = thyroid function tests; TSH = thyroid-stimulating hormone; T_4 = thyroxine; S-A = sinoatrial; ECG = electrocardiogram.
Sources.   Data from Arana and Hyman 1991; Shader 1994.

Drug-Drug Interactions

Table 4–9. Drug-drug interactions with lithium

Agent added to lithium	Potential interaction	Clinical management
Acetazolamide	Decreased lithium level due to increased renal excretion	Close monitoring of lithium level with this combination
Carbamazepine	Increased neurotoxic effect despite therapeutic lithium and carbamazepine levels (mechanism unknown)	Usually this combination is well tolerated; toxicity may be more likely in patients with medical illness, previous history of lithium neurotoxicity; monitor carefully for clinical signs/symptoms when this combination used
Fluoxetine	Increased lithium serum levels and/or lithium toxicity; tremor common, neurotoxicity may progress to ataxia, serotonin syndrome, confusion	Consider reducing lithium dosage, changing to different SSRI, although sertraline plus lithium may lead to tremor
Haloperidol, other antipsychotics	Reported increased neurotoxic effects, despite therapeutic lithium levels, similar to NMS (confusion, rigidity)	Not clear that haloperidol is more likely than other neuroleptics to interact in this way with lithium; any antipsychotic may increase extrapyramidal side effects associated with lithium and vice versa; dosage reduction of one or both agents indicated

(continued)

Table 4–9. Drug-drug interactions with lithium *(continued)*

Agent added to lithium	Potential interaction	Clinical management
Methyldopa	Increased lithium level or increased lithium toxicity without change in level	Avoid combination
NSAIDs	Increased lithium level, perhaps due to effect of NSAIDs on renal prostaglandin synthesis	Monitor lithium level closely and use sulindac if NSAIDs must be used; consider aspirin instead
Theophylline	Decreased lithium level due to increased renal excretion	Monitor lithium level closely with this combination
Thiazide diuretic	Increased serum lithium level due to decreased renal lithium clearance; possible lithium toxicity	50% reduction in lithium dose indicated with use of 50 mg qd hydrochlorothiazide, or use furosemide instead
Tricyclics	A few reports of lithium plus tricyclic (amitriptyline, imipramine, ?others) leading to increased likelihood of seizures, tremor, ?cardiac toxicity	Usually this combination is well tolerated and may be good strategy for refractory depression; monitor for signs and symptoms of neurotoxicity and consider reduced lithium dose if neurotoxicity present; ECG is prudent with this combination

Note.   SSRI = selective serotonin reuptake inhibitor; NMS = neuroleptic malignant syndrome; NSAIDS = nonsteroidal anti-inflammatory drugs; ECG = electrocardiogram; ? = possibly.
Sources.   Data from Brodie and Dichter 1996; Ciraulo et al. 1995; Drug Facts and Comparisons 1995; Ketter et al. 1995a, 1995b; Krishnan et al. 1996; Popli et al. 1995.

Table 4–10. Drug-drug interactions with carbamazepine

Agent added to carbamazepine	Potential interaction	Clinical management
Anticoagulants	Carbamazepine may increase metabolism of anticoagulants, thus reducing their effects	Adjustment of warfarin dose may be necessary when carbamazepine coadministered (or discontinued)
Bupropion	Carbamazepine may decrease plasma bupropion level while greatly increasing hydroxybupropion; this may lead to toxicity in some patients	If bupropion used with carbamazepine, get plasma level of both bupropion and metabolite; watch for signs of confusion, psychosis secondary to high hydroxybupropion levels
Calcium channel blockers	Increased carbamazepine levels and neurotoxicity, probably due to inhibition of CYP3A4 system	Seems to occur with use of verapamil or diltiazem but not nifedipine, which is calcium channel blocker of choice in this context
Cimetidine	Transient increase in carbamazepine levels, with possible increase in carbamazepine side effects during first 3–5 days of treatment	When possible, use ranitidine, famotidine, or other antacid in patients taking carbamazepine

(continued)

Table 4–10. Drug-drug interactions with carbamazepine (*continued*)

Agent added to carbamazepine	Potential interaction	Clinical management
Clozapine, haloperidol (?other antipsychotics)	Carbamazepine induces metabolism of clozapine and haloperidol, thus reducing levels of both agents; reduction of haloperidol may be clinically significant in some cases; reduction of antipsychotic effect in some but not all cases (*Note:* Theoretically, increased risk of agranulocytosis when carbamazepine used with clozapine)	Monitor clozapine levels, consider dosage increase when carbamazepine coadministered; if carbamazepine discontinued, may need to reduce clozapine dose; monitor haloperidol levels and clinical response if carbamazepine used concomitantly
Isoniazid	Increased carbamazepine level and toxicity and possible increased risk of isoniazid-induced hepatotoxicity	Monitor carbamazepine levels, LFTs carefully with this combination
Lamotrigine	Neurotoxicity possible due to increased levels of carbamazepine's epoxide metabolite	Avoid coadministration of lamotrigine and carbamazepine if possible

Macrolide antibiotics (erythromycin, troleandomycin)	Carbamazepine toxicity, probably due to inhibition of CYP systems by macrolides	May be more likely with larger doses of macrolides; if possible, use different type of antibiotic; monitor carbamazepine levels and clinical signs of weakness, lethargy, ataxia
Oral contraceptives	Effectiveness of oral contraceptives reduced in presence of carbamazepine via induction of metabolism	Breakthrough bleeding may be warning of interaction; avoid carbamazepine in patients taking oral contraceptives and using Norplant
Phenobarbital, primidone	Reduced carbamazepine levels via enhanced hepatic metabolism; apparently no loss of seizure control; carbamazepine may increase levels of phenobarbital (which is metabolite of primidone)	Monitor carbamazepine levels
Phenytoin	Reduced carbamazepine levels via enhanced hepatic metabolism of carbamazepine; effect of carbamazepine on phenytoin highly variable	Monitor carbamazepine and phenytoin levels
SSRIs	Studies inconsistent, but fluoxetine and perhaps other SSRIs (e.g., fluvoxamine) may impair carbamazepine metabolism, leading to carbamazepine toxicity and/or serotonin syndrome	Monitor carbamazepine levels closely when SSRIs used concomitantly, especially fluoxetine and fluvoxamine; in theory, nefazodone also may increase carbamazepine levels via inhibition of CYP3A4

(continued)

Table 4–10. Drug-drug interactions with carbamazepine *(continued)*

Agent added to carbamazepine	Potential interaction	Clinical management
Valproate	Increased ratio of carbamazepine epoxide to carbamazepine via inhibition of epoxide hydroxylase (possible neurotoxicity); valproate may cause displacement of carbamazepine from plasma-binding proteins; carbamazepine reduces valproate levels but increases levels of 2-propyl-4-pentanoic acid metabolite, which is hepatotoxic and teratogenic	Avoid this combination if possible; if carbamazepine and valproate used together, monitor levels of both closely; obtain level of carbamazepine epoxide if possible, and closely monitor patient for signs of neurotoxicity; check LFTs more frequently than with either agent alone

Note. CYP = cytochrome P450; LFTs = liver function tests; SSRIs = selective serotonin reuptake inhibitors.
Sources. Brodie and Dichter 1996; Ciraulo et al. 1995; Drug Facts and Comparisons 1995; Ketter et al. 1995a, 1995b; Krishnan et al. 1996; Popli et al. 1995.

Table 4–11. Drug-drug interactions with valproate

Agent added to valproate	Potential interaction	Clinical management
Aspirin, naproxen	Aspirin and naproxen may displace valproate from its binding sites on plasma proteins[a]; aspirin also inhibits valproate metabolism; some clinical evidence suggests aspirin/valproate toxicity	Use nonaspirin pain relievers, if possible, with valproate
Bupropion	Valproate does not affect bupropion concentration but increases hydroxybupropion level	Consider reducing bupropion dose if signs of toxicity develop
Carbamazepine	Carbamazepine reduces valproate levels but increases levels of 2-propyl-4-pentanoic acid metabolite, which is hepatotoxic and teratogenic	May need to monitor LFTs more closely; adjust one or both anticonvulsant doses and follow levels periodically
Chlorpromazine (?other antipsychotics)	Increased valproate levels due to competitive inhibition of metabolism	Monitor valproate levels closely when valproate and phenothiazines used concomitantly; haloperidol may not have this effect on valproate

(continued)

Table 4–11. Drug-drug interactions with valproate *(continued)*

Agent added to valproate	Potential interaction	Clinical management
Cimetidine	Increased valproate levels due to decreased clearance	Use ranitidine or famotidine with valproate
Fluoxetine	Increased valproate levels via inhibition of hepatic metabolism	Monitor valproate levels and adjust dose
Lamotrigine	Increased lamotrigine levels due to valproate inhibition of hepatic metabolism; may lead to neurotoxicity, increased incidence of Stevens-Johnson syndrome	Reduce dose of lamotrigine and/or valproate; avoid coadministration
Magnesium/aluminum hydroxide antacids	Increased valproate levels	Adjust dosage of valproate if side effects occur
Phenobarbital	Increased phenobarbital levels	Reduce phenobarbital dose

Note. LFTs = liver function tests; ? = possibly.
[a]Probably leads to very transient effects.
Sources. Ciraulo and Slattery 1995; Drug Facts and Comparisons 1995.

Potentiating Maneuvers

Table 4–12. Augmenting agents for mood stabilizers

Primary agent	Augmenter	Comments
Carbamazepine	Lithium	Carbamazepine plus lithium may have synergistic effects in treatment of refractory bipolar illness; some additive neurotoxicity.
		Both drugs may reduce thyroid activity; lithium may mitigate carbamazepine-induced decrease in neutrophils but does not protect against myelosuppression/aplastic anemia
	Valproate	May result in sustained prophylactic response in patients poorly responsive to carbamazepine or valproate alone; valproate inhibits epoxide hydrolase, leading to increased plasma levels of carbamazepine-epoxide and potential neurotoxicity
	Gabapentin	Little experience with this combination; no known adverse interactions
	Lamotrigine	Carbamazepine induces lamotrigine metabolism and thus reduces levels; lamotrigine increases levels of epoxide metabolite of carbamazepine, increasing risk of neurotoxicity
Lithium	Carbamazepine	As above (carbamazepine plus lithium)
	Valproate	Valproate may augment mood-stabilizing effects of lithium, especially in rapid-cycling patients.
		Usually well tolerated; increased tremor may result from combination

(continued)

Table 4–12.   Augmenting agents for mood stabilizers (*continued*)

Primary agent	Augmenter	Comments
Lithium (*continued*)	Thyroxine (T$_4$)	May decrease cycling frequency and severity in rapid-cycling patients unresponsive to lithium alone
	Lamotrigine	Lamotrigine may be effective either alone or in combination with other mood stabilizers for patients with refractory bipolar illness, including those with depression or rapid cycling
		Not clear how useful for mania, and may cause some patients to switch from depression to mixed or manic state
		Begin lamotrigine as 25–50 mg/day, with total daily dose increased by 50 mg every 2 weeks to target dose of 100–400 mg/day
		Generally avoid lamotrigine use with either carbamazepine or valproate, because of risks of neurotoxicity and skin rash, respectively. Lamotrigine side effects include dizziness, diplopia, somnolence, headache, ataxia, asthenia; rash seen in 5%–10% of cases, sometimes severe (Stevens-Johnson syndrome in 1/1,000 adults, 1/50 children)
		No well-validated therapeutic blood levels in bipolar disorder

Gabapentin		Anecdotal reports suggest that gabapentin may be a useful adjunct in acutely manic patients, usually in combination with lithium, valproate, and antipsychotics
		May reduce depression in bipolar patients but may also induce more rapid cycling in some patients
		Dosage begins with 300–600 mg/day; effective range seems to be 500–3,600 mg/day in divided doses
		Gabapentin does not have significant interactions with valproate or other anticonvulsants
		Gabapentin generally well tolerated, but side effects may include somnolence, dizziness, ataxia, fatigue, nystagmus
		No well-validated therapeutic blood levels in bipolar disorder
Valproate (divalproex)	Lithium	As above (lithium plus valproate)
	Carbamazepine	As above (carbamazepine plus valproate)
		Carbamazepine leads to decreased valproate levels but may increase levels of valproate metabolite, and this metabolite may cause hepatotoxicity
	Lamotrigine	Increased risk of skin rash
		Valproate raises lamotrigine levels; best to avoid concomitant use
	Gabapentin	Gabapentin may augment mood-stabilizing effects of valproate; no adverse interactions reported

Sources. Ayd 1995; Ciraulo et al. 1995; Drug Facts and Comparisons 1995; Keck et al. 1992a; Sussman 1997; Sporn and Sachs 1997.

▌ Use in Special Populations

Table 4–13.   Mood stabilizers in special populations

Population	Special concerns
Women of child-bearing age, pregnant patients	Risk of Ebstein's anomaly in infants exposed to lithium in first trimester; exposure to carbamazepine, valproate linked to craniofacial defects, spinal cord malformations
Children, young adolescents	Very few controlled studies of mood stabilizers in young populations; lithium appears to be well tolerated; valproate can cause hepatotoxicity in children younger than age 3 years; carbamazepine may be eliminated more rapidly than in adults
Elderly, medically/ neurologically ill	Elderly brain more sensitive to drugs; lithium elimination half-life increased in elderly (especially those with renal dysfunction) and neurotoxicity may occur at lower plasma levels; carbamazepine may be more likely to produce neurotoxicity in older populations; valproate may be effective at lower dosage/plasma levels than in younger populations; valproate may be useful in aggressive, disinhibited dementia patients

Sources.   Dubovsky 1994; Dulcan et al. 1995.

Questions and Answers

▮ Drug Class

Q. Are the anticonvulsants lamotrigine (Lamictal) and gabapentin (Neurontin) considered mood stabilizers?

A. As of this writing, it is too soon to say whether these agents are mood stabilizers in the same robust sense that applies to lithium and valproate. Preliminary indications are that both lamotrigine and gabapentin are useful as adjunctive agents in patients with refractory bipolar illness. Thus far, lamotrigine seems promising in the depressed phase of bipolar illness; its effects on manic and mixed presentations are still unclear. Lamotrigine apparently has the potential to "switch" patients from a depressive into a manic or mixed state (Sporn and Sachs 1997). Gabapentin appears to have both antimanic and antidepressant properties, and, like LTG, also has the potential to produce euphoria or increased cycling rates (Sussman 1997). Randomized, placebo-controlled studies of both lamotrigine and gabapentin will be needed to sort out the complex effects of these agents. At present, I recommend their use only in bipolar patients who have not responded to more traditional treatments.

▮ Indications

Q. What is the role of mood stabilizers versus antidepressants in the treatment of the depressed phase of bipolar illness?

A. In a review of the literature on the treatment of acute bipolar depression, Srisurapanont et al. (1995) conclude that lithium, monoamine oxidase inhibitors (MAOIs), cyclic antidepressants (an umbrella term these authors use to describe all non-MAOIs), and electroconvulsive therapy (ECT) are all effective in treating bipolar depression. Therefore, the side effect profile of these agents—including their propensity to induce a hypomanic-manic switch—should be a crucial determinant in choosing the most appropriate form of treatment for bipolar depression. Mood stabilizers should be considered the *first-line agents* for acute bipolar depression, in view of the fact that their efficacy may be equal to antidepressant treatment and that their use is rarely associated with hypomanic switch. Thus, in the algorithm of Srisurapanont et al. (1995), if a bipolar patient not already taking a mood stabilizer (lithium, valproate, carbamazepine) is in the depressed phase of illness, the first step is to use a *mood stabilizer alone.* If the patient is already taking a mood stabilizer, *plasma levels should be increased* and the patient observed for 2–3 weeks. Thus, if a patient with bipolar depression enters the hospital with a lithium level of 0.8 mEq/L, dosage might be increased to achieve a level of 1.1 mEq/L, for example, *before use of any antidepressant.* If this strategy does not work, Srisurapanont et al. (1995) recommend adding an MAOI for anergic bipolar depression, a selective serotonin reuptake inhibitor (SSRI) or bupropion (in preference to a tricyclic) for nonanergic bipolar depression, or an antipsychotic plus an antidepressant for psychotic bipolar depression. Alternatively, ECT is one of the few interventions that may quickly and effectively treat *both* the manic and depressed phases of bipolar disorder—but many patients and their families remain fearful of ECT and are unwilling to try it. Srisurapanont et al. (1995) note that seven of eight double-blind, placebo-controlled studies of 116 patients with bipolar depression showed lithium superior to placebo, with a mean response rate of 76%. The only double-blind study comparing lithium with imipramine for bipolar depression found a 32% mean reduction in scores for depression with lithium versus 58% with imipramine (Fieve et al. 1968). Of course, imipramine can propel some bipolar patients into mania. Unfortunately, lithium may not be effective in patients with bipolar depression for 3–4 weeks, and neither valproate nor carbamazepine has proved terribly effective in acute bipolar depression. If an antidepressant must be used, bupropion (Sachs 1996) and perhaps SSRIs seem less likely to provoke hypomania/mania than tricyclics; however, in moderate-to-high doses (150–400 mg/day), bupropion may provoke hallucinations or other psychotic symptoms in a few patients (Ames et al. 1992). Some clinicians recommend discontinuing antidepressants within 2 weeks of achieving remission of the acute depressive bout; however, a slow taper over 3 weeks may be more prudent because sudden withdrawal of antidepressants may occasionally *provoke* hypomania/mania.

Q. What is the most *rapidly effective* treatment for an acute manic episode?

A. A recent retrospective, nonrandomized study of 78 acutely manic bipolar patients (Frye et al. 1996) examined the length of hospital stay in relation to four drug regimens: 1) lithium alone, 2) carbamazepine alone, 3) divalproex alone, and 4) lithium plus carbamazepine. The mean length of stay was about 40% shorter for the divalproex group (around 10 days) and the lithium plus carbamazepine group (around 12 days), compared with lithium alone (around 18 days) or carbamazepine alone (around 18 days). Although this study has some methodological problems (including what may have been suboptimal blood levels of lithium), it does suggest that divalproex may be a time-efficient treatment for acute mania. It is usually better tolerated than a combination of lithium plus carbamazepine. A valproate *loading-dose strategy* also has been found to be rapidly effective, whereby divalproex is used in divided doses of 20 mg/kg/day (Keck et al. 1993); in contrast, lithium and carbamazepine cannot be loaded without significant side effects. Of course, ECT also may be rapidly effective in acute mania.

Q. What factors differentially predict response to lithium, valproate, and carbamazepine in the treatment of acute mania?

A. High likelihood of response to lithium is predicted by the presence of a milder manic episode, one with pure manic symptomatology (e.g., elation and grandiosity without a mix of depressive features), prior good response to lithium, and a history of fewer manic episodes. Patients with complicated types of mania (e.g., secondary to substance abuse, brain pathology) and mixed manic states generally have poorer responses to lithium (Bowden 1995b). Valproate seems to be a broader-spectrum mood stabilizer in that mixed mania responds as well to divalproex as does pure mania and better than it responds to lithium. There is preliminary evidence that valproate is effective in rapidly cycling and secondary bipolar disorders. Predictors of response to carbamazepine are less clear, although carbamazepine appears to be more effective than lithium in secondary mania and may work in patients who have not responded to lithium (Bowden 1995b). The data on carbamazepine in mixed and rapid-cycling bipolar disorder are contradictory at this time (Bowden 1995b).

Q. What are the risks of stopping lithium therapy in bipolar patients?

A. Withdrawing lithium from long-term, stable bipolar patients is associated with a high risk of early recurrence, an increased mortality from suicide, and possibly a rebound treatment-refractory state (Faedda et al. 1993; G. M. Goodwin 1994; Osser 1996; Suppes et al. 1991). *Rapid* discontinuation produces the worst outcome, with a 50% relapse rate (within 6 months) associated with lithium discontinuation over a 2-week period or less. More gradual tapering improves 6-month outcome but not relapse rate over a 5-year period. Relapse rates for bipolar patients taken off lithium actually may be worse than for patients *never treated* with lithium (G. M. Goodwin 1994); therefore, lithium treatment may not be prudent if there is a high probability the patient will discontinue it within the first year or two. (We do not know the long-term effect of switching from lithium to an anticonvulsant mood stabilizer, although clinical experience would suggest a much more favorable outcome. We also do not know whether the same problems associated with lithium discontinuation will appear if a patient is taken off long-term anticonvulsant treatment [Osser 1996].)

Q. Besides their use in bipolar disorder, what other indications exist for valproate and carbamazepine?

A. With respect to off-label uses (nonapproved by the FDA), valproate has been found variably effective in the treatment of *acute major depression, aggressive behavior in dementia patients, panic disorder, posttraumatic stress disorder,* and *borderline personality disorder.* Carbamazepine also has been used in these conditions, as well as in *alcohol* or *sedative-hypnotic withdrawal* and *trigeminal neuralgia* (Keck et al. 1992b). Most of the data for use of valproate and carbamazepine in these conditions are derived from open studies and case reports. It appears that the use of valproate in panic disorder is better substantiated than use of carbamazepine; conversely, the use of carbamazepine in the treatment of behavioral dyscontrol appears to be better supported than use of valproate (Keck et al. 1992b). Carbamazepine also appears comparable to standard agents (e.g., benzodiazepines) for treatment of alcohol and sedative withdrawal and has been used to facilitate withdrawal from alprazolam (Klein et al. 1986). Finally, valproate also has been used in migraine prophylaxis.

Q. In what psychiatric conditions (besides bipolar disorder) is lithium useful?

A. Lithium has been found useful as an adjunctive agent (i.e., added to a primary antidepressant) in both unipolar and bipolar depression. In unipolar depression, response to adjunctive lithium may be evident within 1–2 weeks and represents a viable alternative to changing the primary agent (Lenox and Manji 1995). Sometimes this response may be seen with relatively low doses of lithium (e.g., 300–600 mg/day), but many patients will require higher doses and plasma levels in the usual therapeutic range (0.5–0.9 mEq/L).

Pope et al. (1988) found lithium useful when added to fluoxetine in five refractory depressed patients, and clinical experience has generally supported the view that lithium may augment response to SSRIs. Lithium also has been found useful in schizoaffective disorder, although this disorder has been defined in various ways over the years. After reviewing virtually the entire literature on schizoaffective disorder as of 1988, Levitt and Tsuang (1988) concluded that the most helpful therapeutic maneuver is to divide the disorder by "polarity" (i.e., whether the patient shows "schizomanic" or "schizodepressive" features). These authors note several studies showing that schizomanic patients respond to lithium. In schizodepressive patients, the benefits of lithium are less clear. Lithium has not been found particularly useful in schizophrenia, but there may be a lithium-responsive subset of psychotic (nonbipolar) patients. Thus, Schexnayder et al. (1995) examined a group of 66 psychotic patients diagnosed with schizophrenia or schizophreniform disorder. These patients were then treated with lithium *alone*. Lithium responders and nonresponders did not differ according to DSM-III (American Psychiatric Association 1980) or Research Diagnostic Criteria (RDC) diagnoses or number of positive schizophrenic symptoms. However, the lithium responders showed a paucity of *negative symptoms* and an absence of *"familial schizophrenic spectrum disorders."* This spectrum was defined as including schizophrenia, schizophreniform disorder, schizotypal personality disorder, and *schizoaffective disorder.* One could argue that including schizoaffective disorder in this spectrum begs the question of the "true nature" of schizoaffective disorder; nevertheless, the results of the study support the clinical impression that lithium response is not robust in psychotic patients with marked emotional withdrawal, blunted affect, and a family history more suggestive of schizophrenia than of affective illness. The study by Schexnayder et al. (1995) does suggest that a paucity of negative symptoms and lack of a family history of schizophrenia-like illness may predict good response to lithium in psychotic patients. Other possible indications for lithium include *impulsive aggression, obsessive-compulsive disorder (as an adjunct to primary agent), borderline personality disorder,* and *alcoholism.* However, with the exception of impulsive aggression, the data for use in the other conditions mentioned is relatively weak.

Q. Can mood stabilizers prevent a bipolar patient from "switching" into mania while taking an antidepressant?

A. The whole notion of antidepressant-induced switching is fraught with controversy because it is difficult to discriminate a patient's "natural" manic periods from those induced by external causes. Nevertheless, some data suggest that among *treatment-refractory* bipolar patients, about a third will have manic episodes probably due to an antidepressant (Altshuler et al. 1995). (Because this population may have contained a large number of *rapid-cycling patients,* the general applicability of this finding is in question.) One study has suggested that mood stabilizers do not offer protection against antidepressant-induced mania, whereas two others found some protective effects. The study by Altshuler et al. (1995) found that the majority of those patients who had a probable antidepressant-induced switch into mania were concurrently taking a mood stabilizer during the switch; thus, the protective effect of mood stabilizers was not dem-

onstrated. In clinical practice, the aim is generally to minimize dose and exposure to antidepressants and to use
concurrent mood stabilizers to buffer the potential for
antidepressant-induced mania. Some data suggest that
SSRIs, MAOIs, and bupropion may be somewhat less likely
to precipitate mania than the tricyclics (Simpson and
DePaulo 1991; Wright et al. 1985), but these claims are hardly
well validated.

Q. How useful are calcium channel blockers in treating bipolar disorder?

A. Initial enthusiasm about calcium channel blockers as antimanic agents (Dubovsky et al. 1986) has been tempered in recent years, although one textbook maintains that "available
data support the use of verapamil for both the short-term
and maintenance treatment of bipolar I disorder," adding
that verapamil "should be considered a fourth-line drug"
(Kaplan et al. 1994, p. 923), following trials on standard mood
stabilizers. In a recent review by Gelenberg (1997), the work
of Walton et al. (1996) is discussed. Walton et al. (1996) con-
ducted a study of acute manic patients, who were randomly
assigned to treatment with either verapamil 230–360 mg/day
or lithium 500–1,000 mg/day (mean serum level = 0.51 mmol/L).
Over the 28 days of the study, patients treated with lithium,
but not those treated with verapamil, showed significant improvement on all rating scales. Gelenberg (1997) concludes
(based on these and other studies) that verapamil "might still
be considered (alone or as an adjunct) for occasional patients
unresponsive to or intolerant of more standard treatments.
Certainly, lithium divalproex, and carbamazepine, alone or
in combination, should be considered first" (p. 7). Other clinicians believe there is little credible evidence supporting the
use of verapamil in mania (F. J. Ayd, Jr., personal communication, September 1997).

Verapamil is usually used at doses of 120–480 mg/day, in divided doses, in the treatment of mania (Arana and Hyman 1991; Dubovsky 1995). Constipation, vertigo, headache, cardiac conduction problems, and hypotension have been reported with verapamil (Arana and Hyman 1991), and drug-drug interactions may occur with lithium and carbamazepine (see Table 4–10 and answer to question about role of calcium channel blockers as adjunctive agents in bipolar disorder in "Potentiating Maneuvers" that follows). A recent report by Goodnick (1995) found nimodipine (up to 60 mg tid) effective as the sole agent in the treatment of two patients with rapidly cycling bipolar disorder, even after 5- to 12-month follow-up (see answer to last question in "Potentiating Maneuvers" that follows).

■ Mechanisms of Action

Q. What are the postulated mechanisms of action of lithium in manic-depressive illness?

A. The exact mechanism is not known, although the answer may be intimately related to the mechanisms underlying bipolar disorder itself. Lithium has a plethora of effects on neurotransmitters, intracellular secondary messenger systems, and even gene expression (Lenox and Manji 1995). The antimanic action of lithium may be related, in part, to its ability to reduce both pre- and postsynaptic dopamine receptor function and perhaps dopamine formation. Its antidepressant action may be related to enhanced presynaptic serotonergic activity, among other mechanisms. Recent interest has focused on lithium's potent inhibition of the intracellular enzyme *inositol monophosphatase* (IMPase), leading to reduced production of free *inositol*—the substrate that fuels intracellular and intercellular signaling (Lenox and Manji 1995). Interestingly, this property does *not* seem to be shared with carbamazepine or valproate, suggesting that IMPase inhibition is not a necessary property for mood stabilization (Vadnal and Parthasarathy 1995). A recent review by Stoll and Severus (1996) also suggests that lithium may reduce "excessive signaling" through the phosphatidylinositol (PI) system, at least during mania. Models of bipolar illness, and a hypothesis focusing on abnormalities in the sodium, potassium-activated adenosine triphosphatase pump (Na,K-ATPase system), are reviewed by El-Mallakh and Wyatt (1995).

Q. What is the mechanism of valproate action in treating psychiatric illnesses?

A. Valproate's mechanism of action is not known. Valproate inhibits breakdown of GABA and also may enhance neuronal sensitivity to GABA (McElroy and Keck 1995). Valproate may exert its antiseizure effects via these effects on GABA and/or via direct neuronal effects on sodium and potassium exchange. It is not known which (if either) of these mechanisms is involved in valproate's effects on mania, depression, and anxiety. In the rat, valproate has *regional* effects on norepinephrine (i.e., valproate *increases* norepinephrine in the hippocampus but *decreases* it in the hypothalamus [Baf et al. 1994]). It is tempting to speculate that such regional modulation might allow valproate to have both antimanic and antidepressive effects in humans, although the latter effects are modest. Other studies in the rat suggest that valproate does not have significant effects on 5-HT_{1A}, 5-HT_2, or β-adrenergic receptor number (Khaitan et al. 1994). Neither does valproate appear to have any significant effect on IMPase (see immediately preceding question and answer regarding lithium) (Vadnal and Parthasarathy 1995). Valproate may decrease dopamine turnover (McElroy and Keck 1995), possibly accounting for its modest antipsychotic effects.

Q. What is the mechanism of action of carbamazepine in treating psychiatric illness?

A. The antiseizure effects of carbamazepines are probably mediated via inactivation of sodium channels, with consequent reduction of sodium influx (into the neuron). The antimanic and mood-stabilizing properties of carbamazepine have not yet been linked to a specific biochemical mechanism (McElroy and Keck 1995), although carbamazepine has effects on numerous neurotransmitters. In theory, carbamazepine's acute effects in mania may relate to its reduction of glutamate release (an excitatory neurotransmitter). Subchronic treatment with carbamazepine may decrease norepinephrine and dopamine turnover, which might have implications for the antimanic properties of carbamazepine. Unlike lithium, which inhibits IMPase, carbamazepine seems to *stimulate* this system in bovine brain preparations (Vadnal and Parthasarathy 1995).

Q. Doesn't the effect of anticonvulsants on "kindling" have something to do with their mood-stabilizing effects?

A. The term *kindling* originally referred to a process whereby in effect it becomes progressively easier to set off neuronal firing. In technical terms, repeated *subthreshold* stimuli progressively increase the responsivity of some brain region until a seizure occurs. Eventually, application of even a *single* subthreshold stimulus can evoke a seizure (Ayd 1995). Kindling occurs most readily in limbic regions and may be pharmacologically induced by substances such as Metrazol or cocaine. This process may explain why alcohol withdrawal symptoms recur more readily with repeated episodes of drinking (Ayd 1995). Kindling is associated with induction of *transcription factors* under the regulation of so-called *immediate early genes,* such as *c-fos.* This induction process may in turn regulate neurotransmitter metabolism and neuronal receptor production. Post (1993) has adduced evidence showing that cycle acceleration in bipolar patients may be related to so-called kindling phenomena: "With sufficient numbers of episodes, the illness may, as in the kindling model, become progressively more 'well grooved' or autonomous" (p. 88). The anticonvulsants carbamazepine and valproate appear to have antikindling properties in animal models of amygdala kindling and may reduce affective cycling via a similar mechanism. The kindling model predicts tolerance (declining clinical effect at the same dose) to anticonvulsants and some degree of cross-tolerance between carbamazepine and valproate, but it is not clear that this occurs in clinical practice. If such tolerance did develop in bipolar patients, theory would predict that *brief interruption* of anticonvulsant treatment might restore responsivity in patients with *loss of efficacy* (Post 1993). To my knowledge, this hypothesis has not been tested in controlled, clinical studies. (*Note:* Strictly speaking, using the term *kindling* in relation to bipolar episodes may not be correct because seizures actually block true kindling phenomena [C. A. Pearlman, personal communication, February 1997]. Therefore, if a manic episode is truly analogous to a seizure, an episode of mania should actually *reduce* the likelihood of further manic episodes—similar to the way that a session of ECT *raises* the seizure threshold, making it harder to induce a subsequent seizure. Thus, *progressive sensitization* may be a better term than *kindling* to describe the putative tendency of repeated mood swings to induce still more mood swings.)

Q. Does response to one mood stabilizer predict response to another?

A. The answer seems to be no, as might be expected because of the differing mechanisms of action of these agents. Although previous response to lithium strongly predicts lithium response for the index episode of mania, response to divalproex is *not* related to previous lithium response (i.e., poor lithium responders often do quite well on valproate [Bowden et al. 1994]). The relationship between lithium and carbamazepine response is less clear, but some lithium non-responders do respond to carbamazepine. Post (1993) cites "many individual cases" of patients who respond to one anticonvulsant but not another, as well as patients who do not respond to either agent alone but who do respond well to a combination of carbamazepine and valproate (Keck et al. 1992a). This combination, however, may produce complex pharmacokinetic interactions (see also the discussion on "Drug-Drug Interactions" that follows).

▌ Pharmacokinetics

Q. How does the "autometabolism" of carbamazepine affect dosing strategy?

A. Because carbamazepine induces its own metabolism when given chronically, its elimination $t\frac{1}{2}$ ranges from 15 to 50 hours initially but from 8 to 20 hours chronically. In practical terms, this means that unless the dosage is adjusted to keep up with dropping plasma levels, the patient may eventually fail to respond to carbamazepine. Carbamazepine is usually started at 200–600 mg/day in divided doses, with increases of about 100–200 mg every 3–5 days as tolerated. This rate may need to be slowed in patients who develop significant side effects (e.g., sedation, dizziness). A typical daily dose after 2 weeks would be about 1,000 mg, but there is wide interpatient variability. Clinical response and adverse effects are more important in dosing than the plasma level, although generally one aims for a level of about 5–12 µg/mL. (Keep in mind that toxicity due to the 10,11-epoxide metabolite will not be evident from looking at routine plasma levels of carbamazepine.) Plasma levels should be monitored every 5–7 days for the first 3 weeks or so. By this time, autometabolism may be starting (Gerner and Stanton 1992), although it is sometimes not evident until weeks 4–8 of treatment (Bowden 1995b). Depending on the individual patient, upward adjustment of carbamazepine dosage will soon become necessary, sometimes requiring *twice* the dose arrived at during the first 2–3 weeks of treatment (Potter and Ketter 1993). As the $t\frac{1}{2}$ of carbamazepine drops, the time to steady state after each dosage change also will drop, because steady state is reached after four to five $t\frac{1}{2}$s. Plasma levels should generally be obtained at each new steady-state level. Assuming a $t\frac{1}{2}$ (after 6 weeks) of about 15 hours, each new steady state would be reached after about 68 hours or approximately 3 days (four to five $t\frac{1}{2}$s). Thus, in theory, if the dosage is still being increased 6 weeks into treatment (to keep up with autometabolism), levels should be checked about *every 3 days*. In clinical practice, weekly levels are probably adequate for most patients during this transitional phase. Once two or three stable levels have been obtained—presumably reflecting maximum autometabolism—plasma levels are usually obtained once every 1–3 months, depending on several variables. If the patient requires a dosage change or is prescribed a medication that may affect carbamazepine metabolism (see also the discussion on "Drug-Drug Interactions" that follows), more frequent checks may be necessary. As always, remember that it is the patient, not laboratory values, that is being treated.

Q. Does the daily dosing schedule of lithium affect the steady-state plasma level and/or therapeutic efficacy (e.g., twice daily versus single dose)?

A. No. The steady-state concentration (plasma level) of a drug with first-order kinetics is chiefly determined by the *total dose* given during a 24-hour period and the rate of the drug's clearance, typically via hepatic and renal elimination. As long as the total dose and rate of clearance remain constant during a given period of administration, the concentration at steady state will not be affected by the daily dosing schedule. This effect can be illustrated by using arbitrary values in the following equation (Magliozzi and Tupin 1988):

$$Css = \frac{D}{\tau \times CL}$$

where D is the fixed dose, Css is the concentration at steady state, τ is the dosing interval per day (e.g., every 4 hours, 8 hours, 24 hours), and CL is the systemic clearance. Let us compare the values for Css if the total daily dose of lithium (1,200 mg) is given according to two different schedules: as a single daily dose versus four doses of 300 mg each (every 6 hours). Let us assume an arbitrary clearance of 20. The equations are now as follows:

1. $Css = \dfrac{1,200}{24 \times 20}$

   2. $Css = \dfrac{300}{6 \times 20}$

The Css in *both* cases is 2.5. However, although the Css does not differ in these two scenarios, there will be a difference in the *peak* plasma levels achieved during a 24-hour period, as well as a difference in the delta (fluctuation) between *peaks* and *troughs*. In effect, a more frequent dosing schedule results in a lower peak plasma level and a smoother plasma level curve (i.e., less interdose fluctuation), often leading to fewer side effects for many patients, including some taking lithium. On the other hand, there may be advantages to a single daily dose of lithium for *some* patients (see the following discussion on "Main Side Effects"). The assumption in these equations, of course, is that clearance is *constant*. In actuality, the renal clearance of lithium is slightly *less* during sleep, leading to somewhat-higher-than-predicted plasma levels if the same total dose is given all at night instead of, for example, as three daily doses.

Q. How are the various preparations of valproate absorbed and metabolized?

A. Valproate is available in four oral preparations: 1) valproic acid (Depakene and others), 2) sodium valproate (Depakene syrup), 3) divalproex sodium (Depakote, an enteric-coated, delayed-release tablet), and 4) divalproex sodium sprinkle capsules (Depakote Sprinkle Capsules) that can be pulled apart and sprinkled on food (McElroy and Keck 1995). In the management of psychiatric disorders, it is primarily the two formulations of *divalproex sodium* that are used. Divalproex sodium tablets reach peak serum concentrations within 3–8 hours. The sprinkle formulation has an *earlier onset of absorption* but a *slower rate of absorption* than the tablets and produces a somewhat *lower* peak plasma level (McElroy and Keck 1995; Wilder 1992). (It is probably these characteristics that result in fewer GI side effects with the sprinkles.) Valproate metabolism is quite complex (Wilder 1992), mediated via two hepatic pathways (one mitochondrial, one via the microsomal CYP route). Numerous metabolites are produced, at least one of which appears to be hepatotoxic (see the following discussion on "Main Side Effects"). Valproate's elimination $t\frac{1}{2}$ is roughly 5–20 hours and (unlike carbamazepine) does not show autometabolism. As the plasma concentration of valproate increases, clearance also increases because of saturation of protein-binding sites and resultant increased availability of unbound valproate. Transient side effects may be more frequent at higher serum concentrations, and laboratory levels may be less useful for purposes of monitoring, probably because of rapid shifts in unbound valproate as plasma proteins become saturated (McElroy and Keck 1995).

■ Main Side Effects

Q. What are the advantages and disadvantages of giving lithium as a single daily or at-bedtime dose?

A. There are some data showing that patients who take lithium as a single daily dose have less *glomerular* pathology than those who receive multiple doses (Hetmar et al. 1987; Plenge et al. 1982); however, these studies did not control for total dosage, since patients receiving the multiple-dose regimen received a higher total daily dose. In a study in which total lithium dosage was kept the same in both the once-daily and multiple-dose groups, 24-hour urine volume fell significantly after 12 days of single-dose treatment (Perry et al. 1981). Furthermore, patients who take lithium in a single at-bedtime dose are *less* likely to develop polyuria than are patients who take lithium in multiple daily doses (Bowen et al. 1991). Severe polyuria, of course, can lead to dehydration and consequent lithium toxicity. Because plasma levels of lithium may increase by approximately 20% on a single-dose regimen, total daily dose may need to be decreased when converting a patient from multiple- to single-dose regimens. Some patients given their entire lithium dose at bedtime may awaken with GI side effects (diarrhea, nausea), probably because of higher (although briefer) peak plasma levels. Patients with lithium-induced tremor may sometimes benefit from taking all or most of their total dose at bedtime.

Q. What side effects from lithium are most likely to produce noncompliance?

A. When patients are asked this question, the most frequent answer involves *cognitive side effects,* such as mental confusion, poor concentration, memory problems, and mental slowness (F. K. Goodwin and Jamison 1990; Lenox and Manji 1995). Lithium may exert some of these cognitive effects via its action on protein kinase C, with consequent effects on neurotransmission (Lenox and Manji 1995). However, not all studies of neuropsychiatric function have demonstrated cognitive impairment from lithium, and in some patients, gradual tolerance to cognitive side effects may develop. (Dosage reduction or multiple dosing also may help.) Many patients also complain of significant weight gain from lithium and may refuse to take it for this reason.

Q. Can lithium cause tardive dyskinesia (TD)?

A. Although fine hand tremor is commonly seen with lithium treatment (perhaps in as many as 45% of patients), lithium per se has rarely been associated with the onset of TD in clinical practice (Lenox and Manji 1995). Indeed, lithium has been reported to delay or ameliorate TD, possibly by reducing dopamine receptor hypersensitivity (Pert et al. 1978). However, a small retrospective review of patients treated with a neuroleptic alone ($n = 20$) or a neuroleptic plus lithium ($n = 13$) showed no evidence that lithium reduced the severity of TD in patients taking neuroleptics (Foti and Pies 1986). A more unsettling finding has emerged from a study of 110 affective disorder outpatients receiving lithium, of whom 37 were receiving it in combination with antidepressants and 19 with neuroleptics (Ghadirian et al. 1996). Surprisingly, 7 of 51 patients taking lithium had symptoms of TD, despite *absence* of neuroleptic use for the previous 6 months. Although there are several possible explanations for this finding (e.g., neuroleptic exposure before 6-month washout predisposes to lithium-induced TD), the authors hypothesize that "lithium may exacerbate the vulnerability of affective disordered patients to dyskinesias" (Ghadirian et al. 1996, p. 22). Larger prospective studies are needed to confirm this finding, but the clinician should be aware that lithium use may be one of several risk factors for the development of TD. (This study also found that tremor was twice as prevalent [42%] in the 19 patients treated with lithium plus a neuroleptic than in those treated with lithium alone [21%].)

Q. What is the acute management of lithium toxicity?

A. Lithium toxicity may exist even within the so-called therapeutic range of roughly 0.5–1.4 mEq/L. Symptoms may include nausea, tremor, muscle fasciculations, twitching, rigidity, hyperreflexia, fever, confusion, and coma. For patients with mild-to-moderate signs of toxicity, normal renal function, and levels *less* than 2 mEq/L, a period of observation and monitoring of vital signs, coupled with substantial dosage reduction, may be all that is necessary (Janicak et al. 1993) (e.g., reducing lithium dose by 75% for 24 hours, resuming at one-half the usual dose for an additional 24 hours, then resuming the usual dose). A repeat serum lithium determination is appropriate after 3–4 days. Because lithium may cause bradyarrhythmias, an electrocardiogram (ECG) should be considered for patients with pulse rates below 55. For more severe toxicity (levels above 2.5 mEq/L), *forced saline diuresis* is indicated. *Hemodialysis* may be necessary in some cases. However, recent concerns have been raised regarding too *rapid* a correction of "hyperlithemia" (Schou 1996; Swartz and Jones 1996). Because rapid diminution of intraneuronal lithium leads to replacement by sodium, the brain may be subject to massive electrolyte shifts when lithium toxicity is corrected too rapidly, possibly leading to increased risk of seizures and delirium (Swartz and Jones 1996).

Q. Can lithium withdrawal lead to mania in some unipolar depressed patients?

A. Two cases reported by Hoaken and Hoaken (1996) suggest that in apparent *unipolar* depressed patients, discontinuation of lithium augmentation may induce hypomanic or manic symptoms. Both patients had a history of recurrent depression without known hypomanic/manic episodes; both had lithium added to their ongoing tricyclic treatment. Their lithium was stopped over periods of 5–14 days. The authors speculate that "some patients with mood disorder have only depressive episodes until lithium, used as monotherapy . . . or as an antidepressant augmenting agent, is withdrawn, causing a temporary destabilization and the eruption of hypomania or mania" (Hoaken and Hoaken 1996, pp. 47–48). This finding would be consistent with the so-called permissive hypothesis of serotonergic function, which holds that both mania and depression are characterized by low central serotonergic function (Mendels and Frazer 1975). In this hypothesis, lithium acts to stabilize serotonin systems and when withdrawn can cause an excursion into *either* depression *or* mania. More recent theories of lithium action, however, might suggest different mechanisms. For example, if lithium acts (in mania) to inhibit excessive signaling through the PI system (Stoll and Severus 1996), it is theoretically possible that sudden discontinuation of lithium might lead to some form of rebound hyperactivity in the PI system, although this theory must remain as speculation at this time. When lithium augmentation is discontinued in patients with recurrent unipolar depression, it may be prudent to do so gradually, over a period of 1–2 months.

Q. What is the treatment approach to carbamazepine-induced hyponatremia?

A. Carbamazepine has been implicated in causing a state of hyponatremia and water intoxication, resembling the syndrome of inappropriate secretion of antidiuretic hormone (SIADH) (Lahr 1985). Because hyponatremia less than 125 mEq/L may lead to anorexia, vomiting, confusion, and coma, recognizing and treating this condition are important, particularly in the elderly. Successful treatment of carbamazepine-induced hyponatremia has been reported with the use of either of two tetracyclic antibiotics, demeclocycline or doxycycline (Boutros et al. 1995). Doxycycline (100 mg bid) has the advantage of not being dependent on renal excretion and also having a longer $t\frac{1}{2}$ than demeclocycline.

Q. What is the risk of hepatotoxicity with valproate and carbamazepine, and how is this managed?

A. Although neither anticonvulsant is highly hepatotoxic, both may cause alterations in liver function tests (LFTs) that may (often unnecessarily) alarm clinicians. Baseline LFTs are indicated, with periodic follow-ups, depending on subsequent LFT values and the patient's *clinical status*. Valproate (divalproex) has been associated with fatal hepatotoxicity in about 1 in 40,000 cases, almost entirely in patients younger than age 2 years who were receiving multiple anticonvulsants (Janicak et al. 1995). Fatal hepatotoxicity is idiosyncratic and *not* related to dose. In contrast, transient alterations in LFTs (particularly transaminases) do occur in a dose-related fashion with valproate but are not generally suggestive of impending hepatic toxicity. Unless the transaminases reach three times normal values, or alkaline phosphatase or bilirubin has risen from baseline (which may suggest an obstructive process), or—perhaps most important—the patient shows *clinical evidence* of hepatotoxicity (malaise, fever, anorexia, vomiting, easy bruising, jaundice), there is no need to discontinue the valproate (dosage reduction and the passage of time may suffice). Janicak et al. (1995) recommend baseline LFTs, a single follow-up during the first few weeks of valproate treatment, then a repeat of LFTs every 6–12 months, under ordinary circumstances. With carbamazepine, elevation of LFTs occurs in 5%–15% of patients (McElroy and Keck 1995), usually a benign dose-related finding. Dosage reduction or brief interruption of carbamazepine treatment followed by rechallenge at a lower dose often suffices.

Q. What is the management of valproate-induced hair loss or thinning?

A. Hair loss from valproate is usually transient; new hair tends to be more curly than before medication. Interruption of valproate treatment is rarely necessary, and multivitamins containing selenium (25 μg/day) and zinc (50 mg/day) are useful in preventing or stabilizing this hair loss (Potter and Ketter 1993).

∎ Drug-Drug Interactions

Q. How does one safely use a combination of valproate and carbamazepine in refractory bipolar patients?

A. As mentioned earlier, addition of valproate to carbamazepine may lead to an increased ratio of carbamazepine epoxide to carbamazepine via inhibition of epoxide hydroxylase; in theory, this could lead to neurotoxicity in some patients. Also, in theory, valproate may cause displacement of carbamazepine from plasma-binding proteins, producing a *transient* increase in carbamazepine effects. Conversely, carbamazepine reduces valproate levels but increases levels of valproate's 2-propyl-4-pentanoic acid metabolite, which is hepatotoxic and teratogenic. Given these concerns, it is reassuring that clinical experience is generally positive regarding carbamazepine-valproate combination therapy in bipolar patients (Tohen et al. 1994). Thus, in the study by Tohen et al. (1994), all 12 *bipolar* patients given this combination showed moderate-to-marked response; only 2 patients had minor side effects (mild drowsiness). (In contrast, none of the four *schizoaffective* patients responded to this combination. Patients with *organic brain syndromes* fared less well on the carbamazepine-valproate combination, showing adverse effects such as slurred speech and oversedation.) In the study by Tohen et al. (1994)—which was based on a review of pharmacy records, not prospective monitoring—patients received an average dose of 1,500 mg/day valproate and 1,200 mg/day carbamazepine. In the seven cases in which carbamazepine was added to valproate, the valproate level declined (as predicted). However, in the cases in which valproate was added to carbamazepine, there was no change in carbamazepine blood levels. *Metabolite levels* were not reported (and are rarely obtained in clinical practice). Although Tohen et al. (1994) did conclude that the carbamazepine-valproate combination is "usually well tolerated," the authors advised reducing carbamazepine dosage to avoid potential toxicity. Furthermore, if carbamazepine and valproate are used together, monitor levels of both closely, obtain the level of carbamazepine epoxide if possible, and closely monitor the patient for signs of neurotoxicity. LFTs should be checked more frequently than with either agent alone. This combination does not seem as useful or safe in schizoaffective and brain-damaged patients. Finally, keep in mind that in some patients maintained on this combination, discontinuing carbamazepine may lead to increased valproate levels (Jann et al. 1988).

Q. How does valproate interact with anticonvulsants other than carbamazepine?

A. Valproate may reduce elimination, and/or raise plasma levels, of *ethosuximide, lamotrigine,* and *phenobarbital,* sometimes leading to significant toxicity (Ciraulo and Slattery 1995). Interactions between valproate and *phenytoin* are quite variable and usually not of clinical significance. *Felbamate* may inhibit metabolism of valproate, possibly leading to toxicity (Ciraulo and Slattery 1995).

Q. Can carbamazepine be used safely with MAOIs in refractory unipolar or bipolar depression?

A. The structural similarities between carbamazepine and tricyclics have led some clinicians to warn against this combination. Theoretical concerns include the development of hypertensive and hyperpyrexic states, postural hypotension, muscle twitching, convulsions, delirium, and coma (Ketter et al. 1995a). Moreover, some data suggest that phenelzine (Nardil) and tranylcypromine (Parnate) could inhibit hepatic metabolism of carbamazepine. Nevertheless, in a small ($n = 10$) double-blind study in which MAOIs were added to carbamazepine, no major adverse reactions occurred (Ketter et al. 1995a). Furthermore, 4 of the 10 patients (7 bipolar, 3 unipolar depressed inpatients) improved substantially on the carbamazepine-MAOI combination. These four patients had previously been refractory to either agent alone. Responder polarity was not discussed, but responders and nonresponders did not differ significantly in polarity of illness. Carbamazepine pharmacokinetics did not seem to be altered in this study.

Q. What precautions are indicated when a patient is taking concomitant lithium and NSAIDs?

A. Several NSAIDs can increase serum lithium levels, apparently by decreasing renal blood flow; thus, *ibuprofen, indomethacin, diclofenac,* and *ketorolac* can significantly increase serum lithium levels, potentially leading to toxicity (Ayd 1995; Sarid-Segal et al. 1995). It appears that *sulindac, aspirin,* and *acetaminophen* do *not* significantly raise serum lithium levels (Ayd 1995; Ragheb 1990) and may be the analgesics of choice for patients taking lithium.

Q. What is the basis for, and management of, *neurotoxicity* associated with combined lithium and neuroleptic use?

A. The degree to which lithium and antipsychotics interact to cause neurotoxicity is still debated. The original report of

W. J. Cohen and Cohen (1974) implicated the combination of lithium and haloperidol in four cases of irreversible neurotoxicity; subsequent reviews have seriously impugned both the basis and the likelihood of this supposed interaction (for a discussion, see Goff and Baldessarini 1995). Still, given lithium's ability to *reduce* both pre- and postsynaptic dopaminergic function (Lenox and Manji 1995), a pharmacodynamic interaction with antipsychotics is plausible. This interaction may be manifest as frank neurotoxicity (e.g., confusion, disorientation, ataxia) or as increased extrapyramidal effects (Ayd 1995). Some cases of apparent lithium-neuroleptic neurotoxicity actually may be cases of neuroleptic malignant syndrome (NMS); interestingly, lithium itself may be a precipitant of NMS (Susman and Addonizio 1987). It is not clear that any particular neuroleptic is especially likely to interact adversely with lithium, although most cases have involved haloperidol—perhaps because haloperidol is so frequently used. The best management strategy entails 1) using low initial and maintenance doses of the neuroleptic when combined with lithium, 2) carefully monitoring mental status and vital signs after one agent is added to the other, 3) avoiding *simultaneous* prescription of lithium and a neuroleptic (i.e., starting both drugs at precisely the same time, thus obfuscating which agent is causing adverse effects), and 4) decreasing the dose of the neuroleptic if signs of neurotoxicity appear in this context (F. Miller and Menninger 1987). The management of NMS is discussed in Chapter 2.

Q. Can angiotensin-converting enzyme (ACE) inhibitors (for hypertension) be used safely with lithium?

A. ACE inhibitors such as captopril, enalapril, and lisinopril are often used in treating hypertension and congestive heart failure. Many elderly bipolar patients may be taking lithium and an ACE inhibitor. A study by DasGupta et al. (1992) found that, overall, enalapril did not significantly affect steady-state lithium levels in nine healthy volunteers tested over 10 days. In contrast, a larger study (Finley et al. 1996) of 20 hypertensive patients previously stabilized with lithium therapy showed that after initiation of an ACE inhibitor, steady-state lithium concentration increased by about 36%. Four patients had signs suggesting lithium toxicity (increased tremor, ataxia, confusion). The increased lithium levels (and decreased lithium clearance) were correlated with increasing age. The authors concluded that elderly patients generally should not be treated with lithium plus an ACE inhibitor. An alternative approach would be to use a reduced dose of lithium in such cases, with frequent monitoring of clinical state and serum lithium level.

Q. Are there any significant interactions between lithium and valproate?

A. There are no clinically significant *pharmacokinetic* interactions, although divalproex (Depakote) levels may be slightly increased by the lithium carbonate preparation; this increase may be due to neutralization of gastric acid by the carbonate form of lithium (Granneman et al. 1996). GI side effects do not appear to be significantly increased by this combination versus lithium alone, but tremor is occasionally worsened.

Potentiating Maneuvers

Q. If a bipolar patient is unresponsive to lithium alone, what might be the best first move in terms of potentiation?

A. The best first move may depend on the target symptoms that are not responding. If a patient shows primarily depressive symptoms, it may be worthwhile raising the lithium level before adding any augmenting agent (e.g., from 0.8 to 1.2 mEq/L) (Srisurapanont et al. 1995). If a patient shows primarily resistant manic symptoms, adding one of the anticonvulsant mood stabilizers may be reasonable, beginning with valproate if there is a mixed presentation (mania with irritable or depressive features). For rapid-cycling patients, adding T_4 to lithium is sometimes helpful. (For treatment of the depressed phase per se, see "Questions and Answers," first question under "Indications.")

Q. What are the guidelines for using T_4 in rapid-cycling bipolar patients?

A. The benefits of T_4 (usually as an adjunctive agent) have not been documented in large-scale, controlled studies of rapid-cycling patients. Nevertheless, T_4 was deemed a useful treatment in such patients by a recent "Expert Consensus Panel for Bipolar Disorder" (Kahn et al. 1996). T_4 is used in doses ranging from 0.1 to 0.3 mg/day, usually as an adjunct to ongoing treatment with lithium or lithium plus another mood stabilizer (Bauer and Whybrow 1991). Behavioral response often occurs before complete suppression of thyroid-stimulating hormone (TSH) and appears to be a function of increased T_4 rather than triiodothyronine (T_3) levels (Bauer and Whybrow 1991). Although rapid cycling is associated with clinical or subclinical hypothyroidism, euthyroid rapid-cycling patients also respond to this T_4 augmentation strategy (Bauer and Whybrow 1991).

Q. How is T_4 tolerated in this group of patients?

A. Based on a fairly small number of patients, T_4 is usually tolerated well (Bauer and Whybrow 1991), although in my experience, some patients will complain of excessive perspiration, mild excitation, or mild, transient tachycardia. (These side effects usually respond to dosage reduction.) There have been concerns about bone demineralization in pre- or postmenopausal women treated with long-term T_4 therapy, but the evidence for this is actually equivocal (Fujiyama et al.

1995; Marcocci et al. 1994). Nevertheless, with T_4 augmentation, the clinician should avoid TSH levels less than 0.35 mIU because long-term suppression of TSH may be associated with osteoporosis (Kahn et al. 1996).

Q. What is the role of calcium channel blockers as adjunctive agents in bipolar disorder?

A. (See also "Questions and Answers," "Indications.") Dubovsky (1995) notes, "clinical experience suggests that combining a calcium channel blocker with another antimanic drug may be helpful for some treatment-refractory patients, but this approach . . . has not been studied formally" (p. 385). Verapamil has been used as an adjunct to lithium in a few patients unresponsive to lithium alone (Brotman et al. 1986), but large controlled studies are lacking. Lenzi et al. (1995) used verapamil in combination with chlorpromazine in 15 female inpatients with acute mania and found that the combination produced global improvement in manic symptoms in most of the patients (see Gelenberg 1997). Calcium channel blockers such as verapamil appear to be most useful for manic patients who are responsive to lithium but cannot tolerate it; indeed, acutely manic patients who do *not* respond to lithium seem less responsive to verapamil (Dubovsky 1995). Calcium channel blocker–lithium interactions include neurotoxicity, parkinsonism, and cardiac slowing (Dubovsky 1995). The usefulness of calcium channel blockers in depression has not been clearly established, and calcium channel blockers have the potential to exacerbate depression. However, Goodnick (1995) found nimodipine (up to 60 mg tid) effective as the sole agent in the treatment of two patients with rapidly cycling bipolar disorder, even after 5- to 12-month follow-up. Larger-scale and better-controlled studies are needed before the role of calcium channel blockers in bipolar disorder is confidently established.

▌ Use in Special Populations

Q. What are the teratogenic risks of various mood stabilizers during pregnancy?

A. Early retrospective data on infants gathered by the International Register of Lithium suggested a rate of Ebstein's anomaly approximately 500 times higher in infants exposed to lithium during the first trimester than in the general population ("The Use of Psychotropic Drugs During Pregnancy and the Puerperium" 1992). But these data were gathered from *physicians' reports,* a method that often leads to overestimation of adverse outcomes. As L. S. Cohen ("The Use of Psychotropic Drugs During Pregnancy and the Puerperium" 1992) has noted, more recent studies point to a *28-fold increase* in the risk of Ebstein's anomaly because of first-trimester lithium exposure—about 1 in 700 lithium-exposed infants versus 1 in 20,000 in the general population. In a recent review of the available data, Altshuler et al. (1996) concluded that Ebstein's anomaly following first-trimester exposure to lithium is roughly 10–20 times the rate in the general population. Thus, although the risk is not insignificant, it is considerably less than once feared. Furthermore, the *risk* of untreated bipolar illness also must be considered (e.g., abrupt discontinuation of lithium will typically lead to relapse of mania or major depression and occasionally to lithium resistance on restarting treatment). Recent studies have linked first-trimester maternal exposure to carbamazepine with higher-than-expected rates of fetal craniofacial defects, fingernail hypoplasia, developmental delay, and spina bifida. There is also a 1% rate of spina bifida in infants exposed to the anticonvulsant mood stabilizer valproate (divalproex [Depakote]); minor dysmorphic syndromes also have been reported (McElroy and Keck 1995). This rate of spina bifida in infants exposed to valproate is clearly much higher than the risk of lithium-induced Ebstein's anomaly, and most clinicians do not advocate substituting valproate for lithium in the pregnant bipolar patient. Folic acid and multivitamins with trace metals (e.g., selenium) may decrease risk in pregnant patients who must be on carbamazepine or valproate (McElroy and Keck 1995).

Q. How is lithium use adjusted for use in the pregnant patient?

A. If lithium is prescribed during pregnancy, it is best to minimize or eliminate use during the first trimester, when organogenesis is proceeding. For pregnant women who have been treated with lithium during the first trimester, a fetal echocardiogram between the 16th and 18th week of gestation is recommended. Because renal clearance of lithium increases during pregnancy and returns to baseline after delivery, dosage and serum levels may need careful adjustment during these periods. Serum lithium levels usually *decrease* as pregnancy progresses, necessitating dosage *increases*. This increase in dosage is best achieved by using divided doses and aiming for the lowest effective level. With the massive fluid loss (and consequent decrease in plasma volume) associated with delivery, maternal lithium levels may rise dramatically. For this reason, as well as to avert lithium toxicity in the neonate, lithium dosage should be decreased by about 50% before delivery. Lithium toxicity in the neonate may appear as flaccidity, lethargy, or poor sucking reflex and may occur at serum levels lower than that of the mother. Transient neonatal hypothyroidism also has been reported (L. J. Miller 1994). Antipsychotics or bilateral ECT may be preferable to lithium for the severely disturbed bipolar patient in the first trimester. Because some manic patients may worsen with unilateral ECT—perhaps due to suboptimal stimulus dosage—bilateral ECT is generally the method of choice in pregnant manic patients (L. J. Miller 1994; Milstein et al. 1987; Pies 1995a; Weiner and Coffey 1988; Zornberg and Pope 1993). However, given the increased cognitive side effects from bilateral ECT, the choice must be individualized and made a part of the informed consent process (for a discussion, see Abrams 1996).

Q. Is the postpartum period one of high risk for female bipolar patients, and does mood-stabilizing medication help reduce this risk?

A. There is a well-established link between bipolar disorder and heightened risk of postpartum mood disorder; one study suggested that the risk of postpartum relapse is around 50% in manic-depressive women (Reich and Winokur 1970). In a study of mood-stabilizer prophylaxis in postpartum bipolar patients (L. S. Cohen et al. 1995), it was found that of 14 patients who received a mood stabilizer postpartum, only 1 demonstrated recurrent mood disturbance in the first 3 months postpartum. Of the 13 women who did *not* receive mood stabilizers in the acute postpartum period, 8 experienced manic or depressive relapse within the first 3 months postpartum. The authors concluded that "women with bipolar disorder appear to benefit from puerperal prophylaxis with mood stabilizers" (L. S. Cohen et al. 1995, p. 1641). It should be remembered that lithium does appear in the breast milk of lactating patients and that breast-feeding is usually best avoided in this population.

Q. What mood stabilizers are indicated for children and adolescents with bipolar disorder, and what special considerations apply?

A. Historically, lithium has been the most commonly prescribed mood stabilizer in these populations, although valproate has become increasingly accepted (Dulcan et al. 1995). Carbamazepine also is used in this population, although much of the literature on carbamazepine relates to the treatment of aggression in younger patients (Dulcan et al. 1995).

There have been few controlled studies of any of the mood stabilizers used in treating children and adolescents; however, clinical experience suggests that lithium is usually well tolerated in this population, with the most common side effects being tremor, weight gain, polyuria, polydipsia, polyphagia, and accentuation of preexisting enuresis (Dulcan et al. 1995; Weller et al. 1986). Lithium does not appear to affect growth in children, but its cognitive side effects have not been well studied. As in adult populations, valproate may produce GI side effects. Valproate can cause hepatotoxicity in children younger than age 3 years, but it is rare in those older than age 10 years (Dulcan et al. 1995). Even more rare in this population are cases of (potentially fatal) valproate-induced pancreatitis (Trimble 1990). Carbamazepine appears to be eliminated more rapidly in children than in adults, with a $t\frac{1}{2}$ around 9 hours (subject to autoinduction). The usual daily dose range of carbamazepine is 10–50 mg/kg, but there is not a good correlation between weight-based dosage and plasma level. The most common carbamazepine-related side effects in younger populations include drowsiness, nausea, rash, diplopia, nystagmus, and dose-related leukopenia (Dulcan et al. 1995). The effective plasma levels for all three mood stabilizers are similar to those used in adult populations.

Q. What concerns arise when mood stabilizers are used in elderly or dementia patients?

A. As a general rule, elderly and dementia patients tend to be more sensitive to both pharmacokinetic and pharmacodynamic factors than do younger patients. Adverse drug reactions may occur in the elderly even at so-called therapeutic plasma levels of mood stabilizers, particularly lithium, whose concentration in the brain may not be accurately reflected in the plasma level. Despite clinical lore, it has not been established that the therapeutic effects of lithium occur at lower levels in the elderly (Dubovsky 1994); however, beginning at lower doses, and using more gradual dosing increments than in younger patients, is often necessary in older patients. Lithium elimination $t\frac{1}{2}$ may be increased (from 24 hours in younger patients to about 40 hours in some elderly patients), resulting in both a longer time to reach steady state (Dubovsky 1994) and a longer washout period when discontinued. In a retrospective study of 114 elderly outpatients taking maintenance doses of lithium, Holroyd and Rabins (1994) found that side effects were correlated with higher mean serum lithium levels; however, delirium—which was the most common side effect (19.3% of patients)—occurred at serum lithium levels ranging from 0.3 to 1.5 mmol/L. In this sample, tremor occurred in 20% of patients and hypothyroidism in 18%. Hypothyroidism was more prevalent than in some other studies and may reflect the long-term use of lithium in this population. Nevertheless, few patients in this elderly population had side effects so serious that discontinuation of lithium was necessary. Lithium distribution in the brain can be nonuniform (Sansone and Ziegler 1985), and patients with underlying brain damage may show selective uptake of lithium in damaged regions of the brain. Uptake in damaged brain regions may lead to focal neurological side effects (such as a unilateral tremor) or to generalized neurotoxicity and impaired mentation. The anticonvulsant mood stabilizers have not been systematically studied in large populations of elderly or dementia patients. Although valproate seems generally well tolerated, lower initial dosage may be necessary in the elderly to avoid side effects. Valproate has been found useful in the management of aggressive, disinhibited behavior in dementia patients. Carbamazepine also may be useful in such populations but may be more likely than valproate to produce neurotoxicity, perhaps via accumulation of its 10,11-epoxide metabolite. Again, dosage and plasma levels probably should be kept in the lower therapeutic ranges in elderly and dementia populations, with slow increases and frequent monitoring of mental status.

Vignettes and Puzzlers

Q. A 70-year-old man with bipolar disorder is admitted to the inpatient unit in the depressed phase of his illness. However, he has some mixed features of irritability and aggressive behaviors. He has been maintained for several years on a regimen of lithium 300 mg bid (level at admission = 0.86 mEq/L) and nortriptyline 35 mg/day (level at admission = 78 ng/mL). Attempts over the years to discontinue nortriptyline inevitably led to recurrent depressive bouts. The patient had taken valproate briefly but had intolerable nausea and diarrhea, despite using the enteric-coated form (divalproex) and the sprinkle formulation. At the time of admission, all laboratory studies, ECG, and physical examination were within normal limits. The patient started taking 100 mg carbamazepine at bedtime, with increases as tolerated to a total of 600 mg/day. Plasma carbamazepine level after 10 days was 7 μg/mL (therapeutic = 4–12 μg/mL). The patient's mood symptoms improved significantly, but he complained of feeling "spacey and dizzy." A nurse noted one episode in which the patient fell backward onto his bed, with transient loss of consciousness. A repeat ECG was markedly abnormal. What is the most likely problem and its cause?

A. Carbamazepine has a tricyclic-like structure and shares with the tricyclic antidepressants quinidine-like properties. Carbamazepine can cause atrioventricular conduction abnormalities, and as in this case, such conduction abnormalities may be more likely when another quinidine-like agent is used simultaneously (e.g., nortriptyline). Such problems can occur even at therapeutic carbamazepine levels. The patient's repeat ECG most likely showed the presence of second-

or third-degree atrioventricular block, with its attendant interruption of cerebrovascular circulation leading to cardiac syncope (Stokes-Adams attack). Carbamazepine has been known to produce intermittent total atrioventricular block and asystole, sometimes requiring insertion of a demand pacemaker (Boesen et al. 1983; Ladefoged and Mogelvang 1982).

Q. A 60-year-old woman with a history of panic disorder had been taking 0.5 mg tid alprazolam with good control of her anxiety. She suddenly developed severe, unilateral, lancinating facial pain, diagnosed as trigeminal neuralgia (tic douloureux), and began taking 200 mg bid carbamazepine. She reported significant pain relief after 4 days but also complained of increased anxiety. Five days later, she experienced two severe panic attacks. What is the most likely explanation?

A. Carbamazepine may increase clearance of both clonazepam and alprazolam, decreasing plasma levels of the latter by as much as 50% (Arana et al. 1988). Patients taking carbamazepine with a benzodiazepine may require increased dosage of the latter.

Q. A 30-year-old woman with unipolar major depression had been taking 40 mg/day fluoxetine. When her depression suddenly worsened, her psychiatrist added 300 mg tid lithium as an augmenting agent. After 1 week, her lithium level had reached 0.8 mEq/L (therapeutic = 0.5–1.4 mEq/L). At the same time, the woman complained of diarrhea, muscle twitching, shivering, and confusion. Her temperature was 100°F. Blood cultures, chest X ray, and urinalysis were all negative. What is the most likely diagnosis?

A. This patient probably has serotonin syndrome (see Chapter 1), brought on by a pharmacodynamic interaction between fluoxetine and lithium (Muly et al. 1993; Sternbach 1991). Other cases suggest that fluoxetine may increase neurotoxicity in patients taking lithium, sometimes (but not always) elevating plasma lithium levels. The mechanism of action underlying this effect is not known (Sarid-Segal et al. 1995).

Q. A 23-year-old man had refractory bipolar disorder that was poorly controlled while taking a combination of lithium 300 mg tid (level = 0.9 mEq/L, therapeutic level = 0.5–1.4 mEq/L) and carbamazepine 400 mg bid (level = 11 µg/mL, therapeutic level 4–15 µg/mL). His psychiatrist added 250 mg bid valproate, with increases up to a total of 1,000 mg/day. A valproate level after 1 week was 78 µg/mL, therapeutic = 50–125 µg/mL). Although the patient's mania was reduced, he showed marked drowsiness, ataxia, and vertigo. A repeat carbamazepine level was 12 µg/mL. What is the likely cause of the patient's new problems?

A. Valproate inhibits the enzyme epoxide hydrolase, leading to increased plasma levels of carbamazepine epoxide—a potentially neurotoxic metabolite. This effect may occur even when levels of the parent compound (carbamazepine) are within the putative therapeutic range (Ciraulo and Slattery 1995; Sovner 1988).

Q. A 24-year-old female bipolar patient has started taking 200 mg tid carbamazepine, with good effects after 1 week. Her baseline total white blood cell count was 5,200 cells/µL (5.2 cells $\times 10^9$/L; normal = 4–11), with 65% neutrophils (normal = 50%–70%). After 1 week, her total white blood cell count is 4, with 60% neutrophils. Is this likely to represent the beginning of an aplastic anemia?

A. No. Transient, benign leukopenia—usually involving the granulocyte fraction—is seen in about 10%–12% of patients taking carbamazepine (McElroy and Keck 1995). This reaction does not predispose the patient to infection, nor is it related to serious blood dyscrasias, such as aplastic anemia. The latter occurs in only about 1 in 575,000 cases, usually after 2–3 months of treatment (Ayd 1995; McElroy and Keck 1995).

Q. A 20-year-old male college student recently was diagnosed as having bipolar I disorder. He initially was seen in the manic phase and began taking 300 mg tid lithium (plasma level 0.9 mEq/L). Because he experienced significant cognitive slowing while taking lithium, he increased his caffeine intake from his usual two cups of caffeinated coffee per day to four cups per day. One week later, he had another manic episode. What is the most likely explanation, other than spontaneous cycling?

A. Caffeine (and related methylxanthines) can increase lithium excretion, sometimes dropping blood levels below the minimum therapeutic range (Ayd 1995). It is also possible, in this case, that the increased caffeine acted directly (i.e., via a pharmacodynamic effect) by increasing neuronal sensitivity to catecholamines, thus increasing the likelihood of mania.

Q. A 37-year-old man with schizoaffective disorder, bipolar type, had been taking clozapine at 350 mg/day for 4 months; his plasma clozapine level was 250 ng/mL, and overall, the patient's psychosis had improved substantially. However, he had significant features of mania, including pressured speech, irritability, and aggression. Attempts to increase clozapine dose and plasma levels had led to intolerable hypotension, sedation, and hypersalivation. Furthermore, the patient had been intolerant of both lithium and valproate in the past. Despite the increased risk of bone marrow suppression, the patient's psychiatrist elected to begin a trial of clozapine in combination with carbamazepine. The latter was begun at 200 mg bid. Within 1 week, the patient's psychotic symptoms had worsened. His psychiatrist increased the clozapine by 100 mg (over a 4-day period) to compensate for these symptoms. The patient improved over the subsequent 2 weeks, taking a total of 450 mg/day clozapine, although he had significant postural hypotension. Carbamazepine was maintained at 200 mg bid, and there was some reduction in manic symptoms. Unfortunately, 3 weeks after initiating carbamazepine, the patient developed a severe rash with some exfoliation. Fearing the development of Stevens-Johnson syndrome, the psychiatrist immediately stopped the carbamazepine but continued the same dose of clozapine. Although the rash cleared up within 5 days, the patient became severely hypotensive, stuporous, and disoriented. What sequence of events led to 1) the initial worsening of psychotic symptoms after initiating carbamazepine and 2) the severe complications after stopping carbamazepine?

A. The initial worsening of psychotic symptoms was probably due to carbamazepine's reduction of plasma clozapine levels (Ciraulo et al. 1995). The severe complications after carbamazepine was stopped probably represented excessive clozapine levels following removal of carbamazepine's enzyme-inducing effect; in effect, the clozapine dose of 450 mg/day was suddenly without a powerful stimulus for its metabolism. This principle was actually demonstrated in the case of a patient who had been taking a regimen of 800 mg/day clozapine and 600 mg/day carbamazepine for several months. After carbamazepine was discontinued, the patient's clozapine level rose from 1.4 to 2.4 µmol/L (Raitasuo et al. 1993).

References

Abrams R: ECT stimulus parameters as determinants of seizure quality. Psychiatric Annals 26:701–704, 1996

Altshuler LL, Post RM, Leverich GS, et al: Antidepressant-induced mania and cycle acceleration: a controversy revisited. Am J Psychiatry 152:1130–1138, 1995

Altshuler LL, Cohen L, Szuba MP: Pharmacologic management of psychiatric illness during pregnancy: dilemmas and guidelines. Am J Psychiatry 153:592–560, 1996

American Psychiatric Association: Diagnostic and Statistical Manual of Mental Disorders, 3rd Edition. Washington, DC, American Psychiatric Association, 1980

Ames D, Wirshing WC, Szuba MP: Organic mental disorders associated with bupropion in three patients. J Clin Psychiatry 53:53–55, 1992

Andrews DG, Schweitzer I, Marshall N: The comparative side effects of lithium, carbamazepine and combined lithium-carbamazepine in patients treated for affective disorders. Human Psychopharmacology 5:41–45, 1990

Arana GW, Hyman SE: Handbook of Psychiatric Drug Therapy. Boston, Little, Brown, 1991

Arana GW, Epstein S, Molloy M, et al: Carbamazepine-induced reduction of plasma alprazolam concentrations: a clinical case report. J Clin Psychiatry 49:448–449, 1988

Ayd FJ: Lexicon of Psychiatry, Neurology, and the Neurosciences. Baltimore, MD, Williams & Wilkins, 1995

Baf MH, Subhash MN, Lakshmana KM, et al: Sodium valproate induced alterations in monoamine levels in different regions of the rat brain. Neurochem Int 24:67–72, 1994

Bauer MS, Whybrow PC: Rapid cycling bipolar disorder: clinical features, treatment, and etiology, in Refractory Depression. Edited by Amsterdam JD. New York, Raven, 1991, pp 191–208

Boesen F, Andersen EB, Jensen EK, et al: Cardiac conduction disturbances during carbamazepine therapy. Acta Neurol Scand 68:49–52, 1983

Boutros NN, Guerra BM, Votolato NA, et al: Carbamazepine-induced hyponatremia resolved with doxycycline. J Clin Psychiatry 56:377–378, 1995

Bowden CL: Predictors of response to divalproex and lithium. J Clin Psychiatry 56 (suppl 3):25–30, 1995a

Bowden CL: Treatment of bipolar disorder, in The American Psychiatric Press Textbook of Psychopharmacology. Edited by Schatzberg AF, Nemeroff CB. Washington, DC, American Psychiatric Press, 1995b, pp 603–614

Bowden CL, Brugger AM, Swann AC, et al: Efficacy of divalproex versus lithium and placebo in the treatment of mania. JAMA 271:918–924, 1994

Bowen RC, Grof P, Grof E: Less frequent lithium administration and lower urine volume. Am J Psychiatry 148:189–192, 1991

Bradwejn J, Shriqui C, Koszycki D, et al: Double-blind comparison of the effects of clonazepam and lorazepam in acute mania. J Clin Psychopharmacol 10:403–408, 1990

Brodie MJ, Dichter MA: Antiepileptic drugs. N Engl J Med 334:168–175, 1996

Brotman AW, Farhadi AM, Gelenberg AJ, et al: Verapamil treatment of acute mania. J Clin Psychiatry 47:136–138, 1986

Calabrese JR, Markowitz PJ, Kimmel SE, et al: Spectrum of efficacy of valproate in 78 rapidly cycling bipolar patients. J Clin Psychopharmacol 12:53S–56S, 1992

Ciraulo DA, Slattery M: Anticonvulsants, in Drug Interactions in Psychiatry, 2nd Edition. Edited by Ciraulo DA, Shader RI, Greenblatt DJ, et al. Baltimore, MD, Williams & Wilkins, 1995, pp 249–310

Ciraulo DA, Shader RI, Greenblatt DJ, et al (eds): Drug Interactions in Psychiatry, 2nd Edition. Baltimore, MD, Williams & Wilkins, 1995

Cohen LS, Sichel DA, Robertson LM, et al: Postpartum prophylaxis for women with bipolar disorder. Am J Psychiatry 152:1641–1645, 1995

Cohen WJ, Cohen NJ: Lithium carbonate, haloperidol, and irreversible brain damage. JAMA 230:1283–1287, 1974

DasGupta K, Jefferson JW, Kobak KA, et al: The effect of enalapril on serum lithium levels in healthy men. J Clin Psychiatry 53:398–400, 1992

DeVane CL: Pharmacogenetics and drug metabolism of newer antidepressant agents. J Clin Psychiatry 55 (suppl):38–45, 1994

Drug Facts and Comparisons. St. Louis, MO, Facts and Comparisons, 1995

Dubovsky SL: Geriatric neuropsychopharmacology, in The American Psychiatric Press Textbook of Geriatric Neuropsychiatry. Edited by Coffey CE, Cummings JL. Washington, DC, American Psychiatric Press, 1994, pp 595–631

Dubovsky SL: Calcium channel antagonists as novel agents for manic-depressive disorder, in The American Psychiatric Press Textbook of Psychopharmacology. Edited by Schatzberg AF, Nemeroff CB. Washington, DC, American Psychiatric Press, 1995, pp 377–388

Dubovsky SL, Franks RD, Allen S, et al: Calcium antagonists in mania: a double-blind study of verapamil. Psychiatry Res 18: 309–312, 1986

Dulcan MK, Bregman JD, Weller EB, et al: Treatment of childhood and adolescent disorders, in The American Psychiatric Press Textbook of Psychopharmacology. Edited by Schatzberg AF, Nemeroff CB. Washington, DC, American Psychiatric Press, 1995, pp 669–706

El-Mallakh RS, Wyatt RJ: The Na,K-ATPase hypothesis for bipolar illness. Biol Psychiatry 37:235–244, 1995

Faedda GL, Tondo L, Baldessarini RJ: Outcome after rapid versus gradual discontinuation of lithium treatment in bipolar disorders. Arch Gen Psychiatry 50:448–455, 1993

Fieve RR, Platman SR, Plutchik RR: The use of lithium in affective disorders, I: acute endogenous depression. Am J Psychiatry 125: 487–491, 1968

Finley PR, O'Brien JG, Coleman RW: Lithium and angiotensin-converting enzyme inhibitors: evaluation of a potential interaction. J Clin Psychopharmacol 16:68–71, 1996

Fogel BS: Combining anticonvulsants with conventional psychopharmacologic agents, in Use of Anticonvulsants in Psychiatry: Recent Advances. Edited by McElroy SL, Pope HG Jr. Clifton, NJ, Oxford Health Care, 1988, pp 77–94

Foti ME, Pies RW: Lithium carbonate and tardive dyskinesia (letter). J Clin Psychopharmacol 6:325, 1986

Frye MA, Altshuler L, Szuba MP, et al: The relationship between antimanic agent for treatment of classic or dysphoric mania and length of hospital stay. J Clin Psychiatry 57:17–21, 1996

Fujiyama K, Kiriyama T, Ito M, et al: Suppressive doses of thyroxine do not accelerate age-related bone loss in late postmenopausal women. Thyroid 5:13–17, 1995

Gelenberg AJ: Verapamil for mania? Biological Therapies in Psychiatry Newsletter 20:6–7, 1997

Gerner RH, Stanton A: Algorithm for patient management of acute manic states: lithium, valproate, or carbamazepine? J Clin Psychopharmacol 12:57S–63S, 1992

Ghadirian A-M, Annable L, Belanger M-C, et al: A cross-sectional study of parkinsonism and tardive dyskinesia in lithium-treated affective disordered patients. J Clin Psychiatry 57:22–28, 1996

Goff DC, Baldessarini RJ: Antipsychotics, in Drug Interactions in Psychiatry, 2nd Edition. Edited by Ciraulo DA, Shader RI, Greenblatt DJ, et al. Baltimore, MD, Williams & Wilkins, 1995, pp 129–174

Goodnick P: Nimodipine treatment of rapid cycling bipolar disorder (letter). J Clin Psychiatry 56:330, 1995

Goodwin FK, Jamison KR: Manic-Depressive Illness. New York, Oxford University Press, 1990

Goodwin GM: Recurrence of mania after lithium withdrawal: implications for the use of lithium in the treatment of bipolar affective disorder. Br J Psychiatry 164:149–152, 1994

Granneman GR, Schneck DW, Cavanaugh JH, et al: Pharmacokinetic interactions and side effects resulting from concomitant administration of lithium and divalproex sodium. J Clin Psychiatry 57:204–206, 1996

Hester RK: Outcome research: alcoholism, in The American Psychiatric Press Textbook of Substance Abuse Treatment. Edited by Galanter M, Kleber HD. Washington, DC, American Psychiatric Press, 1994, pp 35–44

Hetmar O, Brun C, Clemmensen L, et al: Lithium: long-term effects on the kidney, II: structural changes. J Psychiatr Res 21:279–288, 1987

Hoaken PCS, Hoaken P: Undue mood elevation in unipolar patients following cessation of lithium augmentation treatment: implications for the understanding of mood disorders. Can J Psychiatry 41:46–48, 1996

Holroyd S, Rabins PV: A retrospective chart review of lithium side effects in a geriatric outpatient population. American Journal of Geriatric Psychiatry 4:346–351, 1994

Janicak PG, Davis JM, Preskorn SH, et al: Principles and Practice of Psychopharmacotherapy. Baltimore, MD, Williams & Wilkins, 1993

Janicak PG, Davis JM, Ayd FJ, et al: Advances in the pharmacotherapy of bipolar disorder. Update: Principles and Practice of Psychopharmacotherapy 1(3):1–20, 1995

Jann MW, Fidone GS, Israel MK, et al: Increased valproate serum concentrations upon carbamazepine cessation. Epilepsia 29:578–581, 1988

Kahn DA, Carpenter D, Docherty JP, et al (eds): The Expert Consensus Guidelines for treatment of bipolar disorder. J Clin Psychiatry 57 (suppl 12A):11–80, 1996

Kaplan HI, Sadock BJ, Grebb JA (eds): Synopsis of Psychiatry, 7th Edition. Baltimore, MD, Williams & Wilkins, 1994

Keck PE, McElroy SL, Vuckovic A, et al: Combined valproate and carbamazepine treatment of bipolar disorder. J Neuropsychiatry Clin Neurosci 4:319–322, 1992a

Keck PE, McElroy SL, Friedman LM: Valproate and carbamazepine in the treatment of panic and posttraumatic stress disorders, withdrawal states, and behavioral dyscontrol syndromes. J Clin Psychopharmacol 12:36S–41S, 1992b

Keck PE, McElroy SL, Tugrul KC, et al: Valproate oral loading in the treatment of acute mania. J Clin Psychiatry 54:305–308, 1993

Ketter TA, Post RM, Parekh PI, et al: Addition of monoamine oxidase inhibitors to carbamazepine: preliminary evidence of safety and antidepressant efficacy in treatment-resistant depression. J Clin Psychiatry 56:471–475, 1995a

Ketter TA, Jenkins JB, Schroeder DH, et al: Carbamazepine but not valproate induces bupropion metabolism. J Clin Psychopharmacol 15:327–333, 1995b

Khaitan L, Calabrese JR, Stockmeier CA: Effects of chronic treatment with valproate on serotonin-1A receptor binding and function. Psychopharmacology (Berl) 113:539–542, 1994

Klein E, Uhde TW, Post RM: Preliminary evidence for the utility of carbamazepine in alprazolam withdrawal. Am J Psychiatry 143:235–236, 1986

Krishnan KRR, Steffens DC, Doraiswamy PM: Psychotropic drug interactions. Primary Psychiatry 3:21–45, 1996

Ladefoged SD, Mogelvang JC: Total atrioventricular block with syncope complicating carbamazepine therapy. Acta Medica Scandinavica 212:185–186, 1982

Lahr MB: Hyponatremia during carbamazepine therapy. Clin Pharmacol Ther 37:693–696, 1985

Lenox RH, Manji HK: Lithium, in The American Psychiatric Press Textbook of Psychopharmacology. Edited by Schatzberg AF, Nemeroff CB. Washington, DC, American Psychiatric Press, 1995, pp 303–349

Lenzi A, Marazziti D, Raffaelli S, et al: Effectiveness of the combination of verapamil and chlorpromazine in the treatment of severe manic or mixed patients. Prog Neuropsychopharmacol Biol Psychiatry 19:519–528, 1995

Levitt JJ, Tsuang MT: The heterogeneity of schizoaffective disorder: implications for treatment. Am J Psychiatry 145:926–936, 1988

Magliozzi JR, Tupin JP: Glossary of pharmacological terms, in Handbook of Clinical Psychopharmacology. Edited by Tupin JP, Shader RI, Harnett DS. Northvale, NJ, Jason Aronson, 1988, pp 455–465

Marcocci C, Golia F, Bruno-Bossio G, et al: Carefully monitored levothyroxine suppressive therapy is not associated with bone loss in premenopausal women. J Clin Endocrinol Metab 78:818–823, 1994

Mattson RH, Cramer JA, Collins JF, et al: A comparison of valproate with carbamazepine for the treatment of complex partial seizures and secondarily generalized tonic-clonic seizures in adults. N Engl J Med 327:765–771, 1992

Maxmen JS: Psychotropic Drugs: Fast Facts. New York, WW Norton, 1991

McElroy SL, Keck PE: Antiepileptic drugs, in The American Psychiatric Press Textbook of Psychopharmacology. Edited by Schatzberg AF, Nemeroff CB. Washington, DC, American Psychiatric Press, 1995, pp 351–375

Mendels J, Frazer A: Reduced central serotonergic activity in mania: implications for the relationship between depression and mania. Br J Psychiatry 126:241–248, 1975

Miller F, Menninger J: Lithium-neuroleptic neurotoxicity is dose dependent. J Clin Psychopharmacol 7:89–91, 1987

Miller LJ: Psychiatric medication during pregnancy: understanding and minimizing risks. Psychiatric Annals 24:69–75, 1994

Milstein V, Small JG, Klapper MH, et al: Uni- versus bilateral ECT in the treatment of mania. Convuls Ther 3:1–9, 1987

Muly EC, McDonald W, Steffens D, et al: Serotonin syndrome produced by a combination of fluoxetine and lithium (letter). Am J Psychiatry 150:1565, 1993

Osser D: Hazards of stopping maintenance pharmacotherapy of bipolar disorder. Lecture presented at the Cambridge Hospital, Boston, January 6, 1996

Perry PJ, Dunner FJ, Hahn RL, et al: Lithium kinetics in single daily dosing. Acta Psychiatr Scand 64:281–294, 1981

Pert A, Rosenblatt JE, Sivit C, et al: Long-term treatment with lithium prevents the development of dopamine receptor supersensitivity. Science 201:171–173, 1978

Physicians' Desk Reference, 50th Edition. Montvale, NJ, Medical Economics, 1996

Pies R: Psychotropic medication during pregnancy and postpartum. Clinical Advances in the Treatment of Psychiatric Disorders 9:4–7, 1995a

Pies R: Women, mood, and the thyroid. Women's Psychiatric Health 4:4–11, 1995b

Pies R, Popli AP: Self-injurious behavior: pathophysiology and implications for treatment. J Clin Psychiatry 56:580–588, 1995

Plenge P, Mellerup ET, Bolwig TG, et al: Lithium treatment: does the kidney prefer one daily dose instead of two? Acta Psychiatr Scand 66:121–128, 1982

Pope HG, McElroy SL, Nixon RA: Possible synergism between fluoxetine and lithium in refractory depression. Am J Psychiatry 145:1292–1294, 1988

Popli AP, Tanquary J, Lamparella V, et al: Bupropion and anticonvulsant drug interactions. Ann Clin Psychiatry 7:99–101, 1995

Post RM: Issues in the long-term management of bipolar affective illness. Psychiatric Annals 23:86–93, 1993

Potter WZ, Ketter TA: Pharmacological issues in the treatment of bipolar disorder: focus on mood-stabilizing compounds. Can J Psychiatry 38 (suppl 2):51–56, 1993

Ragheb M: The clinical significance of lithium–nonsteroidal anti-inflammatory drug interactions. J Clin Psychopharmacol 10:350–354, 1990

Raitasuo V, Lehtovaara R, Huttunen MO: Carbamazepine and plasma levels of clozapine (letter). Am J Psychiatry 150:169, 1993

Reich T, Winokur G: Postpartum psychosis in patients with manic depressive disease. J Nerv Ment Dis 151:60–68, 1970

Rifkin A, Quitkin F, Curillo C, et al: Lithium carbonate in emotionally unstable character disorders. Arch Gen Psychiatry 27:519–523, 1972

Sachs GS: Bipolar mood disorder: practical strategies for acute and maintenance phase treatment. J Clin Psychopharmacol 16 (suppl 1):32S–47S, 1996

Sansone MEG, Ziegler DK: Lithium toxicity: a review of neurologic complications. Clin Neuropharmacol 8:242–248, 1985

Sarid-Segal O, Creelman WL, Shader RI: Lithium, in Drug Interactions in Psychiatry, 2nd Edition. Edited by Ciraulo DA, Shader RI, Greenblatt DJ, et al. Baltimore, MD, Williams & Wilkins, 1995, pp 175–213

Schexnayder LW, Hirschowitz J, Sautter FJ, et al: Predictors of response to lithium in patients with psychoses. Am J Psychiatry 152:1511–1513, 1995

Schou M: Hyperlithemia correction: an untraditional view (letter). J Clin Psychiatry 57:42, 1996

Shader RI: Approaches to the treatment of manic-depressive states, in Manual of Psychiatric Therapeutics, 2nd Edition. Edited by Shader RI. Boston, Little, Brown, 1994, pp 247–258

Sillanpaa M: Carbamazepine: pharmacology and clinical uses. Acta Neurol Scand 64 (suppl 88):139–161, 1981

Simpson SG, DePaulo JR: Fluoxetine treatment of bipolar II depression. J Clin Psychopharmacol 11:52–54, 1991

Sovner R: A clinically significant interaction between carbamazepine and valproic acid. J Clin Psychopharmacol 8:448–449, 1988

Sovner R, Davis JM: A potential drug interaction between fluoxetine and valproic acid (letter). J Clin Psychopharmacol 11:389, 1991

Sporn J, Sachs G: The anticonvulsant lamotrigine in treatment-resistant manic-depressive illness. J Clin Psychopharmacol 17:185–189, 1997

Srisurapanont M, Yatham LN, Zis AP: Treatment of acute bipolar depression: a review of the literature. Can J Psychiatry 40:533–544, 1995

Sternbach H: The serotonin syndrome. Am J Psychiatry 148:705–713, 1991

Stoll AL, Severus WE: Mood stabilizers: shared mechanisms of action at postsynaptic signal-transduction and kindling processes. Harvard Review of Psychiatry 4:77–89, 1996

Suppes T, Baldessarini RJ, Faedda GL, et al: Risk of recurrence following discontinuation of lithium treatment in bipolar disorder. Arch Gen Psychiatry 48:1082–1088, 1991

Susman VL, Addonizio G: Reinduction of neuroleptic malignant syndrome by lithium. J Clin Psychopharmacol 7:339–341, 1987

Sussman N: Gabapentin and lamotrigine: alternative agents for the treatment of bipolar disorder. Primary Psychiatry 4:25–41, 1997

Swartz CM, Jones P: Drs. Swartz and Jones reply (to letter of M Schou). J Clin Psychiatry 57:42–43, 1996

Tohen M, Castillo J, Pope HG, et al: Concomitant use of valproate and carbamazepine in bipolar and schizoaffective disorders. J Clin Psychopharmacol 14:67–70, 1994

Trimble MR: Anticonvulsants in children and adolescents. Journal of Child and Adolescent Psychopharmacology 1:107–124, 1990

The use of psychotropic drugs during pregnancy and the puerperium: an interview with Lee S. Cohen, M.D. Currents in Affective Illness, September 1992, pp 5–13

Vadnal R, Parthasarathy R: Myo-inositol monophosphatase: diverse effects of lithium, carbamazepine, and valproate. Neuropsychopharmacology 12:277–285, 1995

Walton SA, Berk M, Brook S: Superiority of lithium over verapamil in mania: a randomized, controlled single-blind trial. J Clin Psychiatry 57:543–546, 1996

Weiner RD, Coffey CE: Indications for use of electroconvulsive therapy, in American Psychiatric Press Review of Psychiatry, Vol 7. Edited by Frances AJ, Hales RE. Washington, DC, American Psychiatric Press, 1988, pp 458–481

Weller E, Weller R, Fristad M: Lithium dosage guide for prepubertal children: a preliminary report. Journal of the American Academy of Child Psychiatry 25:92–95, 1986

Wilder BJ: Pharmacokinetics of valproate and carbamazepine. J Clin Psychopharmacol 12:64S–68S, 1992

Wright G, Galloway L, Kim J, et al: Bupropion in the long-term treatment of cyclic mood disorders: mood-stabilizing effects. J Clin Psychiatry 46:22–25, 1985

Zornberg GL, Pope HG: Treatment of depression in bipolar disorder: new directions for research. J Clin Psychopharmacol 13:397–408, 1993

Index

*Page numbers printed in **boldface** type refer to tables or figures.*

role in metabolism of
antipsychotics,
115–116, **131–132**
role in metabolism of
benzodiazepines, 213,
256–257
role in metabolism of
carbamazepine, 286,
295
SSRI effects on, **22,** 92
steroidogenic, 3
xenobiotic, 3

Dalmane. *See* Flurazepam
Dantrolene sodium
for malignant hyperthermia,
47, 142
for neuroleptic malignant
syndrome, **47, 142,**
178
Delirium, 198
Delusional disorder
antipsychotics for, **125,** 166
SSRIs for, 166
Demeclocycline, 337
Dementia
Alzheimer's, 114, **127,** 161,
198
buspirone for agitation
related to, 212
Lewy body, 165
multi-infarct, 161
use of antidepressants in, 2,
13, 15
use of antipsychotics in, **127,**
160–161, 190–191,
198–199
use of mood stabilizers in,
348–350

Demerol. *See* Meperidine
Dental caries, 170
Depakene, Depakote, Depakote
Sprinkle. *See* Valproate
Dependence on
benzodiazepines, 213
L-Deprenyl, **10**
Depression, 2
antidepressants for, 1–100
(*See also*
Antidepressants)
atypical, 61–62
benzodiazepines and,
212–214, **225, 232, 234,**
251–253
buspirone and, 212, **232**
effect of calcium channel
blockers in, 344
lithium for, 322, 335–336
in medically ill patients,
89–92
mixed anxiety-depressive
states, 61
multiple episodes of, 57–58
with psychotic features, 114,
127
treatment of depressed
phase of bipolar
illness, 317–319
treatment-resistant, 6, 82–86
carbamazepine combined
with MAOI for,
339–340
Desalkylflurazepam, 259
N-Desalkyl-2-oxoquazepam
(DOQ), 259
Desipramine
interaction with alprazolam,
265

Slurred speech,
    benzodiazepine-induced,
    233
Social phobic disorder
    benzodiazepines for, 212,
    223
    SSRIs for, **12**
    TCAs for, **14**
Sodium bicarbonate, **47,**
    142
Sodium chloride, **32**
Sodium valproate, 332. *See also*
    Valproate
Somatoform disorders,
    antidepressants for, 2, **13,**
    15
Sparine. *See* Promazine
Special populations
    antidepressants for, 6–7,
    54–56, 89–95
    antipsychotics for, 119–120,
    152–155, 186–192
    anxiolytics and
        sedative-hypnotics for,
        214–215, **240–243,**
        268–271
    mood stabilizers for,
        289–290, **316,**
        345–350
Spina bifida, mood stabilizers
    and, 290, 345
SSRIs. *See* Selective serotonin
    reuptake inhibitors
St.-John's-wort, 87–88
Stelazine. *See* Trifluoperazine
Stevens-Johnson syndrome, 96,
    354
Stokes-Adams attacks, 351
Substance abuse

abuse liability of
    benzodiazepines,
    259–260
benzodiazepines for
    withdrawal
    symptoms, 212, **226**
    psychosis secondary to, **126**
Succinylcholine, interaction
    with phenelzine, **40**
Suicidal patients, alprazolam
    for, 252
Sulindac, interaction with
    lithium, 340
Sumatriptan, interaction with
    MAOIs, **40**
Surmontil. *See* Trimipramine
Sweating,
    antidepressant-induced,
    26, 28
Symmetrel. *See* Amantadine
Sympathomimetic amines,
    interactions with
    antidepressants, 5, 6, **36,**
    49, 79
Syncope
    cardiac, 351
    risperidone-induced, 176
Syndrome of inappropriate
    secretion of antidiuretic
    hormone (SIADH),
    drug-induced
    carbamazepine, 336
    fluoxetine, 7

T_4. *See* Thyroxine
Tachycardia, drug-induced. *See*
    also Arrhythmias
    antipsychotics
        clozapine, 174, 192

Tachycardia, drug-induced
(continued)
antipsychotics (continued)
in fetus, 187
benzodiazepines, **231**
buspirone, **231**
TCAs, 4
management of, **32**
Tacrine, **38**
Tagamet. See Cimetidine
Tamoxifen, interaction with
antidepressants, 81
Tapering
of antidepressants, 68–69,
319
of benzodiazepines, **235**,
261–262, 266
of lithium, 320–321
Taractan. See Chlorprothixene
Tardive dyskinesia (TD), 114,
117, **136**, 161, 193
in elderly persons, 117
incidence of, 117
induced by atypical
antipsychotics,
135
lithium and, 334–335
TCAs. See Tricyclic
antidepressants
TD. See Tardive dyskinesia
Tegretol. See Carbamazepine
Temazepam
cost of, **222**
dosage equivalent to 5 mg
diazepam, **221**
pharmacokinetics of, 213,
229, 230, 256
tablet sizes and dosage of,
217

Teratogenicity. See also
Pregnancy and drug use
of antipsychotics, 120, **155**,
187–188
of benzodiazepines, 214–215,
240, 268–269
of fluoxetine, 7, 93
of mood stabilizers, 287,
289–290, **316**, 345–346
of TCAs, 93
Terfenadine, interaction with
antidepressants, 6, **39**, 92
Tetracyclines
for carbamazepine-induced
hyponatremia, 337
interaction with lithium, 288
Theophylline (Theo-Dur)
drug interactions with
antidepressants, **38**, 80–81,
99–100
carbamazepine, 288
lithium, 288, **306**
seizures induced by, 187
"Therapeutic window"
for clozapine, 116
for haloperidol, 116
for TCAs, 4, **23**
Thermoregulation. See also
Hyperthermia
problems in infants exposed
to benzodiazepines in
utero, 215, 269
Thiazide diuretic interactions
with lithium, 288, **306**
with MAOIs, **40**
Thienobenzodiazepine, **121**
Thioridazine, 197
for dementia with psychosis,
198